Study Guide for

FOCUS ON Nursing Pharmacology

Wolters Kluwer | Lippincott Williams & Wilkins
Health
Philadelphia · Baltimore · New York · London
Buenos Aires · Hong Kong · Sydney · Tokyo

D1417504

Acquisitions Editor: Hilarie Surrena
Product Manager: Helene T. Caprari
Marketing Manager: Amy Giuffi
Editorial Assistant: Laura Scott
Design Coordinator: Joan Wendt
Illustration Coordinator: Karin Duffield
Production Service: Aptara, Inc.

Copyright © 2011 Wolters Kluwer Health | Lippincott Williams & Wilkins

All rights reserved. This book is protected by copyright. No part of this book may be reproduced or transmitted in any form or by any means, including as photocopies or scanned-in or other electronic copies, or utilized by any information storage and retrieval system without written permission from the copyright owner, except for brief quotations embodied in critical articles and reviews. Materials appearing in this book prepared by individuals as part of their official duties as U.S. government employees are not covered by the above-mentioned copyright. To request permission, please contact Lippincott Williams & Wilkins at 530 Walnut Street, Philadelphia, PA 19106, via email at permissions@lww.com, or via our website at lww.com (products and services).

9 8 7 6 5 4 3

Printed in the United States of America

978-1-5825-5919-3

Care has been taken to confirm the accuracy of the information presented and to describe generally accepted practices. However, the author, editors, and publisher are not responsible for errors or omissions or for any consequences from application of the information in this book and make no warranty, expressed or implied, with respect to the currency, completeness, or accuracy of the contents of the publication. Application of this information in a particular situation remains the professional responsibility of the practitioner; the clinical treatments described and recommended may not be considered absolute and universal recommendations.

The author, editors, and publisher have exerted every effort to ensure that drug selection and dosage set forth in this text are in accordance with the current recommendations and practice at the time of publication. However, in view of ongoing research, changes in government regulations, and the constant flow of information relating to drug therapy and drug reactions, the reader is urged to check the package insert for each drug for any change in indications and dosage and for added warnings and precautions. This is particularly important when the recommended agent is a new or infrequently employed drug.

Some drugs and medical devices presented in this publication have Food and Drug Administration (FDA) clearance for limited use in restricted research settings. It is the responsibility of the health care provider to ascertain the FDA status of each drug or device planned for use in his or her clinical practice.

LWW.com

Preface

This Study Guide was created by Maryann Foley, RN, BSN, for the fifth edition of *Focus on Nursing Pharmacology,* by Amy M. Karch. The Study Guide is designed to help you practice and retain the knowledge you've gained from the textbook, and it is structured to integrate that knowledge and give you a basis for applying it in your nursing practice. The following types of exercises are provided in each chapter of the Study Guide.

■ ASSESSING YOUR UNDERSTANDING

The first section of each Study Guide chapter concentrates on the basic information of the textbook chapter and helps you to remember key concepts, vocabulary, and principles.

■ Fill in the Blanks

Fill in the blank exercises test important chapter information, encouraging you to recall key points.

■ Labeling

Labeling exercises are used where you need to remember certain visual representations of the concepts presented in the textbook.

■ Match the Following

Matching questions test your knowledge of the definition of key terms.

■ Sequencing

Sequencing exercises ask you to remember particular sequences or orders, for instance testing processes and prioritizing nursing actions.

■ Short Answers

Short answer questions will cover facts, concepts, procedures, and principles of the chapter. These questions ask you to recall information as well as demonstrate your comprehension of the information.

■ Crossword Puzzles

Crossword Puzzles also cover important facts, concepts, procedures, and principles of the chapter in a diverting exercise.

■ APPLYING YOUR KNOWLEDGE

The second section of each Study Guide chapter consists of case study–based exercises that ask you to begin to apply the knowledge you've gained from the textbook chapter and reinforced in the first section of the Study Guide chapter. A case study scenario based on the chapter's content is presented, and then you are asked to answer some questions, in writing, related to the case study. The questions cover the following areas:

■ Assessment
■ Planning Nursing Care
■ Communication
■ Reflection

■ PRACTICING FOR NCLEX

The third and final section of the Study Guide chapters helps you practice NCLEX-style questions while further reinforcing the knowledge you have been gaining and testing for yourself through the textbook chapter and the first two sections of the study guide chapter. In keeping with the NCLEX, the questions presented are multiple-choice and scenario-based, asking you to reflect, consider, and apply what you know and to choose the best answer out of those offered.

■ ANSWER KEYS

The answers for all of the exercises and questions in the Study Guide are provided at the back of the book, so you can assess your own learning as you complete each chapter.

We hope you will find this Study Guide to be helpful and enjoyable, and we wish you every success in your studies toward becoming a nurse.

The Publishers

Contents

v

CHAPTER **1**

Introduction to Drugs

LEARNING OBJECTIVES

Upon completion of this chapter, you will be able to:

1. Define the word *pharmacology*.

2. Outline the steps involved in developing and approving a new drug in the United States.

3. Describe the federal controls on drugs that have abuse potential.

4. Differentiate between generic and brand name drugs, over-the-counter drugs, and prescription drugs.

5. Explain the benefits and risks associated with the use of over-the-counter drugs.

■ ASSESSING YOUR UNDERSTANDING

MATCHING

Select the description from column 2 that best describes the term in column 1.

Column 1

___ **1.** Pharmacology

___ **2.** Brand name

___ **3.** Chemical name

___ **4.** Generic name

___ **5.** Adverse effects

Column 2

a. The original drug designation given when the drug company applies for approval

b. The study of the biologic effects of a chemical

c. Undesirable or possibly dangerous result of a drug

d. The trade name of a drug

e. The designation for a drug that reflects chemical structure

SEQUENCING

Each of the following statements reflects a step in the process of drug evaluation. Place the number of the statement in the boxes below based on the order in which they occur.

1. Healthy male volunteers are used to test the drugs.

2. The Food and Drug Administration (FDA) approves the drug.

3. Patients with the disease receive the drug.

4. The drug is tested in the laboratory using animals.

5. Prescribers administer the drug reporting any unexpected adverse effects.

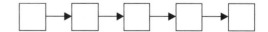

FILL IN THE BLANKS

Provide the missing term or terms in the blanks provided.

1. _____ is the branch of pharmacology that uses drugs to treat, prevent, and diagnose disease.

2. Morphine is an example of a drug derived from a _____ source.

3. Scientists produce human insulin by altering the DNA of *Escherichia coli* via a process called _____ _____.

4. During preclinical trials, a drug is considered _____ if it is found to cause adverse effects on the fetus.

5. A drug in pregnancy category _____ is considered safe for use during pregnancy because studies have shown it not to be at risk to the fetus in the first trimester or in later trimesters.

6. An _____ drug is one that has been discovered but is not considered financially viable and has not been adopted by any drug company.

■ APPLYING YOUR KNOWLEDGE

CASE STUDY

A 66-year-old man comes to the clinic for a routine visit. He has brought along a brown paper bag that contains numerous medicines. The nurse empties the bag on the table and begins to review the bottles. The patient states, "I've got so many bottles of pills here, I'm not sure what I'm supposed to take and not take." The nurse observes that several of the bottles contain the same medication.

a. How would knowledge of generic and brand names be helpful in this situation?

b. What other information would be important to obtain when taking this patient's drug history?

■ PRACTICING FOR NCLEX

Circle the letter that corresponds to the best answer for each question.

1. After administering a medication to a patient, the patient complains of an upset stomach. The nurse interprets this as a negative effect of the drug and identifies it as which of the following?
   a. Adverse effect
   b. Intended effect
   c. Teratogenic effect
   d. Therapeutic effect

2. Which of the following is a key concern related to clinical pharmacology?
   a. The biologic effect of a drug
   b. The body processes used to eliminate a drug
   c. The drug's effects on the body
   d. The proper method for administering a drug

3. Which of the following drugs may be derived from an animal source?
   a. Digitalis
   b. Opium
   c. Morphine
   d. Insulin

4. A group of students are reviewing information about the natural sources of drugs. The students demonstrate understanding of the information when they identify which of the following as a drug derived from inorganic compounds?
   a. Thyroid hormone
   b. Ferrous sulfate (iron)
   c. Codeine
   d. Castor oil

5. During a phase II study, a drug may be removed from testing for which reason?
   a. Greater than anticipated effectiveness
   b. Low risk of toxicity
   c. High benefit-to-risk ratio
   d. Unacceptable adverse effects

Copyright © 2011 by Wolters Kluwer Health | Lippincott Williams & Wilkins. *Study Guide for Focus on Nursing Pharmacology.*

6. During which stage of drug development is the drug tested on laboratory animals?
   a. Preclinical trial
   b. Phase I study
   c. Phase II study
   d. Phase III study

7. While reviewing a package insert for a drug, which of the following would the nurse identify as the drug's generic name?
   a. L-thyroxine
   b. Levothyroxine sodium
   c. Levothroid
   d. Synthroid

8. Which phase of drug development is associated with continual evaluation of the drug?
   a. Phase I study
   b. Phase II study
   c. Phase III study
   d. Phase IV study

9. A nurse reviews the pregnancy risk categories for several drugs. A drug belonging to which category would the nurse identify as being safest to administer to a pregnant woman?
   a. Category X
   b. Category A
   c. Category B
   d. Category C

10. Male volunteers are usually selected for drug testing during a phase I study for which reason?
    a. Women are more unreliable in terms of adhering to the terms of the study.
    b. Men typically have a greater consistency in body build and makeup.
    c. The risk for damaging or destroying ova is too great.
    d. Men are less likely to develop toxic effects related to the drug.

11. A nurse is preparing to administer a cough syrup containing codeine to a patient. The nurse understands that this drug would be classified as which schedule of a controlled substance?
    a. C-II
    b. C-III
    c. C-IV
    d. C-V

12. Regulatory control over drug testing and evaluation by the FDA resulted from which legislation?
    a. Pure Food and Drug Act of 1906
    b. Federal Food, Drug, and Cosmetic Act of 1938
    c. Durham-Humphrey Amendment of 1951
    d. Kefauver-Harris Act of 1962

13. Which agency is responsible for the enforcement of controlled substances?
    a. FDA
    b. U.S. Department of Justice
    c. Drug Enforcement Agency
    d. Department of Health and Human Services

14. After studying the various sources of drugs, a group of students demonstrate a need for additional study when they identify which of the following as an example of a synthetic source for a drug?
    a. Plants
    b. Animals
    c. Inorganic compounds
    d. Genetic engineering

15. A nurse is administering a drug to patients who have the disease for which a drug is designed to treat. The nurse is most likely participating in which of the following?
    a. Preclinical trial
    b. Phase I study
    c. Phase II study
    d. Phase III study

Copyright © 2011 by Wolters Kluwer Health l Lippincott Williams & Wilkins. *Study Guide for Focus on Nursing Pharmacology.*

Drugs and the Body

LEARNING OBJECTIVES

Upon completion of this chapter, you will be able to:

1. Describe how body cells respond to the presence of drugs that are capable of altering their function.

2. Outline the process of dynamic equilibrium that determines the actual concentration of a drug in the body.

3. Explain the meaning of half-life of a drug and calculate the half-life of given drugs.

4. List at least six factors that can influence the actual effectiveness of drugs in the body.

5. Define drug–drug, drug–alternative therapy, drug–food, and drug–laboratory test interactions.

■ ASSESSING YOUR UNDERSTANDING

SEQUENCING

The four steps of pharmacokinetics are listed below. Place the number of the step in the boxes below based on the order in which they occur.

1. Metabolism

2. Excretion

3. Absorption

4. Distribution

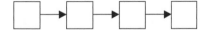

MATCHING

Select the description from column 2 that best describes the term in column 1.

Column 1

___ 1. Critical concentration

___ 2. Loading dose

___ 3. First-pass effect

___ 4. Half-life

Column 2

a. The time it takes for amount of drug in the body to decrease 50% of the peak level

b. The use of a higher dose than that which is usually used for treatment

c. The amount of drug that must be reached in tissues to cause the desired effect

d. Inactivation of an orally administered drug by liver enzymes before entering the general circulation

FILL IN THE BLANKS

Provide the missing term or terms in the blanks provided.

1. _____ refers to how a drug affects the body.

2. _____ refers to how the body acts on a drug.

3. A drug that interacts directly with receptor sites causing the same activity that natural chemicals would cause at that site is called

an _____.

4. The major process through which drugs are absorbed into the body is _____ _____.

5. Drug metabolism or _____ is the process by which drugs are changed into new, less-active chemicals.

■ APPLYING YOUR KNOWLEDGE

CASE STUDY

A 72-year-old woman comes in for a follow-up visit after being diagnosed with high blood pressure. The woman is obese and has a history of kidney disease. Her blood pressure remains elevated despite lifestyle changes. Medications to control her blood pressure are being ordered.

a. When assessing this patient, which factors possibly influencing drug effects would be most important to consider?

b. What other factors might play a role for this patient?

■ PRACTICING FOR NCLEX

Circle the letter that corresponds to the best answer for each question.

1. Which of the following would be a key element associated with pharmacodynamics?
   a. Enzyme systems
   b. Critical concentration
   c. Dynamic equilibrium
   d. Protein binding

2. When administering a drug, the nurse understands that a drug administered by which route would be absorbed most rapidly?
   a. Oral
   b. Intramuscular
   c. Intravenous
   d. Subcutaneous

3. When researching information about a drug, the nurse finds that the drug tightly binds to protein. The nurse would interpret this to mean which of the following?
   a. The drug will be released fairly quickly.
   b. The drug will have a long duration of action.
   c. The drug will be excreted quickly.
   d. The drug will lead to toxicity when given.

4. Which of the following most commonly occurs first when an oral drug is being absorbed?
   a. Liver enzymes break down the drug into metabolites.
   b. The drug is delivered to the circulatory system for transport.
   c. The drug moves from the small intestine directly into the portal venous system.
   d. A portion of the drug reaches the tissues before getting to the liver.

5. When describing biotransformation to a group of students, which of the following would the instructor include as part of phase II biotransformation?
   a. Oxidation
   b. Reduction
   c. Hydrolysis
   d. Conjugation

6. Which of the following substances would most likely inhibit the cytochrome P450 enzyme system?
   a. Nicotine
   b. Alcohol
   c. Ketoconazole
   d. Cortisone

7. Which of the following plays the largest role in drug excretion?
   a. Skin
   b. Kidneys
   c. Feces
   d. Lungs

Copyright © 2011 by Wolters Kluwer Health I Lippincott Williams & Wilkins. *Study Guide for Focus on Nursing Pharmacology.*

8. A patient is receiving 250 mg of a drug that has a half-life of 8 hours. How much drug would remain after 24 hours?

   a. 125 mg

   b. 62.5 mg

   c. 31.25 mg

   d. 15.625 mg

9. A nurse administers a prescribed loading dose of digoxin based on the understanding that doing so will result in which of the following?

   a. Critical concentration being reached more quickly

   b. Enhanced absorption for effectiveness

   c. Prevention of drug breakdown by stomach acid

   d. Prolonged half-life of the administered drug

10. A nurse is preparing to administer a prescribed drug to a patient who has liver disease. The nurse expects a reduction in dosage based on the understanding that which of the following might be altered?

    a. Absorption

    b. Distribution

    c. Metabolism

    d. Excretion

11. Which mechanism is primarily responsible for drug absorption in the body?

    a. Active transport

    b. Passive diffusion

    c. Protein binding

    d. Filtration

12. When assessing a patient for possible factors that may affect the pharmacokinetics of a drug, a patient with a history of which of the following would lead the nurse to suspect that the patient may experience an alteration in the distribution of a drug?

    a. Gastrointestinal disease

    b. Liver disease

    c. Kidney disease

    d. Vascular disease

13. A nurse is reading an article that describes predictable differences in the effects of drugs in people of particular culture backgrounds due to their genetic makeup. The nurse is reading about which of the following?

    a. Pharmacogenomics

    b. Pharmacodynamics

    c. Pharmacokinetics

    d. Pharmacology

14. An instructor is describing a specific area on a cell membrane where most drugs are thought to act. The students demonstrate understanding of this information when they identify this area as which of the following?

    a. Lock

    b. Enzyme system

    c. Receptor site

    d. Agonist

15. Penicillin causes bacterial cell death without disrupting normal human cell functioning. This is an example of which of the following?

    a. Critical concentration

    b. Selective toxicity

    c. First-pass effect

    d. Enzyme induction

Copyright © 2011 by Wolters Kluwer Health I Lippincott Williams & Wilkins. *Study Guide for Focus on Nursing Pharmacology.*

CHAPTER 3

Toxic Effects of Drugs

LEARNING OBJECTIVES

Upon completion of this chapter, you will be able to:

1. Define the term *adverse drug reaction* and explain the clinical significance of this reaction.

2. List four types of allergic responses to drug therapy.

3. Discuss five common examples of drug-induced tissue damage.

4. Define the term *poison*.

5. Outline the important factors to consider when applying the nursing process to selected situations of drug poisoning.

■ ASSESSING YOUR UNDERSTANDING

MATCHING

Select the description from column 2 that best describes the term in column 1.

Column 1

_____ **1.** Anaphylactic reaction

_____ **2.** Cytotoxic reaction

_____ **3.** Serum sickness reaction

_____ **4.** Delayed allergic reaction

Column 2

a. Reaction involving antibodies that are bound to specific white blood cells

b. Reaction involving antibodies circulating in the blood and attacking antigens on cell sites, causing cell death

c. Reaction involving antibodies circulating in the blood and causing damage to tissues via deposition in blood vessels

d. Reaction involving antibody with specific sites in the body causing the release of chemicals to produce an immediate reaction

SHORT ANSWER

Supply the information requested.

1. List two reasons why adverse effects can occur.

2. Explain why it is important to always review the contraindications and cautions associated with a drug before administering it.

3. Identify the most common reason for the development of adverse effects related to drug therapy.

4. List the four main classifications of drug allergies.

5. Describe how superinfections occur with drug administration.

6. Define *blood dyscrasia*.

7. Name the electrolyte that when altered due to drug therapy can cause the most serious effects.

8. List four assessment findings associated with anticholinergic effects.

■ APPLYING YOUR KNOWLEDGE

CASE STUDY

The nurse is obtaining a history from a 35-year-old woman who is being scheduled for outpatient surgery. During the interview, the patient reports using an over-the-counter antihistamine for her hay fever. The nurse also asks the patient about any allergies to food or medications. The patient responds, "I'm allergic to codeine."

a. What effects might the nurse expect the patient to report with the use of antihistamines?

b. What information would the nurse need to obtain to determine if the patient has a "true allergy" to codeine?

■ PRACTICING FOR NCLEX

Circle the letter that corresponds to the best answer for each question.

1. When instructing a patient who is taking an antibiotic about the possibility of nausea and diarrhea, the nurse understands that these effects are examples of which of the following?
   a. Primary actions
   b. Secondary actions
   c. Drug allergy
   d. Hypersensitivity

2. A patient develops a cytotoxic reaction to a drug. Which of the following would the nurse expect to do?
   a. Administer prescribed epinephrine subcutaneously
   b. Encourage the use of Medic-alert identification
   c. Discontinue the drug immediately as ordered
   d. Administer antipyretics as ordered

3. When assessing a patient who has developed a serum sickness reaction, which of the following would the nurse expect to find?
   a. Hives
   b. Difficulty breathing
   c. Decreased white blood cell count
   d. Facial edema

4. A patient develops stomatitis from drug therapy. Which measure would be most appropriate for the nurse to suggest?
   a. Consumption of three large meals per day
   b. The use of an astringent mouthwash
   c. Frequent rinsing with cool liquids
   d. Brushing of teeth with a firm toothbrush

5. The nurse would assess a patient receiving which medication for possible superinfection?
   a. Antibiotics
   b. Antihistamines
   c. Antihypertensives
   d. Antineoplastics

Copyright © 2011 by Wolters Kluwer Health l Lippincott Williams & Wilkins. *Study Guide for Focus on Nursing Pharmacology.*

6. Which of the following would lead the nurse to suspect that a patient has developed a blood dyscrasia related to drug therapy? Select all that apply.

   a. Thrombocytopenia

   b. Anemia

   c. Leukocytosis

   d. Dilute urine

   e. Headache

   f. Sore throat

7. The nurse is reviewing the laboratory test results of a patient receiving drug therapy. Which of the following would the nurse suspect if the results reveal an elevation in the blood urea nitrogen level and creatinine concentration?

   a. Liver injury

   b. Hypoglycemia

   c. Hyperkalemia

   d. Renal injury

8. Which of the following would the nurse include in the teaching plan for a patient who is to receive a drug that is associated with anticholinergic effects?

   a. Try to stay as warm as possible to prevent chilling.

   b. Be sure to drink plenty of fluids to prevent dehydration.

   c. Try using hard candy or lozenges to prevent dry mouth.

   d. Eat a low-fiber diet to prevent constipation.

9. Which of the following would the nurse expect to assess if a patient develops neuroleptic malignant syndrome?

   a. Mental confusion

   b. Hypothermia

   c. Hypertension

   d. Hyperactive reflexes

10. A patient exhibits muscular tremors, drooling, gait changes, and spasms. When reviewing the patient's medication history, which of the following would the nurse most likely find?

    a. Antipsychotic agent

    b. Antidiabetic agent

    c. General anesthetic

    d. Anticholinergic agent

11. An instructor is preparing a class that describes the toxic effects of drugs. Which of the following would the instructor expect to include?

    a. Many drugs are potentially harmless if used correctly.

    b. Any effect results from the alteration of several chemical factors.

    c. Most reactions occurring with present-day therapy are less severe than before.

    d. Drugs cause unexpected or unacceptable reactions despite screening and testing.

12. Which of the following is an example of a secondary action?

    a. Anticoagulant that leads to excessive and spontaneous bleeding

    b. Dizziness and weakness with a recommended dose of antihypertensive

    c. An antihistamine causes the patient to experience drowsiness

    d. Urinary retention develops in a patient with an enlarged prostate who is taking an anticholinergic

13. Which of the following would the nurse expect to assess in a patient experiencing an anaphylactic reaction? Select all that apply.

    a. Dilated pupils

    b. Feeling of panic

    c. High fever

    d. Swollen joints

    e. Difficulty breathing

14. Which of the following would the nurse expect the physician to order for a patient with a delayed allergic reaction?

    a. Epinephrine

    b. Antipyretic

    c. Anti-inflammatory

    d. Topical corticosteroid

15. A patient is receiving a drug to lower his blood glucose level. Which of the following would lead the nurse to suspect that his blood glucose level was too low?

    a. Cold, clammy skin

    b. Increased urination

    c. Fruity breath odor

    d. Increased hunger

Copyright © 2011 by Wolters Kluwer Health I Lippincott Williams & Wilkins. *Study Guide for Focus on Nursing Pharmacology.*

CHAPTER 4

The Nursing Process in Drug Therapy and Patient Safety

Upon completion of this chapter, you will be able to:

1. List the responsibilities of the nurse in drug therapy.

2. Explain what is involved in each step of the nursing process as it relates to drug therapy.

3. Describe key points that must be incorporated into the assessment of a patient receiving drug therapy.

4. Describe the essential elements of a medication order.

5. Outline the important points that must be assessed and considered before administering a drug, combining knowledge about the drug with knowledge of the patient and the environment.

6. Describe the role of the nurse and the patient in preventing medication errors.

■ ASSESSING YOUR UNDERSTANDING

MATCHING

Select the description from column 2 that best describes the term in column 1.

Column 1

___ **1.** Assessment

___ **2.** Nursing diagnosis

___ **3.** Implementation

___ **4.** Evaluation

___ **5.** Nursing process

Column 2

a. Actions undertaken to meet a patient's needs

b. Information gathering

c. Determination of effectiveness

d. Problem-solving method

e. Actual or potential problem statement

SHORT ANSWER

Supply the information requested.

1. Explain what the nurse accomplishes when applying the nursing process to drug therapy.

2. List two major aspects associated with assessment.

3. Identify the seven rights to ensure safe and effective drug administration.

4. Name two areas that need to be addressed when obtaining a patient's history related to drug therapy.

5. Describe one reason why a patient may not reveal the use of over-the-counter drugs or alternative therapies during a history.

6. Explain why it is important to obtain a patient's weight before beginning drug therapy.

7. Describe the rationale for assessing physical parameters related to disease or drug effects before drug therapy begins.

8. Explain the term *placebo effect*.

LABELING

On the chart below, place the letter of the statement or phrase in the column that corresponds to the correct step of the nursing process.

Assessment	Nursing Diagnosis
Implementation	Evaluation

a. Deficient knowledge related to possible adverse effects of antihypertensive therapy

b. Diagnosed with type 2 diabetes 5 years ago

c. Administer the drug with food to minimize gastric upset

d. Takes omega-3 fish oil three times per week

e. Patient lives with husband in a two-bedroom apartment

f. Patient demonstrates independence in administering subcutaneous insulin administration

g. Obtain serum drug levels as ordered

h. Risk for injury related to drug's effect on balance and alertness

■ APPLYING YOUR KNOWLEDGE

CASE STUDY

An older adult patient is to begin drug therapy for treatment of a bacterial infection. The nurse completes an assessment and notes that the patient has a history of heart disease and diabetes. The patient, who is also somewhat underweight for his height, lives alone in a small apartment. His closest relative lives about an hour away. The patient is a native of Poland and speaks little English. He is accompanied by an older adult friend who helps explain information to him.

a. How might the patient's history of heart disease and diabetes impact his drug therapy?

Copyright © 2011 by Wolters Kluwer Health I Lippincott Williams & Wilkins. *Study Guide for Focus on Nursing Pharmacology.*

b. Would the nurse expect the patient to be prescribed the typical recommended dosage? Why or why not?

c. What issues might affect the patient's ability to comply with the drug therapy regimen?

■ PRACTICING FOR NCLEX

Circle the letter that corresponds to the best answer for each question.

1. A nurse is gathering information about a patient. The nurse is participating in which step of the nursing process?
   a. Assessment
   b. Nursing diagnosis
   c. Implementation
   d. Evaluation

2. Which of the following would the nurse expect to do during implementation?
   a. Develop statements about a patient's actual problem
   b. Obtain baseline information about the patient's pattern of health care
   c. Identify the patient's social support network
   d. Provide patient teaching about a drug therapy regimen

3. A group of students are reviewing information about the nursing process and drug therapy in preparation for an examination on the material. The students demonstrate understanding of the material when they state which of the following about the nursing process?
   a. A continuous linear approach to problem solving
   b. A set of sequential steps that are dynamic in nature
   c. A method for determining a patient's priority needs
   d. A means to gather information about a patient's current status

4. During assessment, a nurse asks a patient about any chronic conditions that might have an impact on the patient's prescribed drug therapy. Which of the following, if reported by the patient, would alert the nurse to a possible problem?
   a. Two episodes of pneumonia over the last 5 years
   b. Kidney disease diagnosed 2 years ago
   c. Nearsightedness for the past 10 years
   d. Episode of gastroenteritis last month

5. Which of the following would be least important to include when teaching a patient about drug therapy?
   a. Alternative therapies to avoid
   b. Timing of administration
   c. Drug toxicity warning signs
   d. How to report a medication error

6. The nurse is reviewing several orders for medications. Which dosage would cause the nurse to be concerned?
   a. 0.5 mg
   b. 50 mg
   c. .5 mg
   d. 500 mg

7. A patient is to receive a topical drug. Which of the following would the nurse need to do?
   a. Check to see if it needs to be reconstituted
   b. Determine the possible need for skin preparation
   c. Question if the drug can be crushed
   d. Use a large amount of the drug to ensure effectiveness

8. Which of the following instructions would be most appropriate for the nurse to teach the patient to reduce the risk of medication errors in the home setting?
   a. Keep a written record of all prescription medications taken.
   b. Store the medications in the bathroom medicine cabinet.
   c. Take the medications according to what works best with the patient's schedule.
   d. Know what each drug is being used for as treatment.

Copyright © 2011 by Wolters Kluwer Health I Lippincott Williams & Wilkins. *Study Guide for Focus on Nursing Pharmacology.*

9. A nurse who is caring for a patient receiving drug therapy performs the actions below. Place the actions in the proper sequence to reflect the steps of the nursing process.

   a. Teaches the patient how to minimize adverse reactions

   b. Identifies pertinent problems related to functioning

   c. Determines that the drug is therapeutically effective

   d. Questions the patient about any chronic conditions

10. After teaching the parents of a child who is receiving drug therapy, which statement indicates the need for additional teaching?

    a. "Some over-the-counter drugs contain the same ingredients, so we need to read each label closely before giving the medication."

    b. "We can use the same medications that we use for similar problems in our child, but we might need to adjust the dosage."

    c. "When measuring a liquid medication, we should use a measured device or spoon rather than a kitchen tablespoon or teaspoon."

    d. "We need to tell each health care provider about all the medications that our child is taking, even nonprescription ones."

11. Assessment of a patient receiving drug therapy reveals that the patient has been experiencing gastrointestinal upset related to the drug. The patient states, "My stomach has been so upset that all I've been able to eat is soup and dry crackers." Which nursing diagnosis would be most likely?

    a. Imbalanced nutrition: Less than body requirements

    b. Risk for imbalanced fluid volume

    c. Feeding self-care deficit

    d. Noncompliance

12. Which of the following would be least likely to occur during the assessment phase of the nursing process for drug therapy?

    a. Obtaining information about the patient's drug use

    b. Determining relevant data about financial constraints

    c. Developing outcomes for effective response to drug therapy

    d. Identifying the patient's level of understanding

13. The following are steps of the nursing process. Place the steps in the proper sequence from beginning to end.

    a. Nursing diagnosis

    b. Assessment

    c. Evaluation

    d. Implementation

14. The nurse questions a patient about the use of alternative therapies based on the understanding of which of the following?

    a. These therapies may lead to possible interactions with other drugs.

    b. The alternative therapies will need to be stopped with the newly prescribed drug.

    c. These therapies can lead to an increased risk for addiction.

    d. Alternative therapies provide information about the patient's health beliefs.

15. A nurse notes a medication error. Which action would be most appropriate?

    a. Notify the drug manufacturer.

    b. Make a report to the institution.

    c. Contact the Food and Drug Administration.

    d. Inform the Institute for Safe Medication Practices.

Copyright © 2011 by Wolters Kluwer Health I Lippincott Williams & Wilkins. *Study Guide for Focus on Nursing Pharmacology.*

CHAPTER 5

Dosage Calculations

LEARNING OBJECTIVES

Upon completion of this chapter, you will be able to:

1. Describe four measuring systems that can be used in drug therapy.

2. Convert between different measuring systems when given drug orders and available forms of the drugs.

3. Calculate the correct dose of a drug when given examples of drug orders and available forms of the drugs ordered.

4. Discuss why children require different dosages of drugs than adults.

5. Explain the calculations used to determine a safe pediatric dose of a drug.

■ ASSESSING YOUR UNDERSTANDING

FILL IN THE BLANKS

Provide the missing term or terms in the blanks provided.

1. One milliliter (mL) is equivalent to one

   _____ _____.

2. _____ rule is a method for determining the correct dose for a child based on the known adult dose.

3. One gram (g) is equivalent to _____ milligrams (mg).

4. All units in the metric system are determined as multiples of _____.

5. A _____ usually reflects the biologic activity of a drug in 1 milliliter (1 mL) of solution.

CROSSWORD

Use the clues to complete the crossword puzzle.

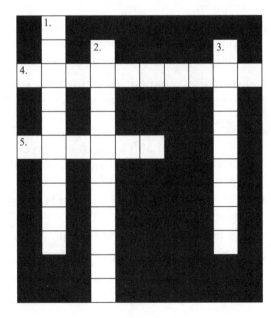

Across

4. Finding equivalent values between two systems
5. Most widely used system of measure

Down

1. Old system of measure used by pharmacists
2. Old system used when compounding medications
3. System of measure found in recipe books

■ APPLYING YOUR KNOWLEDGE

CASE STUDY

A mother brings her 3-year-old child to the clinic for evaluation of ear pain and fever. The child is diagnosed with an ear infection that is to be treated with oral antibiotics. The health care provider orders the antibiotic in suspension form. The nurse is preparing to teach the mother how to administer the antibiotic.

a. What information would be important for the nurse to obtain to ensure that the child receives the proper medication dosage?

b. What instructions would the nurse need to stress to ensure that the child receives the proper dose each time?

■ PRACTICING FOR NCLEX

Circle the letter that corresponds to the best answer for each question.

1. A group of students are reviewing the various measuring systems used for drug therapy. The students demonstrate understanding of these systems when they identify which of the following as the system used by pharmacists when they had to compound their own medications?

    a. Household system
    b. Avoirdupois system
    c. Apothecary system
    d. Metric system

2. Which of the following units of measure would a nurse expect to find when using the apothecary system?

    a. Liters
    b. Kilograms
    c. Drams
    d. Pounds

3. After teaching a group of students about measuring systems and drug calculations, the instructor determines that the teaching was successful when the students identify which system as most widely used?

    a. Metric system
    b. Apothecary system
    c. Household system
    d. Avoirdupois system

4. A nurse is using the metric system for dosage calculations. Which unit would the nurse use as the basic unit for measuring liquids?

    a. Gram
    b. Kilogram
    c. Liter
    d. Minim

5. A drug label reads "1 tablet equals 1 gr." The nurse understands that this one tablet is equivalent to how many milligrams?

    a. 30
    b. 60
    c. 240
    d. 1,000

6. A nurse needs to convert 3 fluid ounces to the metric system equivalent. The nurse performs the calculation to find which result?

    a. 90 mL
    b. 180 mL
    c. 240 mL
    d. 360 mL

7. A health care provider orders "aspirin gr x." The label on the bottle states that one tablet contains 5 grains. How many tablets would the nurse administer?

    a. 1
    b. 2
    c. 3
    d. 4

Copyright © 2011 by Wolters Kluwer Health | Lippincott Williams & Wilkins. *Study Guide for Focus on Nursing Pharmacology.*

8. A physician orders 250 mg of an antibiotic suspension. The label on the suspension reads "500 mg/5 mL." How much would the nurse administer?

   a. 2.5 mL

   b. 5 mL

   c. 7.5 mL

   d. 10 mL

9. A nurse is to administer 500 mg of a drug intramuscularly. The label on the multidose vial reads 250 mg/mL. How much of the medication would the nurse prepare in the syringe?

   a. 0.5 mL

   b. 1 mL

   c. 1.5 mL

   d. 2 mL

10. The physician orders a patient to receive 1000 mL of intravenous fluid over the next 8 hours. The intravenous delivery set is a macrodrip system. The nurse would set the infusion to run at which rate?

    a. 16 gtts/min

    b. 32 gtts/min

    c. 64 gtts/min

    d. 125 gtts/min

11. A nurse needs to calculate a safe dose of medication for a child. Which of the following would be most appropriate for the nurse to use?

    a. Clark's rule

    b. Fried's rule

    c. Young's rule

    d. Body surface area

12. As part of a class exercise, an instructor asks the students to calculate a pediatric dosage using Clark's rule. Which information would be important for the students to know? Select all that apply.

    a. Weight of child in pounds

    b. Child's age in years

    c. Average adult dose

    d. Body surface area

    e. Child's height in centimeters

13. A child weighs 22 kilograms. The physician orders a drug as follows: "1.1 mg/kg by intramuscular injection." The nurse determines the proper dose as which of the following?

    a. 1.2 mg

    b. 2.4 mg

    c. 12 mg

    d. 24 mg

14. Which of the following established standards require all prescriptions to include the metric measure for quantity and strength?

    a. Food and Drug Administration

    b. U.S. Pharmacopeia Convention

    c. Drug Enforcement Agency

    d. Institute of Safe Medication Practices

15. An instructor is describing the units of measure associated with household system. Which of the following would the nurse include? Select all that apply.

    a. Teaspoon

    b. Quart

    c. Dram

    d. Ounce

    e. Cup

    f. Milliliter

Copyright © 2011 by Wolters Kluwer Health I Lippincott Williams & Wilkins. *Study Guide for Focus on Nursing Pharmacology.*

Challenges to Effective Drug Therapy

LEARNING OBJECTIVES

Upon completion of this chapter, you will be able to:

1. Discuss the impact of the media, the Internet, and direct-to-consumer advertising on drug sales and prescriptions.

2. Explain the growing use of over-the-counter drugs and the impact it has on safe medical care.

3. Discuss the lack of controls on herbal or alternative therapies and the impact this has on safe drug therapy.

4. Define the off-label use of a drug.

5. Describe measures being taken to protect the public in cases of bioterrorism.

■ ASSESSING YOUR UNDERSTANDING

MATCHING

Match the street name of the drug in column 2 with the appropriate drug in column 1.

Column 1

___ **1.** Amyl nitrate

___ **2.** Barbiturates

___ **3.** Benzodiazepines

___ **4.** Cocaine

___ **5.** MDA

___ **6.** Heroin

___ **7.** Methamphetamine

___ **8.** Gamma-hydroxybutyrate

___ **9.** Ketamine

___ **10.** LSD

Column 2

a. Acid

b. Ecstasy

c. Blow

d. Boppers

e. Downers

f. Liquid X

g. Uncle Milty

h. Speed

i. Special K

j. Crank

SHORT ANSWER

Supply the information requested.

1. Name the one factor involved in the process for reviewing prescription drugs for possible over-the-counter (OTC) status.

2. State two reasons why patients may not mention the use of alternative therapies to health care providers.

3. Describe three areas that have impacted health care including drug therapy during the 21st century.

4. List two possible health consequences associated with the abuse of anabolic steroids.

5. Explain the term *biological weapon*.

■ APPLYING YOUR KNOWLEDGE

CASE STUDY

A patient comes to the health care clinic for a follow-up visit to evaluate his medications and control of his hypertension. During the visit he states, "My neighbor who is taking the same pills as I am for his high blood pressure has been telling me about all this information that he's gotten about his medicines on the Internet. He even said that he's found some herbs that work better than his medicines. I'm wondering if I should try these herbs too. Maybe they'll work better than what I'm using now."

a. How should the nurse respond to this patient?

b. What guidance should the nurse give to the patient about the Internet as a resource for information?

c. How should the nurse advise the patient about the use of herbs for his blood pressure?

■ PRACTICING FOR NCLEX

Circle the letter that corresponds to the best answer for each question.

1. A nurse is preparing a presentation for a local community group about various influences on drug therapy in today's health care climate. When addressing the impact of the media on drug therapy, which of the following would the nurse include?
   a. Television ads for prescription drugs is a recent development over the past 2 to 3 years.
   b. There currently are no federal guidelines as to what a company can say in an advertisement.
   c. Current medical research or reports are commonly making their way into headlines as news.
   d. Talk shows that include medical information typically present thorough and accurate information.

2. Which practice has contributed to the problem of resistant bacteria?
   a. Patients saving remaining antibiotics for the next time they feel sick
   b. The creation of matrix delivery systems for many medications
   c. The increased availability of generic-type drugs
   d. The use of drugs ordered through the Internet from foreign countries

3. A group of students ask an instructor about where to find the most updated information on biological weapons. Which of the following would the instructor recommend?
   a. Food and Drug Administration (FDA)
   b. Drug Facts and Comparisons
   c. National Center for Complementary and Alternative Medicine
   d. Centers for Disease Control

Copyright © 2011 by Wolters Kluwer Health | Lippincott Williams & Wilkins. *Study Guide for Focus on Nursing Pharmacology.*

4. When describing off-label use, which of the following would the nurse need to keep in mind?

   a. Liability related to off-label use is clearly defined.

   b. Off-label drug use may lead to the discovery of a new use for the drug.

   c. Off-label drug use often involves drugs for treating heart disease.

   d. Off-label use indicates that the drug is awaiting FDA approval.

5. After reviewing the various types of street drugs frequently abused, a group of students demonstrate understanding of the information when they identify gamma-hydroxybutyrate as which class?

   a. Stimulant

   b. Hallucinogen

   c. Depressant

   d. Opioid

6. When discussing the various reasons why patients may order drugs via the Internet from other countries, which of the following would be least likely?

   a. The drugs are commonly less costly.

   b. The patient does not need to see a health care provider.

   c. The medications are delivered directly to the patient's doorstep.

   d. The drugs are the same as those the patient would get at home.

7. Which of the following would a nurse include when teaching a patient about proper drug disposal?

   a. Keep any unused or unneeded drugs in their original containers.

   b. Flush any unused medications down the toilet.

   c. Mix leftover prescription drugs with coffee grounds in a sealable bag.

   d. Crush the remaining medications in kitty litter before throwing into the trash.

8. A patient reports that he takes St. John's wort. When reviewing the patient's medication history, which of the following would be a cause of concern?

   a. Insulin

   b. Digoxin

   c. Ibuprofen

   d. Acetaminophen

9. A nurse is watching television and sees an ad for a drug. The drug's indication is mentioned in the ad. Which of the following would the nurse identify as also being required to include in the ad? Select all that apply.

   a. Adverse effects

   b. Contraindications

   c. Precautions

   d. Typical doses

   e. Route of administration

10. When describing the characteristics of the patient who comes into the health care system today, which of the following would apply?

   a. Limited exposure to other sources of health information

   b. Continued acceptance of the health care provider as omniscient

   c. Eager acceptance of the medications selected for the patient

   d. The use of a complex array of OTC and alternative therapies

11. After teaching a patient about how to evaluate an Internet site for information about health care and drug, which statement indicates that the teaching was successful?

   a. "A site is accurate if it has been updated in the last 10 years."

   b. "A commercial-type site is often the best one to use for current information."

   c. "A site that allows for feedback is more reputable than one that doesn't."

   d. "A site that gives me the information that I need is worthwhile."

Copyright © 2011 by Wolters Kluwer Health l Lippincott Williams & Wilkins. *Study Guide for Focus on Nursing Pharmacology.*

12. Which of the following would be most appropriate to teach a patient about OTC drugs?

    a. They are safe when you use them as directed.

    b. There is little interaction between OTC drugs and prescription medications.

    c. Most OTC drugs have undergone stringent testing for use.

    d. OTC drugs often alert the health care provider to an underlying condition.

13. A patient arrives at the emergency department after abusing ketamine. Which of the following would the nurse expect to assess?

    a. Hallucinations

    b. Loss of sensation

    c. Memory loss

    d. Hypotension

14. A group of students are role-playing scenarios involving biological weapon exposure. Which of the following medications would the students identify as using for a patient with cutaneous anthrax?

    a. Ribavirin

    b. Ciprofloxacin

    c. Streptomycin

    d. Gentamicin

15. Which of the following drugs would be classified as a hallucinogen?

    a. Amyl nitrate

    b. Heroin

    c. Rohypnol

    d. PCP

Copyright © 2011 by Wolters Kluwer Health | Lippincott Williams & Wilkins. *Study Guide for Focus on Nursing Pharmacology.*

Introduction to Cell Physiology

LEARNING OBJECTIVES

Upon completion of this chapter, you will be able to:

1. Identify the parts of the human cell.

2. Describe the role of each organelle found within the cell cytoplasm.

3. Explain the unique properties of the cell membrane.

4. Describe three processes used by the cell to move things across the cell membrane.

5. Outline the cell cycle, including the activities going on within the cell in each phase.

MATCHING

Select the description from column 2 that best describes the term in column 1.

Column 1

____ **1.** Passive transport

____ **2.** Diffusion

____ **3.** Osmosis

____ **4.** Facilitated diffusion

____ **5.** Active transport

Column 2

a. Substance moves against a concentration gradient with the use of energy.

b. Substance moves from a region of higher concentration to a lower one via a carrier molecule.

c. Water moves from an area of low solute concentration to a higher solute concentration.

d. Substance moves across any semipermeable membrane without the use of energy.

e. Substance moves from a region of higher concentration to a lower concentration.

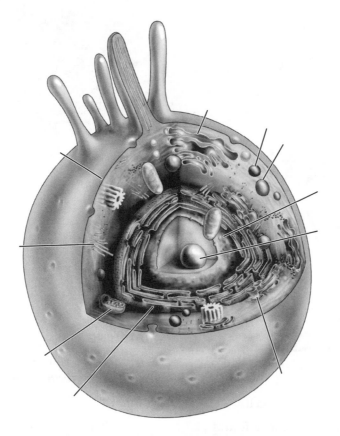

FILL IN THE BLANKS

Provide the missing term or terms in the blanks provided.

1. The _____ is the basic structural unit of the body.

2. Sequences of DNA that allow for cell division are called _____.

3. The cell membrane is composed of _____ and _____.

4. The cytoplasm of a cell contains many structures, called _____, which have specific functions.

5. The mitochondria produces _____ in the form of ATP for use by the cell.

6. The main goal of a cell is to maintain _____, which keeps the cytoplasm stable within the cell membrane via movement of solutes and water into and out of the cell.

7. The cell cycle consists of _____ active phases and a resting phase.

8. The _____ of a cell contains DNA and genetic material.

■ ASSESSING YOUR UNDERSTANDING

LABELING

Use the list of terms below to label the cell.

  Cell membrane
  Centrioles
  Cilia
  Golgi apparatus
  Lysosomes
  Microtubules
  Mitochondria
  Nuclear membrane
  Nuclear pore
  Nucleolus
  Perioxsomes
  Polyrivosomes
  Rough endoplasmic reticulum
  Smooth endoplasmic reticulum

Copyright © 2011 by Wolters Kluwer Health l Lippincott Williams & Wilkins. *Study Guide for Focus on Nursing Pharmacology.*

■ APPLYING YOUR KNOWLEDGE

CASE STUDY

A group of students are working on a class assignment in which they are to present a visual demonstration of the cell cycle and events in each phase. They decide that one student will explain the cell cycle and its phases, while each of the other students will act out the events for a specific phase.

a. What events would the students need to demonstrate for each phase?

b. How might a student demonstrate the G_0 phase?

c. How might the students demonstrate the M phase?

■ PRACTICING FOR NCLEX

Circle the letter that corresponds to the best answer for each question.

1. Which of the following would be found in a cell membrane?
   a. Ribosomes
   b. Genes
   c. Cholesterol
   d. Mitochondria

2. When describing the DNA necessary for cell division, which of the following would be most accurate?
   a. It is found in long strains called *chromatin*.
   b. It is encapsulated in its own membrane.
   c. It is a series of dense fibers and proteins.
   d. It is composed of lipids and proteins.

3. The body uses which of the following to identify a cell as belonging to that individual?
   a. Receptor sites
   b. Histocompatibility antigens
   c. Channels
   d. Organelles

4. The mitochondria is responsible for which of the following functions?
   a. Protein production
   b. Cholesterol production
   c. Hormone processing
   d. Energy production

5. When preparing a class discussion about the various organelles of a cell, the instructor plans to include a description of the structure that contains digestive enzymes. Which of the following would the instructor be describing?
   a. Free ribosomes
   b. Lysosomes
   c. Golgi apparatus
   d. Endoplasmic reticulum

6. A group of students are studying for a test on cellular transport systems. The students demonstrate a need for additional study when they identify which mechanism as requiring no energy?
   a. Facilitated diffusion
   b. Osmosis
   c. Active transport
   d. Diffusion

7. A substance attaches itself to an enzyme in order to move in and out of a cell. This substance is moving via which transport mechanism?
   a. Diffusion
   b. Active transport
   c. Osmosis
   d. Facilitated diffusion

8. A solution contains the same concentration of solutes as human plasm. This solution would be classified as which of the following?
   a. Hypertonic
   b. Isotonic
   c. Hypotonic
   d. Osmotic

Copyright © 2011 by Wolters Kluwer Health l Lippincott Williams & Wilkins. *Study Guide for Focus on Nursing Pharmacology*.

9. Which of the following would occur to a red blood cell if it were placed in a hypotonic solution?

   a. Burst

   b. Shrivel

   c. Shrink

   d. Remain the same

10. Which of the following statements best reflects the cell cycle?

    a. The secretion of enzymes determines the rate at which cells multiply.

    b. The reproductive rate of each cell determines the cell's life cycle.

    c. The cells found in breast tissue characteristically reproduce quickly.

    d. The life cycle of the cell involves four active phases and a resting phase.

11. Which of the following signals the end of the G_1 phase of the cell cycle?

    a. Formation of two identical daughter cells

    b. Formation of DNA

    c. Doubling of DNA

    d. Stimulation of the cell

12. Which transport mechanism is primarily used by the kidneys for drug excretion?

    a. Osmosis

    b. Facilitated diffusion

    c. Active transport

    d. Diffusion

13. A group of students are reviewing material about cell membranes in preparation for a quiz. Which statement indicates the need for additional study?

    a. The freely movable cell membrane allows the cell to repair itself.

    b. The polar regions of the cell membrane repel water.

    c. Receptor sites are located on the cell membrane.

    d. Cholesterol is found in large quantities in the cell membrane.

14. A substance being removed from a cell is being pushed through the cell membrane. What is the name of this process?

    a. Endocytosis

    b. Pinocytosis

    c. Phagocytosis

    d. Exocytosis

15. During which phase of the cell cycle is the cell at rest?

    a. G_0

    b. G_1

    c. S

    d. G_2

Copyright © 2011 by Wolters Kluwer Health I Lippincott Williams & Wilkins. *Study Guide for Focus on Nursing Pharmacology.*

CHAPTER 8

Anti-Infective Agents

Upon completion of this chapter, you will be able to:

1. Explain what is meant by selective toxicity and discuss its importance in anti-infective therapies.

2. Differentiate between broad-spectrum and narrow-spectrum drugs.

3. Define bacterial resistance to antibiotics and discuss the emergence of resistant strains.

4. Explain three ways to minimize bacterial resistance.

5. Describe three common adverse reactions associated with the use of antibiotics.

■ ASSESSING YOUR UNDERSTANDING

MATCHING

Select the drug action from column 2 that best describes the drug in column 1.

Column 1

_____ 1. Penicillins

_____ 2. Sulfonamides

_____ 3. Aminoglycosides

_____ 4. Fluoroquinolones

_____ 5. Antifungals

Column 2

a. Interference with DNA synthesis in the cell

b. Interference with bacterial cell wall biosynthesis

c. Interference with protein synthesis

d. Prevention of invading organisms from using cellular substances

e. Alteration in the cell membrane permeability

SHORT ANSWER

Supply the information requested.

1. Identify the overall goal of anti-infective agents.

2. Explain the terms *bactericidal* and *bacteriostatic*.

3. Describe what is meant by "spectrum of activity."

4. Identify the first step in determining which anti-infective agent should be used.

5. List three ways that health care providers can help prevent the emergence of resistant strains of organisms.

■ APPLYING YOUR KNOWLEDGE

CASE STUDY

A patient comes to the clinic for a follow-up visit. On the previous visit about a week ago, the patient was prescribed penicillin to treat a staphylococcal infection of a wound on the patient's lower left leg. On this visit, the wound appears slightly smaller in size, but there is a moderate amount of purulent drainage oozing from the wound. The patient states, "It was better several days ago, about 3 days after I started taking the penicillin. Since it was better, I stopped taking the medicine."

a. What would the nurse suspect as a potential problem with the patient's wound?

b. What teaching would be most important for this patient?

■ PRACTICING FOR NCLEX

Circle the letter that corresponds to the best answer for each question.

1. A nurse is preparing a teaching plan for a patient who is receiving trimethoprim-sulfamethoxazole. Which of the following would the nurse need to keep in mind when describing how this drug works?
   a. Interfering with the bacterial cell wall
   b. Preventing the organism's cells from using substances
   c. Interfering with protein synthesis
   d. Altering the permeability of the cell membrane

2. Which of the following occurs when the normal flora is destroyed by the use of anti-infectives?
   a. Neurotoxicity
   b. Hypersensitivity
   c. Superinfection
   d. Resistance

3. A patient asks a nurse why the health care provider has prescribed two anti-infective agents. Which response by the nurse would be most appropriate?
   a. "You have a resistant strain of organism that requires the use of more than one drug."
   b. "The one drug doesn't come in a strong enough strength to clear the infection."
   c. "You need larger amounts of both drugs so you'll have fewer adverse effects."
   d. "Your infection, like many infections, is caused by more than one organism."

4. Which of the following would a nurse least expect as an adverse reaction to anti-infective agents?
   a. Kidney damage
   b. Hypersensitivity
   c. Respiratory toxicity
   d. Neurotoxicity

5. A patient is receiving an aminoglycoside antibiotic for an infection. The nurse would monitor the patient closely for which of the following?
   a. Hearing loss
   b. Lethargy
   c. Visual changes
   d. Hallucinations

6. A female patient comes to the clinic complaining of a vaginal discharge with itching. When obtaining the patient's medication history, which of the following would the nurse consider as significant?
   a. Inhaled bronchodilator for asthma
   b. Broad spectrum anti-infective for recent infection
   c. Oral contraceptive use
   d. Daily multivitamin supplement

7. A group of students are reviewing information about anti-infective agents. The students demonstrate a need for additional review when they identify which of the following as an anti-infective agent?
   a. Antibiotic
   b. Anthelmintic
   c. Antiprotozoal
   d. Anticoagulant

Copyright © 2011 by Wolters Kluwer Health l Lippincott Williams & Wilkins. *Study Guide for Focus on Nursing Pharmacology.*

8. When describing an anti-infective agent with a narrow spectrum of activity, which of the following would the nurse include?

    a. The drug is effective against many different organisms.

    b. The drug is highly aggressive in killing the pathogen.

    c. The drug is selective in its action on organisms.

    d. The drug is effective in interfering with the cell's reproduction.

9. After teaching a group of students about resistance, the instructor determines that the students need additional teaching when they identify which of the following as a way that microorganisms develop resistance?

    a. Production of an enzyme that deactivates the drug

    b. Change in cellular permeability preventing drug entrance

    c. Altered binding sites that no longer accept the drug

    d. Production of a chemical to act as an agonist

10. Which of the following would contribute to drug resistance?

    a. High dosage to eradicate the organism

    b. Antibiotic prescription for viral illness

    c. Around-the-clock scheduling

    d. Prescribed duration of therapy

11. A patient is to receive penicillin. The nurse understands that this drug achieves it effect by which action?

    a. Interfering with the bacterial cell wall

    b. Not allowing the organism to use the substances it needs

    c. Disrupting the steps of protein synthesis

    d. Interfering with DNA synthesis

12. To ensure that the most appropriate drug is being used to treat a pathogen, which of the following would need to be done first?

    a. Using combination therapy

    b. Obtaining sensitivity testing

    c. Checking patient allergies

    d. Evaluating the bactericidal effects

13. A patient who is receiving anti-infective therapy is experiencing gastrointestinal toxicity. Which of the following would the nurse expect to assess?

    a. Dizziness

    b. Rash

    c. Diarrhea

    d. Vertigo

14. A patient is receiving chloroquine as part of her treatment for a rheumatic disorder. Which complaint would lead the nurse to suspect that the patient is experiencing neurotoxicity?

    a. "I'm having trouble hearing."

    b. "My vision is getting really poor."

    c. "I feel like the room is spinning."

    d. "I get so dizzy sometimes."

15. An older adult patient is prescribed an anti-infective agent. Which of the following would the nurse need to keep in mind?

    a. Signs and symptoms of infection are the same as those for a younger patient.

    b. The patient has a lower risk for developing gastrointestinal toxicity and neurotoxicity.

    c. Liver and kidney function may be reduced, requiring cautious use.

    d. The patient will most likely want to have a rapid cure for his problem.

Copyright © 2011 by Wolters Kluwer Health | Lippincott Williams & Wilkins. *Study Guide for Focus on Nursing Pharmacology.*

Antibiotics

LEARNING OBJECTIVES

Upon completion of this chapter, you will be able to:

1. Explain how an antibiotic is selected for use in a particular clinical situation.

2. Describe therapeutic actions, indications, pharmacokinetics, contraindications, most common adverse reactions, and important drug–drug interactions associated with each of the classes of antibiotics.

3. Discuss the use of antibiotics as they are used across the life span.

4. Compare and contrast prototype drugs for each class of antibiotics with other drugs in that class.

5. Outline nursing considerations for patients receiving each class of antibiotic.

■ ASSESSING YOUR UNDERSTANDING

FILL IN THE BLANKS

Provide the missing term or terms in the blanks provided.

1. _____ bacteria can survive without oxygen.

2. Bacteria that are _____ - _____ are frequently associated with infections of the respiratory tract.

3. Some antibiotics are given in combination because they are _____.

4. Aminoglycosides are _____, inhibiting protein synthesis and ultimately leading to cell death.

5. The prototype cephalosporin is _____.

LABELING

Place the name of the following drugs in the appropriate box under the correct drug class.

Amikacin

Azithromycin

Erythromycin

Gemifloxacin

Gentamicin

Norfloxacin

Streptomycin

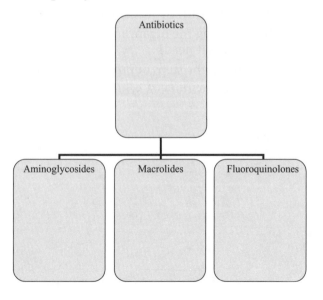

■ APPLYING YOUR KNOWLEDGE

CASE STUDY

A patient comes to the clinic complaining of urinary frequency, urgency, and pain on urination. A urine culture reveals an infection with a *Escherichia coli*. The health care provider prescribes ciprofloxacin to be taken twice daily. The patient also has a history of acid reflux for which she uses an antacid as needed.

a. Would the nurse consider this an appropriate choice for the patient's condition? Please explain.

b. When teaching the patient about this drug, how would the nurse describe the drug's action?

c. What adverse effects would the nurse need to address with this patient?

d. Would the use of antacids interfere with the prescribed drug therapy? Why or why not?

■ PRACTICING FOR NCLEX

Circle the letter that corresponds to the best answer for each question.

1. Which of the following drugs would be classified as an aminoglycoside?
   a. Levofloxacin
   b. Clarithromycin
   c. Gentamicin
   d. Cefaclor

2. A patient is receiving telithromycin. The nurse understands that this drug is structurally related to which of the following?
   a. Penicillins
   b. Macrolides
   c. Cephalosporins
   d. Lincosamides

3. A patient is prescribed streptomycin. The nurse understands that this drug can be given only by which route?
   a. Oral
   b. Intravenous
   c. Ophthalmic
   d. Intramuscular

4. A patient is to receive gentamicin for treatment of an infection. Which of the following would be most important for the nurse to assess to establish a baseline?
   a. Nutritional status
   b. Auditory function
   c. Gastrointestinal function
   d. Muscle strength

5. A group of students are reviewing information about drugs used to treat tuberculosis. The students demonstrate understanding of the material when they identify which of the following drugs as a first-line treatment option?
   a. Rifampin
   b. Kanamycin
   c. Ciprofloxacin
   d. Capreomycin

6. After teaching a group of students about carbapenems, the instructor determines the need for additional teaching when the students identify which of the following as an example?
   a. Doripenem
   b. Imipenem-cilastatin
   c. Cefuroxime
   d. Ertapenem

Copyright © 2011 by Wolters Kluwer Health I Lippincott Williams & Wilkins. *Study Guide for Focus on Nursing Pharmacology*.

7. The nurse is preparing a teaching plan for a patient who is receiving cephalosporins. Which of the following would the nurse identify as the most commonly occurring adverse effects?

   a. Vomiting and diarrhea

   b. Headache and dizziness

   c. Superinfections

   d. Phlebitis

8. A patient comes to the emergency department complaining of a throbbing headache, nausea, vomiting, chest pain, dyspnea, vertigo, and blurred vision. The patient reveals that he has been taking cefaclor for an infection. Which question would the nurse ask next?

   a. "Have you had any alcohol to drink in the past 72 hours?"

   b. "Are you taking an oral anticoagulant such as warfarin?"

   c. "Did the doctor prescribe any other antibiotics with this one?"

   d. "Have you been drinking enough fluids with the medicine?"

9. A group of students are reviewing material for a test on antibiotics. They demonstrate an understanding of the material when they identify which of the following as the first antibiotic introduced for clinical use?

   a. Erythromycin

   b. Ampicillin

   c. Cephalexin

   d. Penicillin

10. After teaching a patient who is prescribed oral erythromycin, the nurse determines that the teaching was successful when the patient states which of the following?

   a. "I need to take the medicine with a meal so I don't get an upset stomach."

   b. "I should drink a full 8-oz glass of water when I take the medicine."

   c. "I might have some bloody diarrhea after using this medicine."

   d. "I only need to take one pill every day for this medicine to work."

11. A patient is receiving rifampin and isoniazid in combination for treatment of tuberculosis. Which of the following would the nurse need to monitor closely?

   a. Liver function studies

   b. Urine culture

   c. Audiometric studies

   d. Pulmonary function studies

12. Which of the following drugs would be classified as a third-generation cephalosporin?

   a. Cefazolin

   b. Cefaclor

   c. Ceftazidime

   d. Cephalexin

13. Which of the following would a nurse identify as the prototype lincosamide drug?

   a. Erythromycin

   b. Clindamycin

   c. Lincomycin

   d. Clarithromycin

14. Which of the following would be considered a penicillinase-resistant antibiotic?

   a. Amoxicillin

   b. Ticarcillin

   c. Carbenicillin

   d. Nafcillin

15. The drug's effect on which of the following best reflects the major reason for avoiding the use of tetracyclines in children under 8 years of age?

   a. Teeth

   b. Hearing

   c. Vision

   d. Kidneys

Copyright © 2011 by Wolters Kluwer Health | Lippincott Williams & Wilkins. *Study Guide for Focus on Nursing Pharmacology*.

CHAPTER 10

Antiviral Agents

LEARNING OBJECTIVES

Upon completion of this chapter, you will be able to:

1. Discuss problems with treating viral infections in humans and the use of antivirals across the life span.

2. Describe characteristics of common viruses and the resultant clinical presentations of common viral infections.

3. Describe the therapeutic actions, indications, pharmacokinetics, contraindications, most common adverse reactions, and important drug–drug interactions associated with each of the types of antivirals discussed in the chapter.

4. Compare and contrast the prototype drugs for each type of antiviral with the other drugs within that group.

5. Outline the nursing considerations for patients receiving each class of antiviral agent.

■ ASSESSING YOUR UNDERSTANDING

LABELING

Place the name of the following drugs in the appropriate box under the correct drug class.

Abacavir

Delavirdine

Indinavir

Nevirapine

Saquinavir

Zidovudine

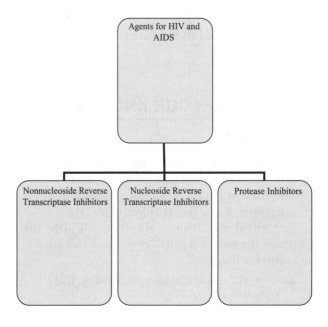

MATCHING

Select the description from column 2 that best describes the drug class in column 1.

Column 1

_____ **1.** CCR5 coreceptor antagonist

_____ **2.** Integrase inhibitor

_____ **3.** Nucleoside reverse transcriptase inhibitor

_____ **4.** Protease inhibitor

_____ **5.** Nonnucleoside reverse transcriptase inhibitor

Column 2

a. Drug that directly binds to the HIV enzyme to prevent the transfer of information that would allow the virus to carry on the formation of viral DNA.

b. Drug that competes with the naturally occurring nucleosides within a human cell that the virus needs in order to develop the DNA chain.

c. Drug that interferes with the enzyme necessary for cell maturation, leaving the HIV particle immature and noninfective and unable to fuse with and inject itself into a cell.

d. Drug that interferes with the virus-specific encoded enzyme needed for viral replication, preventing the formation of the HIV-1 provirus.

e. Drug that blocks the receptor site that the HIV virus needs to interact with in order to enter the cell.

■ APPLYING YOUR KNOWLEDGE

CASE STUDY

A woman is diagnosed with genital herpes and receives a prescription for valacyclovir. The patient is visibly anxious, asking many questions about her condition and the prescribed medication. She states, "I hope this medicine works. I don't ever want this to come back again."

a. How should the nurse respond to the patient's statement?

b. What information would the nurse need to include in the teaching plan for this patient?

■ PRACTICING FOR NCLEX

Circle the letter that corresponds to the best answer for each question.

1. A patient is diagnosed with cytomegalovirus infection and is to receive foscarnet. The nurse would expect to administer this drug by which route?

  a. Oral

  b. Intramuscular

  c. Intravenous

  d. Topical

2. A patient comes to the health care facility complaining of flulike symptoms. After a thorough assessment, the patient is diagnosed with influenza and is to receive oseltamivir. The nurse understands that this drug has been prescribed because the patient been symptomatic for less than:

  a. 2 days

  b. 4 days

  c. 6 days

  d. 8 days

3. Which drug would a nurse least likely expect to be prescribed for a patient with chronic hepatitis B?

  a. Entecavir

  b. Telbivudine

  c. Adefovir

  d. Fosamprenavir

4. Which of the following was the first class of drugs developed to treat HIV infections?

  a. Protease inhibitors

  b. Nucleoside reverse transcriptase inhibitors

  c. Nonnucleoside reverse transcriptase inhibitors

  d. Fusion inhibitors

5. A nurse is explaining the rationale for the use of combination therapy in the treatment of HIV infections. Which of the following would the nurse include as the primary reason?

   a. More than one drug is needed to ensure sensitivity to the different forms of the virus.

   b. The use of multiple drugs allows attack on the virus at different points in its life cycle.

   c. One drug helps to control the virus, while the other drugs help to alleviate the adverse effects.

   d. Using several drugs at once helps to improve the patient's immune response.

6. A patient with HIV is pregnant. Which of the following agents would the nurse expect to be prescribed?

   a. Tenofovir

   b. Lamivudine

   c. Zidovudine

   d. Zalcitabine

7. A patient is receiving nevirapine as part of a treatment for HIV infection. The nurse would instruct the patient about which of the following adverse effects as most commonly experienced?

   a. Dry mouth and dyspepsia

   b. Light-headedness and dizziness

   c. Buffalo hump and thin extremities

   d. Paresthesias and fever

8. A patient is receiving zanamivir. When describing this drug, the nurse understands that it is absorbed through which mechanism?

   a. Gastrointestinal tract

   b. Bloodstream

   c. Respiratory tract

   d. Skin

9. Which of the following would be least likely to cause a drug interaction when rimantadine is prescribed?

   a. Atropine

   b. Acetaminophen

   c. Aspirin

   d. Ibuprofen

10. Assessment of a patient who is receiving nelfinavir reveals a severe life-threatening arrhythmia. The nurse would check the patient's history for use of which of the following?

    a. Midazolam

    b. Warfarin

    c. Clarithromycin

    d. Quinidine

11. Which of the following would a nurse identify as a CCR5 coreceptor antagonist?

    a. Enfuvirtide

    b. Maraviroc

    c. Raltegravir

    d. Didanosine

12. Which of the following would be most important to stress with a patient who is receiving adefovir for treatment of chronic hepatitis B?

    a. Possible adverse effects such as headache and dizziness

    b. Periodic follow-up renal function studies

    c. Maintenance of a continuous adequate supply of drug

    d. Measures to reduce the risk of infection transmission

13. A patient is being treated with docosanol. After teaching the patient about the drug, the nurse determines that additional instruction is needed when the patient states which of the following?

    a. "I should apply the medicine to any new open lesions that arise near the area."

    b. "I might have some burning or stinging in the area when I use the medicine."

    c. "There is little risk for absorbing the drug into my system this way."

    d. "I realize the drug won't cure me, but it should help with the discomfort."

Copyright © 2011 by Wolters Kluwer Health I Lippincott Williams & Wilkins. *Study Guide for Focus on Nursing Pharmacology.*

14. A group of students are reviewing information about antiviral agents used to treat influenza and respiratory virus infections. The students demonstrate understanding of the material when they identify which drug as appropriate for treating Avian flu?

   a. Amantadine

   b. Oseltamivir

   c. Ribavirin

   d. Zanamivir

15. A patient with AIDS develops cytomegalovirus retinitis. The physician orders cidofovir. The nurse would prepare the patient for administration of the drug by which route?

   a. Oral

   b. Topical

   c. Subcutaneous

   d. Intravenous

CHAPTER 11

Antifungal Agents

LEARNING OBJECTIVES

Upon completion of this chapter, you will be able to:

1. Describe the characteristics of a fungus and a fungal infection.

2. Discuss the therapeutic actions, indications, pharmacokinetics, contraindications, proper administration, most common adverse reactions, and important drug–drug interactions associated with systemic and topical antifungals.

3. Compare and contrast the prototype drugs for systemic and topical antifungals with the other drugs in each class.

4. Discuss the impact of using antifungals across the life span.

5. Outline the nursing considerations for patients receiving a systemic or topical antifungal.

■ ASSESSING YOUR UNDERSTANDING

CROSSWORD

Use the clues to complete the crossword puzzle.

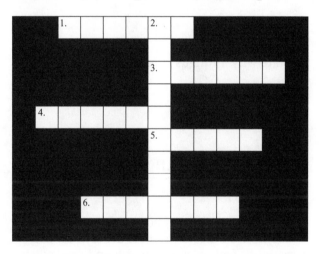

Across

1. A group of drugs used to treat fungal infections
3. An enzyme present in the fungal cell wall but not in human cells
4. A cellular organism with a hard cell wall
5. Ringworm that causes athlete's foot
6. A disease caused by a fungus

Down

2. A steroid-type protein found in fungal cell membranes

SHORT ANSWER

Supply the information requested.

1. Identify the enzyme system that is affected by ketoconazole and fluconazole.

2. Explain the reason why topical antifungals should not be used over open or draining areas.

3. Describe why the incidence of fungal infections has increased.

4. Name the three major types of local fungal infections.

5. State why a fungus is resistant to antibiotics.

■ APPLYING YOUR KNOWLEDGE

CASE STUDY

During a routine physical examination of a client, the nurse notes that the skin on the patient's feet is extremely dry and cracked with areas where the skin is scaly. The area between the toes is slightly reddened, and the skin appears to be peeling. Several round 1- to 2-mm vesicles are also observed. The patient states that his feet perspire quite a bit, and they recently have become itchy. Tinea pedis is diagnosed, and topical clotrimazole as a cream is recommended.

a. How would the nurse instruct the patient to use the topical agent, and why would this be important?

b. What precautions would the nurse include about using this drug?

c. What additional instructions would be appropriate for this patient?

■ PRACTICING FOR NCLEX

Circle the letter that corresponds to the best answer for each question.

1. When describing the action of ketoconazole, which of the following would be most accurate?
   a. It inhibits the production of ergosterol.
   b. It interferes with formation of the fungal cell wall.
   c. It blocks sterol activity of the fungal cell wall.
   d. It inhibits a cytochrome P2D6 enzyme system.

2. A patient states, "My doctor said that I had mycosis, but I thought I had a fungal infection." Which response would be most appropriate?
   a. "You're both correct because mycosis means a disease is caused by a fungus."
   b. "Mycosis means that you have an underlying immune disease."
   c. "Let's talk to the doctor so that we can find out what really is going on here."
   d. "Don't worry, because mycosis is only a minor infection that is easily treatable."

3. Which of the following antifungal agents is available for systemic and topical use?
   a. Butoconazole
   b. Clotrimazole
   c. Voriconazole
   d. Ketoconazole

4. Which of the following would be most important for the nurse to monitor in a patient receiving amphotericin B?

    a. Coagulation studies

    b. Complete blood count

    c. Bowel sounds

    d. Respiratory status

5. The nurse is administering fluconazole intravenously. When would the nurse expect the drug to peak?

    a. 30 minutes

    b. 60 minutes

    c. 90 minutes

    d. 120 minutes

6. A patient is suspected of having a serious fungal infection for which systemic antifungal therapy is planned. Which of the following should be done first?

    a. Obtain a specimen for culture and sensitivity testing.

    b. Assess the patient's nutritional status.

    c. Check the results of the patient's renal function studies.

    d. Insert an intravenous access device for administration.

7. Which of the following statements best reflects topical antifungal agents?

    a. They are most effective when applied in a thick manner.

    b. They rarely cause local irritation and burning.

    c. They are too toxic to be used systemically.

    d. They are associated with many drug–drug interactions.

8. A group of students are studying for a test on antifungal agents. The students demonstrate understanding of the material when they identify which of the following as an example of an echinocandin antifungal?

    a. Terbinafine

    b. Amphotericin B

    c. Nystatin

    d. Caspofungin

9. A patient with a systemic fungal infection and a history of diabetes is to receive an antifungal agent. Based on the nurse's understanding about these agents, which agent would the nurse expect as being the least appropriate?

    a. Ketoconazole

    b. Fluconazole

    c. Itraconazole

    d. Terbinafine

10. A patient is receiving itraconazole. Which of the following drugs should be avoided? Select all that apply.

    a. Simvastatin

    b. Midazolam

    c. Warfarin

    d. Pimozide

    e. Digoxin

    f. Cyclosporine

11. A patient with migraine headaches typically uses ergot for relief. The patient now has a systemic fungal infection for which voriconazole is prescribed. Which of the following suggestions would be most appropriate for the nurse to give?

    a. "You can continue to take the ergot, but separate it from the voriconazole by at least 2 hours."

    b. "Wait until you've finished the regimen of voriconazole before using the ergot again."

    c. "Take the voriconazole with a large glass of water to promote excretion of the ergot."

    d. "The dosage of the voriconazole will need to be decreased when you take the ergot."

12. A patient is receiving flucytosine. The nurse is reviewing the patient's serum drug level. Which serum drug level would lead the nurse to suspect that the patient is developing toxicity?

    a. 22 mcg/mL

    b. 45 mcg/mL

    c. 88 mcg/mL

    d. 110 mcg/mL

13. Which of the following drugs would be contraindicated for a patient who is receiving amphotericin B?

    a. Penicillin

    b. Amantadine

    c. Gentamicin

    d. Aztreonam

14. A patient taking an oral antifungal agent reports gastrointestinal upset. Which of the following would be most appropriate to suggest?

    a. Calling the prescriber to change the drug

    b. Having the patient take the drug with food

    c. Advising the patient to sit upright after taking the drug

    d. Telling the patient to eat three large meals a day

15. The nurse cautions a patient taking sulconazole to limit therapy to which duration?

    a. 2 weeks

    b. 4 weeks

    c. 6 weeks

    d. 8 weeks

CHAPTER 12

Antiprotozoal Agents

LEARNING OBJECTIVES

Upon completion of this chapter, you will be able to:

1. Outline the life cycle of the protozoan that causes malaria.

2. Describe the therapeutic actions, indications, pharmacokinetics, contraindications, proper administration, most common adverse reactions, and important drug–drug interactions associated with drugs used to treat malaria.

3. Describe other common protozoal infections, including their cause and clinical presentation.

4. Compare and contrast the antimalarials with other drugs used to treat protozoal infections.

5. Outline the nursing considerations for patients receiving an antiprotozoal agent across the life span.

■ ASSESSING YOUR UNDERSTANDING

FILL IN THE BLANKS

Provide the missing term in the blanks provided.

1. A _____ is a developing stage of a parasite.

2. *Plasmodium* is the protozoan that causes _____ in humans.

3. _____ is an infestation with a protozoan that causes vaginitis in women.

4. African sleeping sickness is called _____.

5. A _____ is a single-celled organism that passes through several stages in its life cycle.

SEQUENCING

The following are the stages in the life cycle of the plasmodium in humans. Place the number of the stage in the boxes below as they occur once a mosquito bites a human.

1. Schizont

2. Trophozoite

3. Sporozoite

4. Merozoite

5. Gametocyte

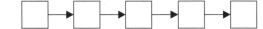

■ APPLYING YOUR KNOWLEDGE

CASE STUDY

A man comes to the urgent care center complaining of gastrointestinal distress. He states, "I've been having a fair amount of diarrhea over the past 2 days, and I have some pain in my belly." A stool specimen is obtained and sent for culture. The stool is loose, watery, and contains mucus. No blood is present. Further investigation reveals that the patient recently was camping in the mountains. Culture reports reveal giardiasis. The health care provider orders tinidazole.

a. What additional questions might the nurse ask to assist in helping the patient understand his condition? Explain why these questions would be important.

b. How would the nurse instruct the patient to take the tinidazole?

c. What specific areas need to be addressed related to this drug therapy?

■ PRACTICING FOR NCLEX

Circle the letter that corresponds to the best answer for each question.

1. Which statement best reflects the use of antimalarial agents for treatment of the protozoan?
   a. Typically, a single drug is sufficient to destroy the sporozoites in the early stages.
   b. Quinine is considered the current mainstay of treatment for malaria.
   c. Combination therapy is used to attack the parasite at various life cycle stages.
   d. The development of resistant strains of the parasite against antimalarial agents is rare.

2. When explaining the action of chloroquine to a patient, the nurse would incorporate knowledge of which of the following about the drug?
   a. Interferes with the parasites ability to reproduce
   b. Causes rupture of the cell, leading to its death
   c. Blocks the use of folic acid needed for protein synthesis
   d. Disrupts the mitochondria of the parasite

3. A patient is receiving mefloquine as part of a treatment for malaria asks the nurse about becoming pregnant. Which response by the nurse would be most appropriate?
   a. "You can plan to become pregnant once you complete the drug therapy regimen."
   b. "You need to avoid pregnancy during the therapy and for 2 months after completion."
   c. "You need to wait at least 6 months after starting the therapy before getting pregnant."
   d. "It's okay to become pregnant during therapy, but just don't plan to breast-feed."

4. A patient taking primaquine develops cinchonism. Which of the following would the nurse assess? Select all that apply.
   a. Tinnitus
   b. Vomiting
   c. Fever
   d. Dyspepsia
   e. Rash
   f. Vertigo

5. Which of the following assessments would be most important to complete for a patient who is to receive an antimalarial agent?
   a. Respiratory status
   b. Ophthalmologic evaluation
   c. Nutritional status
   d. Pupillary response

Copyright © 2011 by Wolters Kluwer Health I Lippincott Williams & Wilkins. *Study Guide for Focus on Nursing Pharmacology.*

6. A patient who is receiving metronidazole therapy for trichomoniasis asks the nurse how this infection occurred. Which response by the nurse would be most appropriate?

   a. "You probably got bitten by a mosquito."

   b. "It is passed to humans by the common housefly."

   c. "The infection is spread during sexual intercourse."

   d. "You probably drank some contaminated water."

7. A patient with amebiasis is to receive metronidazole. The patient also takes warfarin for atrial fibrillation. The nurse would instruct the patient to report which of the following immediately?

   a. Abdominal cramps

   b. Ataxia

   c. Paresthesias

   d. Increased bleeding

8. A patient with *Pneumocystis carinii* pneumonia is to receive pentamidine. The nurse would expect to administer this drug most likely by which route?

   a. Oral

   b. Inhalation

   c. Transdermal

   d. Subcutaneous

9. A patient receiving which agent should be instructed to avoid alcohol consumption?

   a. Pentamidine

   b. Atovaquone

   c. Metronidazole

   d. Nitazoxanide

10. Atovaquone is indicated for use in which of the following?

    a. *Pneumocystis carinii* pneumonia

    b. Amebiasis

    c. Giardiasis

    d. Trypanosomiasis

11. Which agent would the nurse expect to administer to a patient with leishmaniasis?

    a. Metronidazole

    b. Nitazoxanide

    c. Atovaquone

    d. Pentamidine

12. A nurse is preparing a presentation for a group of individuals who are receiving prophylactic treatment for malaria in preparation for a trip to an endemic area. Which of the following would the nurse include as the underlying cause of this disorder?

    a. Bite of an infected mosquito

    b. Consumption of food from contaminated soil

    c. Consumption of unpurified spring water

    d. Bite of an infected tsetse fly

13. Which of the following would a nurse include as a major contributing factor to the development of protozoal infections?

    a. Widely scattered housing

    b. Tropical climate

    c. Adequate sanitary facilities

    d. Insect control

14. When a person is infected with malaria, the person receives which of the following?

    a. Sporozoites

    b. Schizonts

    c. Trophozoites

    d. Merozoites

15. Which agent would a nurse identify as being most schizonticidal?

    a. Chloroquine

    b. Primaquine

    c. Pyrimethamine

    d. Hydroxychloroquine

Copyright © 2011 by Wolters Kluwer Health l Lippincott Williams & Wilkins. *Study Guide for Focus on Nursing Pharmacology.*

Anthelmintic Agents

LEARNING OBJECTIVES

Upon completion of this chapter, you will be able to:

1. List the common worms that cause disease in humans.

2. Describe the therapeutic actions, indications, pharmacokinetics, contraindications, most common adverse reactions, and important drug–drug interactions associated with the anthelmintics.

3. Discuss the use of anthelmintics across the life span.

4. Compare and contrast the prototype drug mebendazole with other anthelmintics.

5. Outline the nursing considerations, including important teaching points to stress, for patients receiving an anthelmintic.

■ ASSESSING YOUR UNDERSTANDING

SHORT ANSWER

Supply the information requested

1. List the five common types of infections by nematodes.

2. Identify the most frequent cause of helminth infection among school-age children in the United States.

3. Describe the difference between nematodes and platyhelminths.

4. Define *helminth*.

5. Name the disease that is caused by the ingestion of encysted roundworm larvae in undercooked pork.

MATCHING

Select the description of manifestations from column 2 that best reflects the infection in column 1.

Column 1

___ 1. Pinworms

___ 2. Whipworms

___ 3. Threadworms

___ 4. Hookworms

___ 5. Cestodes

Column 2

a. Pneumonia, liver abscess

b. Weight loss, abdominal distention

c. Perianal itching, vaginal itching

d. Colic, bloody diarrhea

e. Anemia, malabsorption

■ APPLYING YOUR KNOWLEDGE

CASE STUDY

A mother brings her 7-year-old son to the office for an evaluation. The mother says that her son has been complaining of intense itching in his buttocks area over the last few days. "It's like he is scratching himself all the time." Further questioning reveals that the child attended an overnight camp about 6 weeks ago. The child is diagnosed with a pinworm infection, and drug therapy with mebendazole is prescribed. The mother says, "Oh, I'm so embarrassed. How did this happen?"

a. What factors may have contributed to the child's condition?

b. How should the nurse respond to the mother?

c. What instructions would the nurse include when teaching the mother about this drug therapy?

■ PRACTICING FOR NCLEX

Circle the letter that corresponds to the best answer for each question.

1. Which of the following would be associated with an infection caused by a flatworm?
   a. Pinworm
   b. Whipworm
   c. Ascaris
   d. Tapeworm

2. When interviewing a patient with a suspected worm infection, which of the following would lead the nurse to suspect trichinosis?
   a. Consumption of unwashed vegetables
   b. Ingestion of undercooked pork
   c. Recent insect bite
   d. Swimming in a contaminated lake

3. After reviewing class information about anthelmintic agents, a group of students demonstrate understanding of the material when they identify which drug as the prototype anthelmintic?
   a. Praziquantel
   b. Albendazole
   c. Mebendazole
   d. Pyrantel

4. Which infection would be associated with intestinal invasion by a worm?
   a. Ascaris
   b. Trichinosis
   c. Filariasis
   d. Schistosomiasis

5. A patient is prescribed pyrantel for the treatment of a roundworm infection. The nurse understands that this drug may be preferred for which reason?
   a. It is administered once a month.
   b. It completely eradicates the infection.
   c. It requires a single dose.
   d. It comes in a chewable form.

Copyright © 2011 by Wolters Kluwer Health | Lippincott Williams & Wilkins. *Study Guide for Focus on Nursing Pharmacology.*

6. When describing mebendazole to a group of students, which of the following would the instructor include?

   a. Complete systemic absorption

   b. Numerous adverse effects

   c. No metabolism in the body

   d. Excretion as unchanged in urine

7. A patient is prescribed praziquantel. Which of the following would the nurse include when teaching the patient about how to take the drug?

   a. "Take the drug every morning and evening for a week."

   b. "Chew the tablet thoroughly each morning for 3 days."

   c. "Take the drug every 6 hours for three doses in 1 day."

   d. "Take the drug once in the morning."

8. Which of the following would the nurse be alert for in a patient receiving albendazole?

   a. Stevens-Johnson syndrome

   b. Bone marrow depression

   c. Diarrhea

   d. Fever

9. A patient with filariasis asks the nurse how he got the infection. The nurse would incorporate an understanding of which of the following when responding to the patient?

   a. The patient swam in a freshwater lake or pond where a snail deposited larvae.

   b. The patient consumed undercooked fish that contained the larvae of cestodes.

   c. The patient ate unwashed vegetables that were grown in contaminated soil.

   d. The patient was bitten by an insect that contained worm embryos.

10. Which drug would the nurse identify as the drug of choice for treating a threadworm infection?

    a. Pyrantel

    b. Praziquantel

    c. Thiabendazole

    d. Ivermectin

11. Which of the following would the nurse expect to assess in a patient with a whipworm infection?

    a. Bloody diarrhea

    b. Pneumonia

    c. Fatigue

    d. Weight loss

12. Which of the following would be most important to obtain for a patient who is suspected of having a helminthic infection?

    a. Complete blood count

    b. Urinalysis

    c. Liver function tests

    d. Stool examination

13. After teaching a local community group of students about measures to help prevent the spread of helminths, the nurse determines the need for additional teaching if the group identifies which measure?

    a. Weekly cleaning of bathroom toilets

    b. Thorough, frequent handwashing

    c. Consistent washing of fresh vegetables

    d. Using chlorine-treated water for laundry

14. Which of the following would the nurse identify as causing more damage to humans than most other helminths?

    a. Ascaris

    b. Threadworm

    c. Schistosomiasis

    d. Pinworm

15. Which of the following activities would be appropriate for a nurse to include when teaching a community group about measures to prevent trichinosis?

    a. Washing hands thoroughly after working with the soil

    b. Avoiding swimming in bodies of water that may be contaminated

    c. Ensuring that any pork products are thoroughly cooked

    d. Protecting oneself from possible insect bites

Copyright © 2011 by Wolters Kluwer Health I Lippincott Williams & Wilkins. *Study Guide for Focus on Nursing Pharmacology.*

Antineoplastic Agents

Upon completion of this chapter, you will be able to:

1. Describe the nature of cancer and the changes the body undergoes when cancer occurs.

2. Describe the therapeutic actions, indications, pharmacokinetics, contraindications, most common adverse reactions, and important drug–drug interactions associated with each class of antineoplastic agents and with adjunctive therapy use with these drugs.

3. Discuss the use of antineoplastic drugs across the lifespan.

4. Compare and contrast the prototype drugs for each class of antineoplastic agents with the other drugs in that class.

5. Outline the nursing considerations and teaching needs for patients receiving each class of antineoplastic agents.

■ ASSESSING YOUR UNDERSTANDING

CROSSWORD

Use the clues to complete the crossword puzzle.

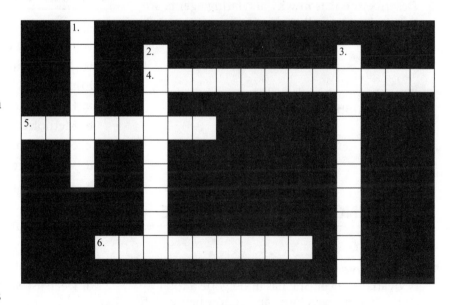

Across

4. Generation of new blood vessels
5. Hair loss
6. Loss of organization and structure

Down

1. Tumor originating in mesenchyme
2. Tumor originating in epithelial cells
3. Ability to enter circulatory or lymphatic system for travel to other areas

SHORT ANSWER

Supply the information requested.

1. Name the two major groups of cancer.

2. Explain how all cancers start.

3. List the two mechanisms by which antineoplastic drugs work.

4. Identify how or when a patient is considered to be cured of cancer.

5. Describe the reason why alkylating agents are said to be non–cell cycle specific.

6. State the phase of the cell cycle in which mitotic inhibitors act.

■ APPLYING YOUR KNOWLEDGE

CASE STUDY

A 75-year-old woman is diagnosed with stage IV ovarian cancer. She has undergone a total abdominal hysterectomy and is now being seen by the oncologist for follow-up chemotherapy. The oncologist plans to use cisplatin and pacli-taxel. While the nurse is working with the patient to set up a schedule for the administration of the chemotherapy, the patient breaks down in tears and says, "I've heard so many horror stories about chemotherapy. I'm worried that I'll be throwing up all the time. And what am I going to do if I lose my hair?"

a. How would the nurse respond to the patient's concerns? What information should the nurse provide to the patient?

b. What issues related to scheduling would the nurse need to work out with the patient about the administration of the drugs? What suggestions would be appropriate for the nurse to make to help the patient during the visit for the chemotherapy administration?

■ PRACTICING FOR NCLEX

Circle the letter that corresponds to the best answer for each question.

1. Which drug would be classified as a mitotic inhibitor?
   a. Fluorouracil
   b. Methotrexate
   c. Chlorambucil
   d. Vincristine

2. A nurse administers ondansetron to a patient receiving chemotherapy for which reason?
   a. Reduce vomiting
   b. Prevent hypersensitivity
   c. Relieve inflammation
   d. Decrease secretions

3. A patient develops leukopenia after receiving chemotherapy. Which nursing diagnosis would be most appropriate?
   a. Disturbed body image
   b. Imbalanced nutrition
   c. Risk for infection
   d. Deficient fluid volume

Copyright © 2011 by Wolters Kluwer Health I Lippincott Williams & Wilkins. *Study Guide for Focus on Nursing Pharmacology.*

4. Which agent would the nurse expect to be administered orally?

   a. Cytarabine

   b. Fluorouracil

   c. Gemcitabine

   d. Methotrexate

5. Which of the following would the nurse expect to administer to counteract the effects of methotrexate?

   a. Alprazolam

   b. Leucovorin

   c. Metoclopramide

   d. Aprepitant

6. Which of the following best reflects the action of antimetabolites?

   a. Reacts chemically with portions of RNA, DNA, or other cellular proteins

   b. Inserts itself between base pairs in the DNA chain, disrupting DNA synthesis

   c. Inhibits DNA production via replacing the natural substances needed for it

   d. Interferes with the ability of the cell to divide by blocking DNA synthesis

7. Which drug would have the least effect on healthy human cells?

   a. Etoposide

   b. Imatinib

   c. Vincristine

   d. Doxorubicin

8. A patient is receiving tamoxifen. Which adverse effect would be most specific to the action of this drug?

   a. Bone marrow suppression

   b. Gastrointestinal toxicity

   c. Hepatic dysfunction

   d. Menopausal effects

9. When planning the care for a patient receiving imatinib, the nurse would identify which nursing diagnosis as most likely?

   a. Excess fluid volume related to fluid retention

   b. Imbalanced nutrition, less than body requirements, related to severe nausea and vomiting

   c. Risk for infection related to bone marrow suppression

   d. Disturbed body image related to hair loss

10. A patient asks the nurse why the chemotherapy is often administered in cycles. Which response by the nurse would be most appropriate?

    a. "The drugs are highly toxic, so the body needs time to recover."

    b. "We want to attack the cells that might be dormant or moving into a new phase."

    c. "The cycles are the only way to guarantee a cure for the cancer."

    d. "The cycles help to prevent the drugs from destroying the healthy cells."

11. Which of the following would the nurse identify as an antineoplastic antibiotic?

    a. Mitomycin

    b. Teniposide

    c. Vinblastine

    d. Docetaxel

12. A patient is receiving bleomycin as part of his chemotherapy regimen. Which of the following would be most important for the nurse to monitor?

    a. Platelet count

    b. Electrocardiogram

    c. Chest x-ray

    d. Serum electrolytes

Copyright © 2011 by Wolters Kluwer Health l Lippincott Williams & Wilkins. *Study Guide for Focus on Nursing Pharmacology.*

13. When describing the use of the various agents for combating chemotherapy-induced nausea and vomiting, the nurse understands that the majority of these agents block which of the following?

a. Neurotransmitters

b. Gastric acidity

c. Gag reflex

d. Chemoreceptor trigger zone

14. A nurse is preparing to administer imatinib to a patient. The nurse expects to administer this drug by which route?

a. Oral

b. Subcutaneous

c. Intramuscular

d. Intravenous

15. When describing the process of cancer cell growth to a patient, the nurse addresses angiogenesis. Which of the following descriptions would the nurse include?

a. A process that involves the cells traveling to other areas of the body to develop new tumors

b. The process of creating new blood vessels to supply oxygen and nutrients to the cells

c. The process of growing without the usual homeostatic restrictions that regulate cells

d. A process in which the cells lose their ability to differentiate and organize

Copyright © 2011 by Wolters Kluwer Health I Lippincott Williams & Wilkins. *Study Guide for Focus on Nursing Pharmacology.*

CHAPTER 15

Introduction to the Immune Response and Inflammation

LEARNING OBJECTIVES

Upon completion of this chapter, you will be able to:

1. List four natural body defenses against infection.

2. Describe the cells associated with the body's fight against infection and their basic functions.

3. Outline the sequence of events in the inflammatory response.

4. Correlate the events in the inflammatory response with the clinical picture of inflammation.

5. Outline the sequence of events in an antibody-related immune reaction and correlate these events with the clinical presentation of such a reaction.

■ ASSESSING YOUR UNDERSTANDING

MATCHING

Select the description from column 2 that best describes the term in column 1.

Column 1

___ **1.** Antibody

___ **2.** Antigen

___ **3.** Calor

___ **4.** Leukocytes

___ **5.** Dolor

___ **6.** Tumor

___ **7.** Rubor

___ **8.** Pyrogen

Column 2

a. Swelling

b. Immunoglobulin

c. Heat

d. Redness

e. Foreign protein

f. Fever-causing substance

g. White blood cells

h. Pain

FILL IN THE BLANKS

Provide the missing term in the blanks provided.

1. The _____ system is activated by Hageman factor as part of the inflammatory response.

2. _____ cells are fixed basophils found in the respiratory and gastrointestinal tracts and in the skin that release chemical mediators.

3. The B-cell plasma cells produce _____ in response to a specific protein.

4. When neutrophils are drawn to an area, _____ is occurring.

5. The process of _____ involves engulfing and digesting foreign material.

■ APPLYING YOUR KNOWLEDGE

CASE STUDY

A patient comes to the clinic for evaluation. The patient is complaining of difficulty swallowing. On inspection, his throat is bright red and swollen. He has a fever and is complaining of an overall feeling of tiredness and general malaise. The patient is diagnosed with a strep throat.

a. How do the patient's signs and symptoms correlate with the events of the inflammatory response?

b. How might the immune system play a role here?

■ PRACTICING FOR NCLEX

Circle the letter that corresponds to the best answer for each question.

1. Which of the following would be considered the body's last barrier of defense?
   a. Skin
   b. Mucous membranes
   c. Gastric acid
   d. Major histocompatibility complex

2. Which of the following would be considered a lymphocyte?
   a. Neutrophils
   b. Monocytes
   c. T cells
   d. Macrophages

3. Which blood cell is responsible for phagocytosis?
   a. Neutrophils
   b. Basophils
   c. Eosinophils
   d. Macrophages

4. A group of students are reviewing class material about lymphoid tissue. The students demonstrate a need for additional teaching when they identify which of the following as lymphoid tissue?
   a. Bone marrow
   b. Thymus gland
   c. Spleen
   d. Histamine

5. Which event in the inflammatory response would the nurse correlate with the action of bradykinin?
   a. Vasoconstriction
   b. Pain
   c. Platelet aggregation
   d. Swelling

Copyright © 2011 by Wolters Kluwer Health I Lippincott Williams & Wilkins. *Study Guide for Focus on Nursing Pharmacology.*

6. When describing the inflammatory response to a group of students, which of the following would the instructor include as the first event that occurs after cell injury?

   a. Activation of Hageman factor

   b. Conversion of kininogen to bradykinin

   c. Release of arachidonic acid

   d. Release of prostaglandins

7. A nurse assesses a patient and notes an area that is reddened and warm. The nurse understands that these findings are related to which of the following?

   a. Activation of nerve fibers

   b. Vasodilation

   c. Fluid leakage into tissues

   d. Release of pyrogen

8. Which cells are responsible for cell-mediated immunity?

   a. T cells

   b. B cells

   c. Neutrophils

   d. Immunoglobulins

9. Which immunoglobulin is released first when a patient encounters an antigen again?

   a. Immunoglobulin M

   b. Immunoglobulin G

   c. Immunoglobulin A

   d. Immunoglobulin E

10. Which substance is responsible for stimulating T and B cells to initiate an immune response?

    a. Thymosin

    b. Tumor necrosis factor

    c. Interleukin-1

    d. Interferons

11. Which of the following occurs when the body produces antibodies against its own cells?

    a. Rejection

    b. Autoimmune disease

    c. Viral invasion

    d. Neoplastic growth

12. Which of the following best explains the role of mucus as a barrier for the body's defense?

    a. It promotes the removal of invaders.

    b. It sweeps away pathogens.

    c. It moves the pathogen to an area for removal.

    d. It traps the foreign material and thus inactivates it.

13. After reviewing information about the various myelocytes, the students demonstrate understanding when they identify mast cells as which of the following?

    a. Mature leukocytes

    b. Circulating myelocytic leukocytes

    c. Fixed basophils

    d. Phagocytic neutrophils

14. Which of the following is responsible for storing a concentrated amount of white blood cells?

    a. Lymph nodes

    b. Thymus

    c. Spleen

    d. Bone marrow

15. A patient who waiting for an organ transplant asks the nurse why the donor organ must be matched. Which response by the nurse would be most appropriate?

    a. "Matching helps ensure that the proper organ is prepared."

    b. "Matching prevents you from having a reaction."

    c. "The closer the match, the less risk there is of rejection."

    d. "Matching is required by law before any transplant."

Copyright © 2011 by Wolters Kluwer Health I Lippincott Williams & Wilkins. *Study Guide for Focus on Nursing Pharmacology.*

Anti-Inflammatory, Antiarthritis, and Related Agents

LEARNING OBJECTIVES

Upon completion of this chapter, you will be able to:

1. Describe the sites of action of the various anti-inflammatory agents.

2. Describe the therapeutic actions, indications, pharmacokinetics, contraindications, most common adverse reactions, and important drug–drug interactions associated with each class of anti-inflammatory agents.

3. Discuss the use of anti-inflammatory drugs across the life span.

4. Compare and contrast the prototype drugs for each class of anti-inflammatory drugs with the other drugs in that class.

5. Outline the nursing considerations and teaching needs for patients receiving each class of anti-inflammatory agents.

■ ASSESSING YOUR UNDERSTANDING

MATCHING

Select the description from column 2 that best describes the term in column 1.

Column 1

_____ 1. Analgesic

_____ 2. Antipyretic

_____ 3. Chrysotherapy

_____ 4. Nonsteroidal anti-inflammatory drug (NSAID)

_____ 5. Anti-inflammatory agent

Column 2

a. Treatment with gold salts

b. Fever blocker

c. Pain blocker

d. Prostaglandin synthesis blocker

e. Inflammatory response blocker

SHORT ANSWER

Supply the information requested.

1. Name the prototype salicylate drug.

2. List two problems associated with the over-the-counter (OTC) use of anti-inflammatory agents.

3. Identify four signs of salicylate toxicity.

4. Describe the actions of cyclooxygenase-1 (COX-1) and cyclooxygenase-2 (COX-2).

5. Define *salicylism*.

■ APPLYING YOUR KNOWLEDGE

CASE STUDY

A 45-year-old man arrives at the clinic because he has noticed that his stools have become darker, almost black, in color and somewhat tarry. He also has noticed that his gums have started to bleed when he brushes his teeth. During the interview, the patient reveals that he takes 600 mg of ibuprofen about three times a day for a back injury that he suffered while working 2 years ago. Inspection reveals several large bruised areas—two on his left arm and one on his lower left leg. "I guess I'm a bit clumsy. I tripped and fell against my refrigerator door."

a. What other assessment information would the nurse need to gather?

b. What would the nurse need to address when teaching this patient?

■ PRACTICING FOR NCLEX

Circle the letter that corresponds to the best answer for each question.

1. Which agent would be least appropriate to administer to a patient with joint inflammation and pain?

a. Ibuprofen

b. Naproxen

c. Acetaminophen

d. Diclofenac

2. A patient is diagnosed with inflammatory bowel disease. Which agent would the nurse expect to administer?

a. Diflunisal

b. Aspirin

c. Choline magnesium trisalicylate

d. Mesalamine

3. After teaching a local community group about the use of OTC anti-inflammatory agents, the nurse determines that the group needs additional teaching when they state which of the following?

a. "These drugs are relatively safe since they don't have adverse effects."

b. "We can easily overdose on them if we don't follow the directions."

c. "Other signs and symptoms of an illness might not appear with these drugs."

d. "The drugs might interact with other drugs and cause problems."

4. A nurse suspects that a patient is experiencing salicylism. Which of the following would the nurse assess?

a. Excitement

b. Ringing in the ears

c. Tachypnea

d. Convulsions

Copyright © 2011 by Wolters Kluwer Health l Lippincott Williams & Wilkins. *Study Guide for Focus on Nursing Pharmacology.*

5. Which instruction would be most important to include when teaching parents about OTC anti-inflammatory agents?
   a. "Be sure to read the label for the ingredients and dosage."
   b. "Aspirin is best for treating your child's flulike symptoms."
   c. "Make sure to give the drug on an empty stomach or before meals."
   d. "Refrain from using acetaminophen for the child's symptoms."

6. A salicylate is contraindicated in patients who have had surgery within the past week for which reason?
   a. Increased risk for allergic reaction
   b. Increased risk for toxicity
   c. Increased risk for bleeding
   d. Increased risk for fluid imbalance

7. Which of the following best describes the action of NSAIDs?
   a. Blocks prostaglandin activity
   b. Acts directly on thermoregulatory cells
   c. Inhibits phagocytosis
   d. Inhibits prostaglandin synthesis

8. A patient is to receive aurothioglucose. The nurse would administer this drug by which route?
   a. Oral
   b. Subcutaneous
   c. Intramuscular
   d. Intravenous

9. Which statement by a patient receiving gold salts indicates understanding of the drug therapy?
   a. "These drugs are used first to try to control my severe disease."
   b. "These drugs will help prevent further damage from my disease."
   c. "These drugs should help because I've had the disease for so long."
   d. "These drugs are safer than most of the other drugs for arthritis."

10. Which of the following would be appropriate to use in combination with gold salts?
    a. Penicillamine
    b. Cytotoxic agents
    c. Immunosuppressants
    d. Low-dose corticosteroids

11. After teaching a group of students about disease-modifying antirheumatic drugs, the instructor determines that the students need additional teaching when they identify which of the following as an example?
    a. Sulindac
    b. Etanercept
    c. Adalimumab
    d. Methotrexate

12. A patient is receiving anakinra as treatment for arthritis. The nurse understands that this drug acts in which manner?
    a. Interferes with free-floating tumor necrosis factor
    b. Inhibits the DHODH enzyme
    c. Blocks interleukin-1
    d. Lowers immunoglobulin M factor levels

13. A patient with severe rheumatoid arthritis of the knees has arrived at the facility for an injection of a drug into the joint. Which agent would the nurse most likely expect to be used?
    a. Aurothioglucose
    b. Penicillamine
    c. Etanercept
    d. Sodium hyaluronate

14. A group of students are reviewing information about cyclooxygenase receptors. The students demonstrate understanding of the information when they identify which of the following as an effect of COX-2 receptors?

   a. Maintenance of renal function

   b. Blockage of platelet clumping

   c. Provision of gastric mucosal integrity

   d. Promotion of vascular hemostasis

15. A black patient is receiving a high dose of NSAID for pain relief. Which of the following would be most important for the nurse to include in the teaching plan?

   a. The need to combine the drug with an OTC salicylate

   b. Signs and symptoms of gastrointestinal bleeding

   c. Avoidance of warm soaks for additional pain relief

   d. Importance of adequate hydration

Copyright © 2011 by Wolters Kluwer Health I Lippincott Williams & Wilkins. *Study Guide for Focus on Nursing Pharmacology.*

CHAPTER 17

Immune Modulators

LEARNING OBJECTIVES

Upon completion of this chapter, you will be able to:

1. Describe the sites of actions of the various immune modulators.

2. Describe the therapeutic actions, indications, pharmacokinetics, contraindications, most common adverse effects, and important drug–drug interactions associated with each class of immune stimulants and immune suppressants.

3. Discuss the use of immune modulators across the life span.

4. Compare and contrast the prototype drugs for each class of immune modulators with the other drugs in that class and with drugs in other classes.

5. Outline the nursing considerations and teaching needs for patients receiving each class of immune modulator.

■ ASSESSING YOUR UNDERSTANDING

LABELING

Place the name of the following drugs in the appropriate box under the correct drug class.

Adalimumab
Aldesleukin
Azathioprine
Cyclosporine
Oprelvekin
Rituximab

Immune Modulators

Interleukins

T- and B-cell Suppressors

Monoclonal Antibodies

SHORT ANSWER

Supply the information requested.

1. Identify the two major classes of immune stimulants.

2. Name the interleukin receptor antagonist.

3. List the typical routes of administration for most monoclonal antibodies.

4. Describe the mechanism of action of the T- and B-cell suppressors.

5. Identify the two most serious risks associated with the use of immune suppressants.

■ APPLYING YOUR KNOWLEDGE

CASE STUDY

A patient who has been diagnosed with multiple sclerosis is experiencing an exacerbation of her symptoms. The patient reports that this has happened several times before, and the symptoms usually resolve without a problem. However, the patient has been noticing that these episodes have been occurring more often and lasting a bit longer. A decision is made to use interferon therapy. The patient asks, "What is this drug, and how will it help me?"

a. How would the nurse respond to the patient?

b. What interferons might be ordered for this patient? How are they similar, and how are they different?

c. What should the nurse include in the teaching plan about the drug therapy?

■ PRACTICING FOR NCLEX

Circle the letter that corresponds to the best answer for each question.

1. Which agent would be classified as an immune stimulant?
   a. Interferon alfa-2b
   b. Abatacept
   c. Mycophenolate
   d. Sirolimus

2. A patient is receiving oprelvekin. Which of the following would suggest that the patient is experiencing a hypersensitivity reaction?
   a. Cardiac arrhythmia
   b. Mental status change
   c. Chest tightness
   d. Fever

3. Which of the following would the nurse expect to administer orally?
   a. Alefacept
   b. Cyclosporine
   c. Glatiramer acetate
   d. Abatacept

4. A patient is experiencing flulike symptoms related to immune stimulant therapy. Which of the following instructions would be most appropriate for the patient?
   a. "Do not use acetaminophen for your fever or aches."
   b. "Keep your environment nice and warm."
   c. "You need to try and stay as busy as possible."
   d. "Drink plenty of fluids throughout the day."

5. Which monoclonal antibody is antibody specific to epidermal growth factor receptor sites?
   a. Muromonab-CD3
   b. Infliximab
   c. Cetuximab
   d. Adalimumab

Copyright © 2011 by Wolters Kluwer Health I Lippincott Williams & Wilkins. *Study Guide for Focus on Nursing Pharmacology.*

6. A patient is to receive erlotinib. The nurse would expect to administer this drug by which route?

   a. Oral

   b. Subcutaneous

   c. Intramuscular

   d. Intravenous

7. Which of the following would lead the nurse to suspect that a patient receiving a monoclonal antibody is experiencing pulmonary edema?

   a. Fever

   b. Chills

   c. Myalgia

   d. Dyspnea

8. Which of the following would be most important for the nurse to do when administering gemtuzumab?

   a. Ensure that the patient's call light is readily available.

   b. Administer adequate fluids for hydration.

   c. Provide the patient with a bedside commode.

   d. Offer small frequent meals and snacks.

9. A patient is receiving mycophenolate after undergoing a liver transplant. Which of the following would be a priority nursing diagnosis?

   a. Acute pain

   b. Imbalanced nutrition

   c. Risk for infection

   d. Deficient knowledge

10. A group of students are reviewing information about immune modulators in preparation for a test. The students demonstrate understanding of the material when they identify which of the following as an immune stimulant?

    a. Monoclonal antibody

    b. Interleukin receptor antagonist

    c. T- and B-cell suppressor

    d. Interferon

11. When describing the production of interferons, the instructor discusses recombinant DNA technology. Which of the following would the instructor include as being produced this way?

    a. Interferon alfa-n3

    b. Interferon alfacon-1

    c. Interferon gamma-1b

    d. Interferon beta-1a

12. The nurse is teaching a patient receiving interferon therapy about measures to combat possible adverse effects. Which statement by the patient indicates the need for more teaching?

    a. "I need to be out in the sun so that I can get vitamin D."

    b. "I should drink plenty of liquids, including water."

    c. "I can use acetaminophen if I get a fever."

    d. "I might need some blood tests to check my blood count."

13. A patient with rheumatoid arthritis has been receiving various drug therapies for treatment but with little effect. Which of the following might the nurse expect to be used?

    a. Alefacept

    b. Azathioprine

    c. Glatiramer

    d. Abatacept

14. The nurse closely monitors a patient who is receiving anakinra and etanercept for which of the following?

    a. Anemia

    b. Severe infection

    c. Bleeding

    d. Hypersensitivity

15. After teaching a group of students about the various monoclonal antibodies, the instructor determines that the teaching was successful when the students identify muromonab-CD3 as specific to which of the following?

    a. T cells

    b. Human tumor necrosis factor

    c. Lymphocyte receptor sites

    d. Interleukin-2 receptor sites

CHAPTER 18

Vaccines and Sera

LEARNING OBJECTIVES

Upon completion of this chapter, you will be able to:

1. Define the terms *active immunity* and *passive immunity*.

2. Describe the therapeutic actions, indications, pharmacokinetics, contraindications, most common adverse effects, and important drug–drug interactions associated with each vaccine, immune serum, antitoxin, and antivenin.

3. Discuss the use of vaccines and sera across the life span, including recommended immunization schedules.

4. Compare and contrast the prototype drugs for each class of vaccine and immune serum with others in that class.

5. Outline the nursing considerations and teaching needs for patients receiving a vaccine or immune serum.

■ ASSESSING YOUR UNDERSTANDING

FILL IN THE BLANKS

Provide the missing term or terms in the blanks provided.

1. Immune sera that contain antibodies to specific poisons produced by invaders are called _____.

2. Biologicals include _____, immune sera, and antitoxins.

3. When a host reacts to injected antibodies or foreign sera, a _____ _____ occurs.

4. _____ immunity results when preformed antibodies are injected into a host who is at high risk for exposure to a specific disease.

5. The process of artificially stimulating active immunity by exposing the body to weakened or less-toxic proteins associated with specific disease-causing organisms is called _____.

6. _____ was one of the first diseases against which children were vaccinated.

7. After an allergy shot, specific _____ antibodies appear in the serum.

8. A person who was bitten by a rattlesnake would most likely receive an _____.

SHORT ANSWER

Supply the information requested.

1. Describe the differences between active and passive immunity.

2. List two manifestations of serum sickness.

3. Describe when the vaccine against the human papilloma virus (HPV) should be given.

4. Identify the recommendations for immunizations for older adults.

5. Name the vaccine that is used throughout the world but is not routinely used in the United States.

■ APPLYING YOUR KNOWLEDGE

CASE STUDY

A mother brings her 14-year-old daughter to the pediatrician's office for a routine physical examination. During the visit, the mother asks the nurse practitioner about the vaccine for HPV. She states, "I've seen all those commercials on television about this vaccine, but I'm still not sure if my daughter should get it. I've heard so many stories about it. My close friend says that she doesn't want her daughter to get it because then her daughter will think that she can have sex sooner."

a. How should the nurse practitioner respond to the mother?

b. What information would be important to discuss with her?

c. If the mother decides that her daughter should be vaccinated, what would the nurse practitioner recommend?

■ PRACTICING FOR NCLEX

Circle the letter that corresponds to the best answer for each question.

1. When describing the use of vaccines to a local community group, which of the following would the nurse include?
   a. Vaccines are used to provide active immunity.
   b. Vaccines promote the development of antigens.
   c. Vaccines can result in signs and symptoms of the full-blown disease.
   d. Vaccines are associated with severe reactions in children.

2. A group of students are reviewing information about immunizations. The students demonstrate a need for additional study when they identify which of the following as a component of an immunization?
   a. Weakened bacterial cell membrane
   b. Viral protein coat
   c. Chemically weakened actual virus
   d. Serum with bacterial antibodies

3. A patient has been bitten by a dog, and the dog's rabies status is unknown. The nurse would expect this patient to receive which of the following?
   a. Vaccine
   b. Immune sera
   c. Antitoxin
   d. Antivenin

4. A nurse is preparing a presentation to a local community group about biological weapons. The nurse would identify which disease as lacking an available vaccine?
   a. Anthrax
   b. Plague
   c. Smallpox
   d. Botulism

5. Which of the following would the nurse identify as a vaccine that is a toxoid?
   a. Haemophilus influenza b
   b. Pneumococcal polyvalent
   c. Tetanus
   d. Hepatitis A

Copyright © 2011 by Wolters Kluwer Health I Lippincott Williams & Wilkins. *Study Guide for Focus on Nursing Pharmacology.*

6. Which of the following would necessitate cautious use of a vaccine in a child? Select all that apply.

   a. Immune deficiency

   b. Allergy to a vaccine component

   c. Blood transfusion within the past 3 months

   d. History of febrile convulsions

   e. History of brain injury

   f. Acute infection

7. The nurse is teaching the parents of a child who is receiving a vaccine about possible adverse effects. Which of the following would the nurse include as necessitating an immediate call to the health care provider?

   a. Pain at the injection site

   b. Moderate fever

   c. Difficulty breathing

   d. Nodule formation at the site

8. A mother asks the nurse what she can do to help with the discomforts that her child may experience due to an immunization. Which of the following would be most appropriate?

   a. "Have him take some time to rest throughout the day."

   b. "Give him aspirin if he develops any fever."

   c. "Apply cold compresses to the injection site every 4 hours."

   d. "Encourage him to move his arm frequently during the day."

9. A patient was bitten by a poisonous snake. Which of the following would be most appropriate to administer?

   a. Antitoxin

   b. Toxoid

   c. Antivenin

   d. Immune sera

10. To prevent meningococcal infections, the nurse would administer which of the following?

    a. Vaccine

    b. Toxoid

    c. Immune globulin

    d. Antivenin

11. A nurse prepares to administer antithymocyte immune globulin. The nurse understands that this is used for which of the following?

    a. Prevent chicken pox

    b. Treat acute renal transplant rejection

    c. Provide postexposure prophylaxis for hepatitis B

    d. Prevent respiratory syncytial virus infection

12. A man who was working on his outside deck comes to the emergency department after sustaining a puncture wound of his hand from a large nail. Which of the following would the nurse expect to administer?

    a. Zoster vaccine

    b. Hepatitis A vaccine

    c. Lymphocyte immune globulin

    d. Tetanus toxoid

13. Which agent would the nurse expect to administer to a pregnant woman to prevent Rh factor sensitization?

    a. Crotalidae polyvalent immune fab

    b. Cytomegalovirus immune globulin

    c. RHO immune globulin

    d. HPV vaccine

14. The nurse is preparing to administer the rotavirus vaccine to an infant. The nurse would expect to administer this vaccine by which route?

    a. Oral

    b. Subcutaneous

    c. Intramuscular

    d. Intradermal

15. A patient who is going to college in the fall is to receive the meningococcal polysaccharide vaccine. The nurse would prepare to administer the vaccine in which site?

    a. Deep into the muscle of the lateral thigh

    b. Into the upper outer quadrant of the buttocks

    c. Directly into the dermis of the skin

    d. Into the fatty tissue of the upper arm

Copyright © 2011 by Wolters Kluwer Health | Lippincott Williams & Wilkins. *Study Guide for Focus on Nursing Pharmacology.*

CHAPTER 19

Introduction to Nerves and the Nervous System

LEARNING OBJECTIVES

Upon completion of this chapter, you will be able to:

1. Label the parts of a neuron and describe the functions of each part.

2. Describe an action potential, including the roles of the various electrolytes involved in the action potential.

3. Explain what a neurotransmitter is, including its origins and functions at the synapse.

4. Describe the function of the cerebral cortex, cerebellum, hypothalamus, thalamus, midbrain, pituitary gland, medulla, spinal cord, and reticular activating system.

5. Discuss what is known about learning and the impact of emotion on the learning process.

■ ASSESSING YOUR UNDERSTANDING

LABELING

Use the list of terms to label the neuron below.

Soma

Dendrite

Nodes of Ranvier

Schwann cells

Axon terminal

Axon

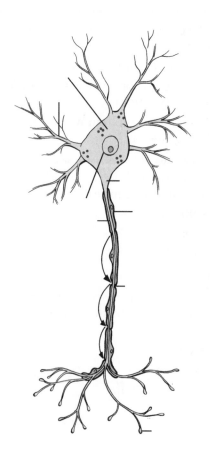

MATCHING

Select the description from column 2 that best describes the term in column 1.

Column 1

____ 1. Hindbrain

____ 2. Engram

____ 3. Dendrite

____ 4. Effector cell

____ 5. Ganglia

____ 6. Neuron

____ 7. Neurotransmitter

____ 8. Synapse

____ 9. Forebrain

____ 10. Axon

Column 2

a. Upper level of the brain consisting of two cerebral hemispheres

b. Short projection on a neuron that transmits information

c. Group of nerve bodies

d. Long projection from a neuron that carries information from one nerve to another

e. Most primitive area of the brain that contains the brain stem

f. Structural unit of the nervous system

g. Short-term memory made up of a reverberating electrical circuit of action potentials

h. Chemical produced by a nerve that reacts with specific receptor site

i. Muscle, gland, or another nerve stimulated by a nerve

j. Junction between a nerve and an effector

■ APPLYING YOUR KNOWLEDGE

CASE STUDY

A patient is admitted to the health care facility after experiencing a cerebrovascular accident due to a completely blocked carotid artery that has resulted in weakness of the patient's right side. His history reveals a narrowing of his carotid artery and several mini-strokes (TIAs) in which he experienced some weakness in his right arm and leg along with some numbness and tingling. These symptoms disappeared after several minutes. The patient says to the nurse, "They said I had a stroke that affected the left side of my brain, but then why is my right side so weak?"

a. How would the nurse respond to the patient?

b. What would the nurse understand about the brain's flow related to the signs and symptoms that the patient experienced with the mini-strokes?

■ PRACTICING FOR NCLEX

Circle the letter that corresponds to the best answer for each question.

1. Which of the following would be identified as the basic unit of the nervous system?

   a. Synapse

   b. Neurotransmitter

   c. Neuron

   d. Soma

2. Which of the following would a nurse identify as being responsible for carrying information from the nerve to the effector cell?

   a. Dendrite

   b. Axon

   c. Soma

   d. Ganglia

3. After teaching a group of students about the functions of the nervous system, the instructor determines that the students need additional teaching when they identify which of the following as a function?

   a. Analysis of incoming stimuli

   b. Control of body functions

   c. Integration of responses

   d. Prevention of stimulus exposure

Copyright © 2011 by Wolters Kluwer Health I Lippincott Williams & Wilkins. *Study Guide for Focus on Nursing Pharmacology.*

4. Which of the following is responsible for carrying nerve impulses from the central nervous system to stimulate a muscle?

   a. Presynaptic nerve

   b. Schwann cell

   c. Efferent fibers

   d. Neurotransmitter

5. Which of the following would be most important for an action potential to occur?

   a. Sodium ions rushing into the cell

   b. Impermeability of the nerve cell membrane to potassium ions

   c. Sufficient strength of a stimulus

   d. Depolarization of the cell

6. Which of the following is considered a neurotransmitter and hormone released by the adrenal medulla?

   a. Dopamine

   b. Gamma-aminobutyric acid (GABA)

   c. Acetylcholine

   d. Epinephrine

7. A nurse is reading an article about sleep and arousal that includes a discussion of a neurotransmitter. Which neurotransmitter would most likely be discussed?

   a. GABA

   b. Serotonin

   c. Norepinephrine

   d. Dopamine

8. Which of the following best describes the blood–brain barrier?

   a. Nonfunctional boundary

   b. Defensive mechanism

   c. Blood delivery mechanism

   d. Vital function control center

9. Which of the following would a nurse identify as a component of the hindbrain?

   a. Thalamus

   b. Limbic system

   c. Brain stem

   d. Cerebrum

10. After studying for a test on the brain and spinal cord, the students demonstrate understanding when they identify the spinal cord as being made up of how many pairs of nerves?

    a. 31

    b. 24

    c. 12

    d. 8

11. When describing the function of the extrapyramidal system, which of the following would the instructor include?

    a. Regulation of motor function control

    b. Coordination of voluntary movement

    c. Processing of emotional information

    d. Coordination of position and posture

12. Stimulation of a nerve results in which of the following?

    a. Membrane potential

    b. Repolarization

    c. Depolarization

    d. Increased sodium outside the cell

13. Which of the following would be associated with the cerebrum? Select all that apply.

    a. Motor neurons

    b. Cranial nerves

    c. Chemoreceptor trigger zone

    d. Speech area

    e. Spinal nerve roots

14. Which of the following would be responsible for the transmission of an electrical impulse along a nerve axon?

    a. Schwann cells

    b. Nodes of Ranvier

    c. Myelin

    d. Synapse

15. Which of the following would be found in the midbrain?

    a. Reticular activating system

    b. Respiratory control center

    c. Hypothalamus

    d. Swallowing center

Copyright © 2011 by Wolters Kluwer Health I Lippincott Williams & Wilkins. *Study Guide for Focus on Nursing Pharmacology.*

Anxiolytic and Hypnotic Agents

LEARNING OBJECTIVES

Upon completion of this chapter, you will be able to:

1. Define the states that are affected by anxiolytic or hypnotic agents.

2. Describe the therapeutic actions, indications, pharmacokinetics, contraindications, most common adverse reactions, and important drug–drug interactions associated with each class of anxiolytic or hypnotic agent.

3. Discuss the use of anxiolytic or hypnotic agents across the life span.

4. Compare and contrast the prototype drugs for each class of anxiolytic or hypnotic drug with the other drugs in that class.

5. Outline the nursing considerations and teaching needs for patients receiving each class of anxiolytic or hypnotic agent.

■ ASSESSING YOUR UNDERSTANDING

FILL IN THE BLANKS

Supply the missing term in the blanks provided.

1. _____ is an unpleasant feeling of tension, fear, or nervousness in response to a real or imagined environmental stimulus.

2. Central nervous system (CNS) depression or sleep that results from extreme sedation is termed _____.

3. Sedation involves a loss of _____ and reaction to environmental stimuli.

4. Anxiety is often accompanied by signs and symptoms of the _____ stress reaction.

5. The most frequently used anxiolytic drugs are _____.

6. Hypnotics react with _____ inhibitory sites to depress the CNS.

7. A patient who consumes alcohol may experience _____ CNS depression if taken with barbiturates.

8. The drug ramelteon stimulates _____ receptors.

SHORT ANSWER

Supply the information requested.

1. Explain the reason why barbiturates are no longer considered a major drug category used to treat anxiety and promote sedation.

2. Describe the rationale for using parenteral forms of benzodiazepines only when absolutely necessary.

3. Identify the common responses that a child may exhibit after receiving an anxiolytic agent.

4. Name the site of action for drugs that are used as hypnotics.

5. Describe why blacks may require a reduced dosage of a benzodiazepine.

■ APPLYING YOUR KNOWLEDGE

CASE STUDY

A 75-year-old man is brought to the health care center by his daughter for a checkup. The daughter says that her father has been having difficulty sleeping lately. She states, "He goes to bed but then he winds up coming back downstairs and watching television. Eventually, he falls asleep a few hours later. Many times, we wake up and find him asleep on the couch." The patient says he just cannot seem to fall asleep when he goes to bed. The patient's physical examination is unremarkable, and the health care provider decides to prescribe zolpidem.

a. What additional information would be important for the nurse to obtain when assessing this patient?

b. Would the nurse expect the patient to receive the usual recommended dose for this drug? Why or why not?

c. What information would be most important for the nurse to include when teaching the patient and his daughter about this drug?

■ PRACTICING FOR NCLEX

Circle the letter that corresponds to the best answer for each question.

1. A patient is receiving ramelteon for insomnia. The nurse would instruct the patient to take the drug at which time?
   a. 2 hours before going to bed
   b. 1 hour before going to bed
   c. ½ hour before going to bed
   d. Immediately before going to bed

2. Which benzodiazepine would a nurse expect to administer as a hypnotic?
   a. Lorazepam
   b. Flurazepam
   c. Diazepam
   d. Alprazolam

3. When describing the action of benzodiazepines as anxiolytics, which of the following would the nurse need to keep in mind?
   a. Enhanced action of gamma-aminobutyric acid
   b. Effect on action potentials
   c. Depression of the cerebral cortex
   d. Depressed motor output

4. A patient received a parenteral benzodiazepine at 11 AM. The nurse would expect to allow the patient out of bed at which time?
   a. 12 PM
   b. 1 PM
   c. 2 PM
   d. 3 PM

Copyright © 2011 by Wolters Kluwer Health I Lippincott Williams & Wilkins. *Study Guide for Focus on Nursing Pharmacology.*

5. Which of the following might occur if a patient inadvertently receives a benzodiazepine intra-arterially?

a. CNS depression

b. Blurred vision

c. Urinary retention

d. Arteriospasm

6. A patient is ordered to receive diazepam as part of the treatment for status epilepticus. The patient has an intravenous (IV) infusion running, which is being used to administer another drug for seizure control. The IV line is in the patient's left arm. Which action by the nurse would be most appropriate?

a. Start another IV line in the patient's right arm.

b. Notify the prescriber that the diazepam cannot be given.

c. Add the diazepam to the current IV infusion.

d. Wait until the other drug is completed to give the diazepam.

7. Which of the following would lead the nurse to suspect that a patient is experiencing withdrawal symptoms associated with benzodiazepine use?

a. Dry mouth

b. Nightmares

c. Hypotension

d. Urinary retention

8. A decrease in dosage of a prescribed benzodiazepine most likely would be necessary if a patient was also taking which of the following?

a. Theophylline

b. Ranitidine

c. Oral contraceptive

d. Alcohol

9. A patient receives a dose of diazepam at 4:00 PM. The nurse would expect to see the maximum effect of this drug at approximately which time?

a. 4:30 PM

b. 5:30 PM

c. 6:30 PM

d. 7:30 PM

10. A nurse is preparing to administer an anxiolytic to a patient. Which of the following would be most appropriate for the nurse to do before administering the drug?

a. Raise the side rails.

b. Institute a bowel program.

c. Dim the lights.

d. Have the patient void.

11. A patient has received a benzodiazepine for sedation before a diagnostic procedure. Which agent would the nurse expect the patient to receive to reverse the sedative effects?

a. Temazepam

b. Triazolam

c. Flumazenil

d. Promethazine

12. After reviewing the various drugs that are classified as barbiturates, a student demonstrates understanding when he identifies which of the following as the prototype?

a. Amobarbital

b. Secobarbital

c. Pentobarbital

d. Phenobarbital

13. A patient is receiving a barbiturate intravenously. The nurse would monitor the patient for which of the following?

a. Hypertension

b. Bradycardia

c. Tachypnea

d. Bleeding

14. A patient is prescribed an anxiolytic agent. Which of the following would be most important for the nurse to include in the teaching?

a. "Be sure not to stop the drug abruptly."

b. "Take the drug with meals if necessary."

c. "Increase the amount of fiber in your diet."

d. "Try other measures to help you relax, too."

15. Which agent has no sedative, anticonvulsant, or muscle relaxant properties but does reduce the signs and symptoms of anxiety?

a. Diphenhydramine

b. Zaleplon

c. Buspirone

d. Meprobamate

Copyright © 2011 by Wolters Kluwer Health | Lippincott Williams & Wilkins. *Study Guide for Focus on Nursing Pharmacology.*

CHAPTER 21

Antidepressant Agents

LEARNING OBJECTIVES

Upon completion of this chapter, you will be able to:

1. Describe the biogenic theory of depression.

2. Describe the therapeutic actions, indications, pharmacokinetics, contraindications, most common adverse reactions, and important drug–drug interactions associated with each class of antidepressant.

3. Discuss the use of antidepressants across the life span.

4. Compare and contrast the prototype drugs for each class of antidepressant with the other drugs in that class and with drugs in the other classes of antidepressants.

5. Outline the nursing considerations and teaching needs for patients receiving each class of antidepressant.

■ ASSESSING YOUR UNDERSTANDING

LABELING

Place the name of the following drugs in the appropriate box under the correct drug class.

Amoxapine

Citalopram

Doxepin

Fluoxetine

Nortriptyline

Phenelzine

Sertraline

Tranylcypromine

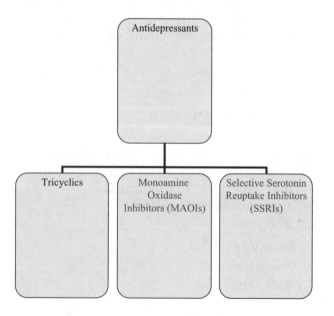

SHORT ANSWER

Supply the information requested.

1. Name the three biogenic amines implicated in depression.

2. Identify the two neurotransmitters that are affected by tricyclic antidepressants.

3. Define *affect*.

4. Describe the effect of combining foods containing tyramine with MAOIs.

5. Identify the tricyclic antidepressant that is associated with the greatest sedative and anticholinergic effects.

6. Explain why SSRIs often are a better choice for treating depression.

■ APPLYING YOUR KNOWLEDGE

CASE STUDY

A patient with a history of major depression comes to the emergency department complaining of a severe occipital headache, nausea, and vomiting. His blood pressure is extremely elevated. During the interview, the patient reports that he has taken several different drugs over the years without any real relief in his depression. He was recently started on phenelzine after having been prescribed imipramine.

a. What might the nurse suspect is happening to the patient?

b. What other assessment findings would help to confirm the suspicions?

c. Once the patient is stabilized, what information would the nurse need to include when teaching this patient about his drug therapy?

■ PRACTICING FOR NCLEX

Circle the letter that corresponds to the best answer for each question.

1. A patient is receiving an antidepressant that also aids in smoking cessation. Which drug would this most likely be?
   a. Venlafaxine
   b. Bupropion
   c. Mirtazapine
   d. Selegiline

2. A nurse is preparing a presentation about the use of antidepressants in children and adolescents. Which of the following would the nurse need to keep in mind?
   a. Studies have shown a clear link between suicide and the use of antidepressants.
   b. The majority of antidepressants approved for use in adults can be used with children.
   c. The smallest amount of drug that is feasible should be dispensed.
   d. Children typically demonstrate a predictable response to the drugs.

Copyright © 2011 by Wolters Kluwer Health l Lippincott Williams & Wilkins. *Study Guide for Focus on Nursing Pharmacology.*

3. Which antidepressant would the nurse identify as being one associated with the least amount of common adverse effects?

   a. Nortriptyline

   b. Amitriptyline

   c. Clomipramine

   d. Doxepin

4. A patient is prescribed a tricyclic antidepressant. The nurse would anticipate administering this drug by which route?

   a. Oral

   b. Topical

   c. Intramuscular

   d. Intravenous

5. A group of students are reviewing information about tricyclic antidepressants and demonstrate understanding of the material when they identify which drug as also being indicated for the treatment of obsessive-compulsive disorder.

   a. Amoxapine

   b. Maprotiline

   c. Clomipramine

   d. Desipramine

6. A patient is to receive a tricyclic antidepressant. The nurse is reviewing the patient's medical record. Which of the following would alert the nurse to a possible contraindication?

   a. Glaucoma

   b. Prostatic hypertrophy

   c. Renal dysfunction

   d. Recent myocardial infarction

7. After teaching a patient who is to receive transdermal selegiline, which patient statement would indicate to the nurse that the patient has understood the instructions?

   a. "I probably won't feel drowsy, dizzy, or nauseous from this drug."

   b. "I should leave the previous patch on for an hour after applying a new one."

   c. "I can apply a new patch to my upper arm, thigh, or torso."

   d. "My skin needs to be a little damp when I apply the patch."

8. Which of the following adverse effects would the nurse instruct a patient to report to his health care provider immediately when taking trazodone?

   a. Hypertension

   b. Dizziness

   c. Sedation

   d. Painful continued erection

9. A patient is prescribed isocarboxazid. The nurse is teaching the patient about foods to avoid. Which of the following would the nurse include in the teaching? Select all that apply.

   a. Aged blue cheese

   b. Red wine

   c. Pepperoni

   d. Whole milk

   e. Fresh shellfish

   f. Sour cream

10. A patient is receiving fluoxetine. The nurse would monitor the patient for which of the following?

    a. Increased salivation

    b. Cough

    c. Improved alertness

    d. Sustained erection

11. A patient is receiving an SSRI. The nurse would inform the patient that the full benefits of the drug may not occur for which time period?

    a. 1 week

    b. 2 weeks

    c. 3 weeks

    d. 4 weeks

12. After reviewing information about the various antidepressants, a group of students demonstrate their understanding of the information when they identify which of the following as an SSRI?

    a. Doxepin

    b. Nefazodone

    c. Sertraline

    d. Bupropion

Copyright © 2011 by Wolters Kluwer Health l Lippincott Williams & Wilkins. *Study Guide for Focus on Nursing Pharmacology.*

13. A patient who was previously taking paroxetine is being switched to phenelzine due to a lack of response. The nurse would expect that the phenelzine will be started at which time?

    a. Concurrently with the paroxetine as it is being tapered

    b. In 4 to 6 weeks after stopping the paroxetine

    c. Immediately upon stopping the paroxetine.

    d. Forty-eight hours after being weaned from the paroxetine

14. When teaching a patient about tricyclic antidepressants, the nurse would include which of the following? Select all that apply.

    a. Taking the drug once a day in the morning for maximum benefit

    b. Using hard candies and gums to combat dry mouth

    c. Eating a low-fiber diet

    d. Keeping the room brightly lit

15. The nurse would assess for which of the following in a patient with type 2 diabetes using an oral antidiabetic agent and receiving an MAOI?

    a. Orthostatic hypotension

    b. Diabetic ketoacidosis

    c. Hypoglycemia

    d. Renal dysfunction

Copyright © 2011 by Wolters Kluwer Health I Lippincott Williams & Wilkins. *Study Guide for Focus on Nursing Pharmacology.*

CHAPTER 22

Psychotherapeutic Agents

LEARNING OBJECTIVES

Upon completion of this chapter, you will be able to:

1. Define the term *psychotherapeutic agent* and list conditions that the psychotherapeutic agents are used to treat.

2. Describe the therapeutic actions, indications, pharmacokinetics, contraindications, most common adverse reactions, and important drug–drug interactions associated with each class of psychotherapeutic agent.

3. Discuss the use of psychotherapeutic agents across the life span.

4. Compare and contrast the prototype drugs for each class of psychotherapeutic agent with other drugs in that class and with drugs in the other classes of psychotherapeutic agents.

5. Outline the nursing considerations and teaching needs for patients receiving each class of psychotherapeutic agent.

■ ASSESSING YOUR UNDERSTANDING

SHORT ANSWER

Supply the information requested.

1. Name the most common type of psychosis.

2. Describe the overall goal of psychotherapeutic agents in comparison to antidepressant agents.

3. Explain why antipsychotic agents are called *neuroleptic agents*.

4. Describe the rationale for no longer calling antipsychotic agents major tranquilizers.

5. Identify the two classifications of antipsychotic drugs.

LABELING

Place the name of each of the drugs listed below in the appropriate column of the table that identifies the neurotransmitter affected by that drug's action. Some drugs may be placed in more than one column.

- Aripiprazole
- Chlorpromazine
- Clozapine
- Lithium
- Molindone
- Pimozide
- Quetiapine
- Ziprasidone

Dopamine	Serotonin	Norepinephrine

■ APPLYING YOUR KNOWLEDGE

CASE STUDY

A 32-year-old woman is brought to the emergency department by the local police after having been called to the scene by several neighbors. The neighbors reported that the patient was talking and laughing extremely loud, banging on doors, and telling everyone that she was the "queen of the world." The patient is dressed in provocative, brightly colored clothing and wearing heavy makeup.

The patient is using exaggerated gestures as she talks, quickly shifting from one topic to another. The patient, who has a history of bipolar disorder, is known to the staff in the emergency department.

a. What information would be most important for the nurse to gather in this situation, and how would the nurse go about obtaining this information?

b. What medications might the nurse expect the physician to prescribe for the patient?

c. How would the nurse approach teaching with this patient?

■ PRACTICING FOR NCLEX

Circle the letter that corresponds to the best answer for each question.

1. A patient with a history of schizophrenia has been receiving antipsychotic therapy for several years. Which of the following would indicate to the nurse that the patient is experiencing pseudoparkinsonism?

- **a.** Cogwheel rigidity
- **b.** Abnormal eye movements
- **c.** Neck spasms
- **d.** Excessive salivation

2. A nurse is reviewing a patient's serum lithium level and determines that the level is therapeutic by which result?

- **a.** 0.2 mEq/L
- **b.** 0.8 mEq/L
- **c.** 1.4 mEq/L
- **d.** 2.0 mEq/L

Copyright © 2011 by Wolters Kluwer Health I Lippincott Williams & Wilkins. *Study Guide for Focus on Nursing Pharmacology.*

3. After reviewing information about antipsychotic agents, a group of students demonstrate understanding of the material when they identify which of the following as an atypical antipsychotic agent?

   a. Haloperidol

   b. Loxapine

   c. Clozapine

   d. Pimozide

4. Which of the following antipsychotics would the nurse identify as a highly potent agent?

   a. Chlorpromazine

   b. Thioridazine

   c. Prochlorperazine

   d. Fluphenazine

5. The nurse administers chlorpromazine intramuscularly to a patient. The nurse would maintain the patient in bed for at least how long after administering the drug?

   a. ½ hour

   b. 1 hour

   c. 2 hours

   d. 3 hours

6. Which of the following would be important for a nurse to include in the teaching plan for a patient taking fluphenazine?

   a. Possible development of fatal arrhythmias

   b. Urine turning pink to reddish-brown

   c. Possible severe rhinorrhea

   d. Development of diabetes mellitus

7. The nurse expects to monitor a patient's white blood count weekly when the patient is prescribed which of the following?

   a. Aripiprazole

   b. Olanzapine

   c. Clozapine

   d. Quetiapine

8. The use of which of the following would a nurse identify as placing a patient receiving lithium therapy at increased risk for toxicity?

   a. Tromethamine

   b. Thiazide diuretic

   c. Psyllium

   d. Antacids

9. A patient has a serum lithium level of 1.8 mEq/L. Which of the following would the nurse assess? Select all that apply.

   a. Electrocardiogram changes

   b. Hypotension

   c. Slurred speech

   d. Hyperreflexia

   e. Polyuria

   f. Seizures

10. A child with attention deficit hyperactivity disorder is to receive methylphenidate twice a day. The nurse would instruct the parents to administer the last dose before which time?

    a. 4 PM

    b. 5 PM

    c. 6 PM

    d. 8 PM

11. Which drug would be indicated for the treatment of narcolepsy?

    a. Atomoxetine

    b. Dexmethylphenidate

    c. Lisdexamfetamine

    d. Modafinil

12. While caring for a patient who is receiving antipsychotic therapy, the nurse observes lip smacking, a darting tongue, and slow and aimless arm movements. The nurse interprets this as which of the following?

    a. Tardive dyskinesia

    b. Akathisia

    c. Pseudoparkinsonism

    d. Dystonia

13. A nurse is assessing a patient who is receiving an antipsychotic agent for possible anticholinergic effects. Which of the following would the nurse assess?

    a. Nasal congestion

    b. Neuroleptic malignant syndrome

    c. Laryngospasm

    d. Arrhythmia

14. The parents of a child receiving a central nervous system stimulant for treatment of attention deficit disorder asks the nurse why they are stopping the drug for a time. Which statement by the nurse would be most appropriate?

    a. "He probably doesn't need the medication anymore since he is getting older."

    b. "We need to check and see if he still has symptoms that require drug therapy."

    c. "The drug should be used for a specified period of time and then switched to another."

    d. "He is prone to developing severe adverse effects if he stays on it any longer."

15. A patient is receiving haloperidol. The nurse would be most especially alert for the development of which of the following adverse effects?

    a. Sedation

    b. Anticholinergic

    c. Extrapyramidal

    d. Hypotension

16. Which of the following would a nurse identify as being used as treatment for mania as well as schizophrenia?

    a. Lithium

    b. Risperidone

    c. Lamotrigine

    d. Aripiprazole

Copyright © 2011 by Wolters Kluwer Health I Lippincott Williams & Wilkins. *Study Guide for Focus on Nursing Pharmacology.*

Anti-seizure Agents

LEARNING OBJECTIVES

Upon completion of this chapter, you will be able to:

1. Define the terms *generalized seizure, tonic-clonic seizure, absence seizure, partial seizure,* and status *epilepticus.*

2. Describe the therapeutic actions, indications, pharmacokinetics, contraindications, most common adverse reactions, and important drug–drug interactions associated with each class of antiseizure agents.

3. Discuss the use of antiepileptic drugs across the life span.

4. Compare and contrast the prototype drugs for each class of antiepileptic drug with the other drugs in that class and with drugs from the other classes.

5. Outline the nursing considerations and teaching needs for patients receiving each class of antiseizure agent.

■ ASSESSING YOUR UNDERSTANDING

MATCHING

Select the description from column 2 that best describes the term in column 1.

Column 1

——— **1.** Absence seizure

——— **2.** Convulsion

——— **3.** Epilepsy

——— **4.** Generalized seizure

——— **5.** Partial seizure

——— **6.** Status epilepticus

——— **7.** Tonic-clonic seizure

Column 2

a. Focal seizure

b. Syndromes characterized by seizures

c. Formerly known as grand mal seizure

d. Beginning in one area of the brain and spreading to both hemispheres

e. Rapidly recurring seizures

f. Muscular reactions to excessive electrical energy arising from nerve cells

g. Sudden temporary loss of consciousness

SHORT ANSWER

Supply the information requested.

1. Name the five types of generalized seizures.

2. Differentiate between simple and complex partial seizures.

3. List the most common adverse effect that results from the drugs used to treat generalized seizures.

4. Identify the drug class most commonly used to treat absence seizures.

5. Explain the underlying reason why phenobarbital has a slow onset and very long duration of action.

6. Identify the two ways that drugs used to control partial seizures stabilize nerve membranes.

■ APPLYING YOUR KNOWLEDGE

CASE STUDY

A 6-year-old child was admitted to the health care facility after experiencing a tonic-clonic seizure. His parents are at his bedside. The child was receiving phenytoin intravenously but is now being switched to oral therapy. It is expected that the child will be discharged home tomorrow. The nurse is talking with the parents about the child's drug therapy when the mother says, "It was so scary watching him like that. I just froze. What if he has another seizure, and what if it happens at school or when his friends are around?"

a. How would the nurse respond to the mother?

b. What suggestions and recommendations would be appropriate in this situation?

■ PRACTICING FOR NCLEX

Circle the letter that corresponds to the best answer for each question.

1. Which of the following agents would a nurse expect to administer intravenously for a partial seizure?
   a. Carbamazepine
   b. Gabapentin
   c. Levetiracetam
   d. Felbamate

2. A patient who is receiving phenytoin has a serum drug level drawn. Which result would the nurse interpret as within the therapeutic range?
   a. 4 mcg/mL
   b. 12 mcg/mL
   c. 22 mcg/mL
   d. 30 mcg/mL

3. A patient is receiving a hydantoin as treatment for tonic-clonic seizures. The nurse includes a discussion of which of the following when teaching the patient about this drug?
   a. Possible leukocytosis
   b. Physical dependence
   c. Withdrawal syndrome
   d. Gingival hyperplasia

4. When describing the action of barbiturates and barbituratelike agents in the control of seizures, which of the following would the nurse include?
   a. Promotion of impulse conduction
   b. Stimulation of the cerebral cortex
   c. Depression of motor nerve output
   d. Maintenance of cerebellar function

5. Phenobarbital is ordered for a child with status epilepticus. The nurse would anticipate administering this drug by which route?
   a. Oral
   b. Rectal
   c. Intramuscular
   d. Intravenous

Copyright © 2011 by Wolters Kluwer Health I Lippincott Williams & Wilkins. *Study Guide for Focus on Nursing Pharmacology.*

6. A patient is receiving lamotrigine as treatment for partial seizures. Which assessment finding would lead the nurse to stop the drug immediately?

   a. Rash

   b. Somnolence

   c. Anorexia

   d. Confusion

7. The nurse is reviewing the medical record of a patient with partial seizures who is prescribed drug therapy. The nurse would question the order for which of the following if the nurse finds that the patient has a history of alcohol abuse?

   a. Topiramate

   b. Pregabalin

   c. Felbamate

   d. Tiagabine

8. The nurse is monitoring the serum carbamazepine level of a patient. Which result would lead the nurse to notify the prescriber that the patient most likely needs an increased dosage?

   a. 2 mcg/mL

   b. 4 mcg/mL

   c. 6 mcg/mL

   d. 8 mcg/mL

9. A patient who is receiving an antiseizure agent complains of feeling sleepy and tired and reports dizziness when standing up. Which intervention would the nurse most likely implement as the priority?

   a. Hydration therapy

   b. Safety precautions

   c. Skin-care measures

   d. Emotional support

10. A child is experiencing febrile seizures for which phenobarbital is ordered to be given intravenously. The dose is administered at 10 AM. The nurse understands that a second dose of the drug may be given at which time?

   a. 2 PM

   b. 4 PM

   c. 6 PM

   d. 10 PM

11. Which drug would the nurse expect to be ordered as the drug of choice for the treatment for myoclonic seizures?

   a. Clonazepam

   b. Diazepam

   c. Valproic acid

   d. Zonisamide

12. After teaching a class on drug classes used to treat seizures, the instructor determines that the teaching has been successful when the students identify which drug as most commonly used in the treatment of absence seizures?

   a. Mephobarbital

   b. Ethotoin

   c. Ethosuximide

   d. Primidone

13. When describing the action of zonisamide, which of the following would the nurse include?

   a. Inhibition of sodium and calcium channels

   b. Decrease in conduction through nerve pathways

   c. Depression of the cerebral cortex

   d. Depression of motor nerve output

14. A patient is to receive ethotoin. The nurse would expect to administer this drug by which route?

   a. Oral

   b. Rectal

   c. Intramuscular

   d. Intravenous

15. Which of the following would be most important to monitor in a patient receiving ethosuximide?

   a. Weight

   b. Nutritional status

   c. Electrocardiogram

   d. Complete blood count

Copyright © 2011 by Wolters Kluwer Health | Lippincott Williams & Wilkins. *Study Guide for Focus on Nursing Pharmacology.*

CHAPTER 24

Antiparkinsonism Agents

LEARNING OBJECTIVES

Upon completion of this chapter, you will be able to:

1. Describe the current theory of the cause of Parkinson's disease and correlate this with the clinical presentation of the disease.

2. Describe the therapeutic actions, indications, pharmacokinetics, contraindications, most common adverse reactions, and important drug–drug interactions associated with antiparkinsonism agents.

3. Discuss the use of antiparkinsonism agents across the life span.

4. Compare and contrast the prototype drugs for each class of antiparkinsonism agent with the other drugs in that class and with drugs from the other classes used to treat the disease.

5. Outline the nursing considerations and teaching needs for patients receiving each class of antiparkinsonism agent.

■ ASSESSING YOUR UNDERSTANDING

FILL IN THE BLANKS

Provide the missing term or terms in the blanks provided.

1. Patients with Parkinson's disease exhibit

   _____ marked by difficulties in performing intentional movements and extreme slowness or sluggishness.

2. In Parkinson's disease, nerve cells begin to degenerate in the dopamine-rich area of the

   brain called the _____ _____.

3. Therapy for Parkinson's disease today aims at restoring the balance between the declining

   levels of _____ and the now-dominant

   _____ neurons.

4. _____ agents have been proven to

   more effective than _____ agents in the treatment of parkinsonism.

5. Patients receiving rasagiline should avoid

   _____-containing foods.

LABELING

Place the name of the following drugs listed below in the appropriate box under the correct drug class.

Amantadine   Entacapone

Benztropine   Levodopa

Biperiden   Ropinirole

Diphenhydramine   Selegiline

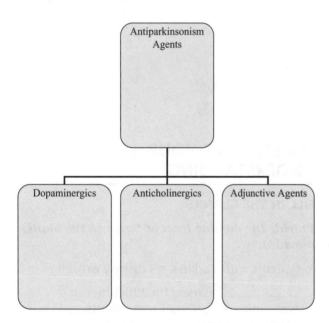

■ APPLYING YOUR KNOWLEDGE

CASE STUDY

A 65-year-old man is brought to the emergency department by his daughter, who reports that her father started complaining of a severe headache several hours ago that has not abated. He also had some nausea and vomiting and was diaphoretic. Examination reveals tachycardia and dilated pupils. The patient also reports some mild chest pain. He states, "The bright lights are really bothering me." The patient has a history of Parkinson's disease for which he takes levodopa. His daughter reports that he just started taking rasagiline about a week ago.

a. How would the nurse interpret the patient's signs and symptoms? What might be happening?

b. What additional information would the nurse need to gather from the patient and his daughter?

■ PRACTICING FOR NCLEX

Circle the letter that corresponds to the best answer for each question.

1. When describing the action of levodopa, which of the following would the nurse include?

   a. Acts like replacement therapy

   b. Increases the release of dopamine

   c. Binds directly with postsynaptic dopamine receptors

   d. Stimulates dopamine receptors

2. A patient asks the nurse why he must take his levodopa in combination with carbidopa. Which response by the nurse would be most appropriate?

   a. "The carbidopa helps the levodopa get into the brain."

   b. "The carbidopa allows a lower dose of levodopa to be used."

   c. "It boosts the action of levodopa to prevent the nerve cells from degenerating."

   d. "The carbidopa prevents too much levodopa from being excreted."

3. A patient is to receive apomorphine as treatment for Parkinson's disease. The nurse would expect to administer this drug by which route?

   a. Oral

   b. Topical

   c. Subcutaneous

   d. Intramuscular

4. When reviewing a patient's history, which of the following would the nurse identify as a contraindication to the use of levodopa?

   a. Myocardial infarction

   b. Bronchial asthma

   c. Peptic ulcer disease

   d. Suspicious skin lesions

Copyright © 2011 by Wolters Kluwer Health I Lippincott Williams & Wilkins. *Study Guide for Focus on Nursing Pharmacology.*

5. Which of the following would a nurse expect to assess as a potential adverse effect of dopaminergic therapy?

   a. Sedation

   b. Muscle flaccidity

   c. Nervousness

   d. Hypertension

6. Which of the following would a nurse identify as least likely to contribute to a decrease in the effectiveness of levodopa?

   a. Pyridoxine

   b. Phenytoin

   c. Multivitamin supplement

   d. St. John's wort

7. A patient is to receive trihexyphenidyl as adjunctive treatment for Parkinson's disease. The nurse would expect to administer this drug by which route?

   a. Oral

   b. Subcutaneous

   c. Intramuscular

   d. Intravenous

8. A nurse is reviewing a patient's history for conditions that would contraindicate the use of anticholinergics for Parkinson's disease. Which of the following would cause the nurse to be concerned?

   a. Hypertension

   b. Myasthenia gravis

   c. Hepatic dysfunction

   d. Cardiac arrhythmia

9. Which of the following would lead the nurse to suspect that a patient is experiencing an adverse effect to an anticholinergic agent?

   a. Diarrhea

   b. Diaphoresis

   c. Excess salivation

   d. Agitation

10. After reviewing the drugs used to treat Parkinson's disease, the students demonstrate understanding when they identify which of the following as a dopaminergic agent?

    a. Diphenhydramine

    b. Biperiden

    c. Bromocriptine

    d. Tolcapone

11. A patient who is receiving biperiden complains of light-headedness, dizziness, and blurred vision. Which nursing diagnosis would be most appropriate?

    a. Risk for impaired thermoregulation

    b. Disturbed thought processes

    c. Deficient knowledge

    d. Risk for injury

12. When administering entacapone, the nurse understands that this drug affects which enzyme?

    a. Lactic dehydrogenase

    b. Catecholamine-O-methyl transferase

    c. Monoamine oxidase

    d. Acetylcholinesterase

13. Which action would be a priority for a patient receiving apomorphine?

    a. Giving the drug with food

    b. Monitoring cardiac status

    c. Checking for skin lesions

    d. Palpating the bladder

14. A patient is experiencing parkinsonism as a result of drug therapy with a phenothiazine. The nurse would anticipate which agent as being prescribed?

    a. Bromocriptine

    b. Pramipexole

    c. Biperiden

    d. Selegiline

15. Which of the following would be considered a peripheral anticholinergic effect of anticholinergic drug therapy?

    a. Delirium

    b. Blurred vision

    c. Agitation

    d. Memory loss

Copyright © 2011 by Wolters Kluwer Health I Lippincott Williams & Wilkins. *Study Guide for Focus on Nursing Pharmacology.*

CHAPTER 25

Muscle Relaxants

LEARNING OBJECTIVES

Upon completion of this chapter, you will be able to:

1. Describe a spinal reflex and discuss the patho-physiology of muscle spasm and muscle spasticity.

2. Describe the therapeutic actions, indications, pharmacokinetics, contraindications, most common adverse reactions, and important drug–drug interactions associated with the centrally acting and the direct-acting skeletal muscle relaxants.

3. Discuss the use of muscle relaxants across the life span.

4. Compare and contrast the prototype drugs baclofen and dantrolene with other muscle relaxants in their classes.

5. Outline the nursing considerations, including important teaching points, for patients receiving muscle relaxants as an adjunct to anesthesia.

■ ASSESSING YOUR UNDERSTANDING

CROSSWORD

Use the clues to complete the crossword puzzle.

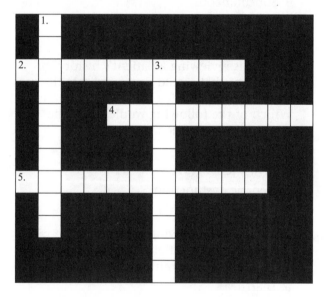

Across

2. Sustained muscle contraction
4. Tract that controls precise intentional movement
5. Structure that communicates with other neurons

Down

1. Excessive muscle response and activity
3. Lower portion of the brain that coordinates muscle movement

SHORT ANSWER

Supply the information requested.

1. Describe the type of movements associated with the pyramidal and extrapyramidal tracts.

2. Explain why muscle spasticity is a permanent condition.

3. Identify the typical cause of muscle spasm.

4. Describe the structures that regulate movement and muscle control.

5. Explain why centrally acting skeletal muscle relaxants are often referred to as spasmolytics.

6. Name the prototype centrally acting skeletal muscle relaxant.

7. Describe the action of direct-acting skeletal muscle relaxants.

8. State the drug that would be used to improve the appearance of moderate to severe glabellar lines.

■ APPLYING YOUR KNOWLEDGE

CASE STUDY

A 27-year-old man comes to the urgent care center for evaluation of his shoulder. He reports that he has been working out at the gym and may have overdone it. He is complaining of pain in the right shoulder and intense muscle spasms in the area. Diagnostic evaluation rules out any tear, dislocation, or fracture. The patient is prescribed cyclobenzaprine as a muscle relaxant.

a. What information would the nurse need to include when teaching the patient about the drug?

b. What additional information would the nurse include to help augment the effects of the prescribed drug therapy?

■ PRACTICING FOR NCLEX

Circle the letter that corresponds to the best answer for each question.

1. An older patient is to receive a centrally acting skeletal muscle relaxant. Which of the following would the nurse expect to be prescribed?
   a. Baclofen
   b. Carisoprodol
   c. Chlorzoxazone
   d. Cyclobenzaprine

2. Simple reflex arcs comprise which of the following?
   a. Pyramidal tract
   b. Extrapyramidal tract
   c. Spindle gamma loop system
   d. Basal ganglia

Copyright © 2011 by Wolters Kluwer Health I Lippincott Williams & Wilkins. *Study Guide for Focus on Nursing Pharmacology.*

3. After reviewing information about skeletal muscle relaxants, a group of students demonstrate understanding of the material when they identify which drug as a direct-acting muscle relaxant?

   a. Botulinum toxin type A

   b. Diazepam

   c. Methocarbamol

   d. Orphenadrine

4. When reviewing a patient's history, which condition would the nurse identify as contraindicating the use of a centrally acting skeletal muscle relaxant?

   a. Epilepsy

   b. Cardiac disease

   c. Hepatic dysfunction

   d. Rheumatic disorder

5. A patient is receiving baclofen at 8 AM. The nurse would monitor the patient for evidence of maximum effect at which time?

   a. 9 AM

   b. 10 AM

   c. 11 AM

   d. 12 PM

6. A patient with amyotrophic lateral sclerosis is experiencing muscle spasticity. Which of the following drugs would the nurse expect the physician to order?

   a. Chlorzoxazone

   b. Metaxalone

   c. Dantrolene

   d. Methocarbamol

7. Which of the following would a nurse include when describing the action of dantrolene?

   a. Interference with calcium release from the muscles

   b. Inhibition of the release of acetycholine

   c. Interference with the reflexes causing the spasm

   d. Inhibition of presynaptic motor neurons in central nervous system

8. The nurse instructs a patient about the possibility of his urine turning orange to purple-red if the patient were receiving which of the following?

   a. Baclofen

   b. Carisoprodol

   c. Chlorzoxazone

   d. Tizanidine

9. A patient comes to the health care provider's office. The patient is to receive botulinum toxin. Which of the following, if assessed, would suggest to the nurse that the drug administration should be postponed?

   a. Recent gastrointestinal upset

   b. Infection at the intended site of administration

   c. Reports of urinary frequency

   d. Difficulty swallowing

10. Signs and symptoms of which of the following would necessitate discontinuation of dantrolene therapy?

    a. Intermittent gastrointestinal upset

    b. Visual disturbances

    c. Urinary retention

    d. Hepatic dysfunction

11. A patient with a history of malignant hyperthermia is scheduled for surgery. Which agent would the nurse most likely expect to administer?

    a. Botulinum toxin type B

    b. Dantrolene

    c. Baclofen

    d. Methocarbamol

12. Which nursing diagnosis most likely would be the priority for a patient who is receiving a centrally acting skeletal muscle relaxant as treatment for acute knee strain?

    a. Deficient knowledge

    b. Risk for injury

    c. Acute pain

    d. Disturbed thought processes

Copyright © 2011 by Wolters Kluwer Health | Lippincott Williams & Wilkins. *Study Guide for Focus on Nursing Pharmacology.*

13. Which of the following would a nurse identify as increasing a patient's risk for hepatic disease with dantrolene use?

    a. Male gender

    b. Age over 35 years

    c. Respiratory disease

    d. Infection

14. A patient is receiving botulinum toxin type A as treatment for her frown lines. The nurse would instruct the patient about which of the following?

    a. Abnormal hair growth

    b. Acne

    c. Photosensitivity

    d. Drooping eyelids

15. A nurse is preparing a teaching plan for a patient who is receiving baclofen therapy. Which of the following would the nurse include as possible adverse effects? Select all that apply.

    a. Drowsiness

    b. Hypertension

    c. Urinary frequency

    d. Agitation

    e. Drooling

    f. Constipation

Copyright © 2011 by Wolters Kluwer Health I Lippincott Williams & Wilkins. *Study Guide for Focus on Nursing Pharmacology.*

26

Narcotics, Narcotic Antagonists and Antimigraine Agents

LEARNING OBJECTIVES

Upon completion of this chapter, you will be able to:

1. Outline the gate theory of pain and explain therapeutic ways to block pain using the gate theory.

2. Describe the therapeutic actions, indications, pharmacokinetics, contraindications, most common adverse reactions, and important drug–drug interactions associated with narcotics and antimigraine agents.

3. Discuss the use of the different classes of narcotics, narcotic antagonists, and antimigraine agents across the life span.

4. Compare and contrast the prototype drugs morphine, pentazocine, naloxone, ergotamine, and sumatriptan with other drugs in their respective classes.

5. Outline the nursing considerations, including important teaching points, for patients receiving a narcotic, narcotic antagonist, or antimigraine drug.

■ ASSESSING YOUR UNDERSTANDING

LABELING

Place the name of the following drugs in the appropriate box under the correct drug classification.

Butorphanol   Naltrexone

Codeine   Pentazocine

Fentanyl   Propoxyphene

Naloxone

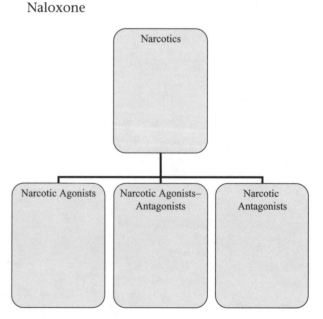

Narcotics

Narcotic Agonists | Narcotic Agonists–Antagonists | Narcotic Antagonists

SHORT ANSWER

Supply the information requested.

1. Identify the two small-diameter sensory nerves involved in the generation of pain sensation.

2. Name the fibers that transmit sensations associated with touch and temperature.

3. Identify the type of receptors that respond to naturally occurring peptins, endorphins, and enkephalins.

4. List three factors that can play a role in pain perception.

5. Identify the functions of narcotic agonists–antagonists.

6. State the action of triptans.

7. Name the four types of opioid receptors.

■ APPLYING YOUR KNOWLEDGE

CASE STUDY

The nurse is visiting the home of a patient with cancer. The patient has been taking morphine for the relief of his pain. However, over the last 2 weeks, the patient reports that he is not experiencing the degree of relief that he had been. The patient also mentions that when he saw the physician last week, a decision was made not to pursue additional treatment.

a. What factors may be contributing to the patient's increase in pain?

b. What possible options might be appropriate for this patient?

c. What measures would the nurse suggest to enhance pain relief?

■ PRACTICING FOR NCLEX

Circle the letter that corresponds to the best answer for each question.

1. A patient is to receive a narcotic that will be applied transdermally. The nurse identifies this as which agent?
   a. Morphine
   b. Fentanyl
   c. Codeine
   d. Hydromorphone

2. A nurse is assessing a patient's pain level. Which of the following would be the most appropriate method?
   a. Ask the patient if he is experiencing any pain.
   b. Have the patient rate it on a scale of 1 to 10.
   c. Palpate the area where the patient says he has pain.
   d. Review the patient's vital signs for changes.

Copyright © 2011 by Wolters Kluwer Health I Lippincott Williams & Wilkins. *Study Guide for Focus on Nursing Pharmacology.*

3. A patient is to receive a narcotic cough syrup. The nurse would expect this preparation to contain which of the following?

   a. Codeine

   b. Fentanyl

   c. Hydromorphone

   d. Meperidine

4. Which instruction would the nurse include for a patient who is prescribed extended-release oxycodone?

   a. Take the tablet as a whole tablet at one time.

   b. Cut the tablet in half, swallowing half a tablet at a time.

   c. Mix it with juice after crushing it.

   d. Chew the tablet thoroughly before swallowing it.

5. A woman who has given birth to a baby girl by cesarean delivery is experiencing abdominal pain. The patient receive a bolus dose of morphine intravenously. The nurse would recommend that the mother refrain from breast-feeding the baby for how long?

   a. 1 to 2 hours

   b. 2 to 4 hours

   c. 4 to 6 hours

   d. 6 to 8 hours

6. The nurse administers an oral dose of morphine to a patient at 3:00 PM. The nurse would expect the drug to peak at which time?

   a. 3:30 PM

   b. 4:00 PM

   c. 4:30 PM

   d. 5:00 PM

7. A patient is receiving a narcotic agonist–antagonist parenterally immediately after surgery but will be switched to the oral form when tolerating fluid and food. Which agent would most likely be preferred?

   a. Buprenorphine

   b. Butorphanol

   c. Nalbuphine

   d. Pentazocine

8. Which of the following would the nurse expect to assess in a patient receiving a narcotic for pain relief?

   a. Dilation of the pupils

   b. Diarrhea

   c. Orthostatic hypotension

   d. Tachypnea

9. A patient is experiencing significant respiratory depression and sedation related to morphine administration. The nurse would anticipate administering which of the following?

   a. Butorphanol

   b. Buprenorphine

   c. Naloxone

   d. Ergotamine

10. A patient is to receive naltrexone. The nurse would expect to administer this drug by which route?

    a. Oral

    b. Subcutaneous

    c. Intramuscular

    d. Intravenous

11. Which assessment finding would support a patient's report of migraine headaches?

    a. Severe unilateral pulsating pain

    b. Sharp steady eye pain

    c. Dull band of pain around the head

    d. Onset occurring during sleep

12. When describing the action of ergot derivatives, the nurse would incorporate understanding of which of the following?

    a. Blockage of alpha-adrenergic receptors

    b. Interference with dopamine

    c. Inhibition of opioid receptors

    d. Interference with cerebral enzyme systems

13. A patient is receiving drug therapy for prevention of an acute migraine attack. Which agent would be the most helpful?

    a. Sumatriptan

    b. Ergotamine

    c. Naloxone

    d. Eletriptan

Copyright © 2011 by Wolters Kluwer Health l Lippincott Williams & Wilkins. *Study Guide for Focus on Nursing Pharmacology.*

14. A patient is prescribed dihydroergotamine. The nurse would instruct the patient to administer this drug most likely by which route?

   a. Oral

   b. Subcutaneous

   c. Intranasal

   d. Sublingual

15. A patient uses sumatriptan for treating her migraine headaches. Which statement by the patient indicates to the nurse that she understands how to take this drug?

   a. "I can repeat a dose in 15 minutes for a total of four doses."

   b. "I should repeat the dose in 30 minutes for a total of three doses."

   c. "I can take another dose 2 hours after the first one."

   d. "I can take another dose in about 4 hours, if needed."

Copyright © 2011 by Wolters Kluwer Health I Lippincott Williams & Wilkins. *Study Guide for Focus on Nursing Pharmacology.*

CHAPTER 27

General and Local Anesthetic Agents

LEARNING OBJECTIVES

Upon completion of this chapter, you will be able to:

1. Describe the concept of balanced anesthesia.

2. Describe the actions and uses of local anesthesia.

3. Describe the therapeutic actions, indications, pharmacokinetics, contraindications, most common adverse reactions, and important drug–drug interactions associated with general and local anesthetics.

4. Outline the preoperative and postoperative needs of a patient receiving general or local anesthesia.

5. Compare and contrast the prototype drugs thiopental, midazolam, nitrous oxide, halothane, and lidocaine with other drugs in their respective classes.

6. Outline the nursing considerations, including important teaching points, for patients receiving general and local anesthetics.

■ ASSESSING YOUR UNDERSTANDING

CROSSWORD

Use the clues to complete the crossword puzzle.

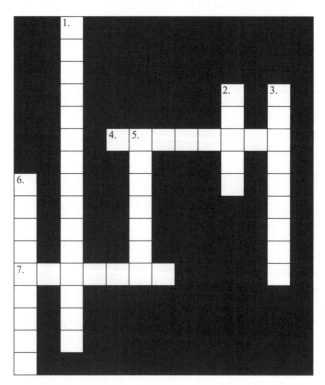

Across

4. Type of anesthesia using several different types of drugs for quick effects
7. Type of anesthesia to create analgesia, unconsciousness, and amnesia

Down

1. Loss of awareness of one's surroundings
2. Type of anesthesia via powerful nerve blockers
3. Time from beginning of anesthesia until achievement of surgical anesthesia
5. Loss of memory
6. Loss of pain sensation

SEQUENCING

Each of the following statements reflects an event in the stages of anesthesia. Place the number of the statement in the boxes below based on the order in which they occur reflecting the depth of anesthesia.

1. Combative behavior with signs of sympathetic stimulation

2. Relaxation of skeletal muscles and return of regular respirations

3. Loss of pain sensation with patient conscious

4. Deep central nervous system (CNS) depression with loss of respiratory and vasomotor center stimuli

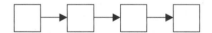

■ APPLYING YOUR KNOWLEDGE

CASE STUDY

A patient is scheduled to undergo abdominal surgery under general anesthesia and is admitted to the health care facility the night before surgery for additional diagnostic testing and preparation. In addition to laboratory tests, a chest x-ray and electrocardiogram are performed. The patient is visited by the anesthesiologist, who obtains a history and physical examination. After the anesthesiologist leaves, the patient presses her call light and wants to talk to the nurse. Upon entering the room, the patient is visibly anxious and upset and says, "Why are they checking my heart and lungs? The problem is in my belly. And who is this doctor that was just here, and why was he asking me all those questions?"

a. How would the nurse respond to the patient?

b. What information would be appropriate to provide to the patient about the events that have happened and are about to happen with surgery?

■ PRACTICING FOR NCLEX

Circle the letter that corresponds to the best answer for each question.

1. When describing the stages of anesthesia, during which stage does pupillary dilation occur?
   a. Stage 1
   b. Stage 2
   c. Stage 3
   d. Stage 4

2. The nurse is reviewing the intraoperative record of a patient who has returned from surgery. The nurse would determine that the patient will most likely need additional analgesia postoperatively due to use of which of the following?
   a. Thiopental
   b. Ketamine
   c. Midazolam
   d. Propofol

3. Which of the following would a nurse expect to assess in a patient who has had general anesthesia using methohexital?
   a. Hypertension
   b. Tachypnea
   c. Increased gastric activity
   d. Vomiting

Copyright © 2011 by Wolters Kluwer Health I Lippincott Williams & Wilkins. *Study Guide for Focus on Nursing Pharmacology.*

4. A patient is receiving a narcotic after having received a barbiturate for general anesthesia. Which of the following would most likely occur?

   a. Bleeding

   b. Apnea

   c. Headache

   d. Delirium

5. After reviewing information about nonbarbiturate anesthestics, a group of students demonstrate understanding of the information when they identify which of the following as an example?

   a. Midazolam

   b. Nitrous oxide

   c. Thiopental

   d. Halothane

6. Which anesthetic is associated with a bizarre state of unconsciousness in which the patient appears to be awake and yet cannot feel pain?

   a. Propofol

   b. Droperidol

   c. Ketamine

   d. Etomidate

7. Which anesthetic would have the fastest onset of action?

   a. Droperidol

   b. Ketamine

   c. Propofol

   d. Etomidate

8. The nurse would monitor the patient for which of the following during recovery from etomidate?

   a. Chills and hypotension

   b. Respiratory depression and CNS suppression

   c. Hallucinations and cardiac arrhythmias

   d. Myoclonic movements and vomiting

9. Which agent would the nurse identify as always being given with oxygen?

   a. Cyclopropane

   b. Nitrous oxide

   c. Halothane

   d. Enflurane

10. After reviewing information about general anesthetics, a group of students demonstrate understanding of the information when they identify which of the following as acting like gas anesthetics?

    a. Volatile liquids

    b. Nonbarbiturate anesthetics

    c. Barbiturate anesthetics

    d. Esters

11. During recovery from general anesthesia, which of the following would be a priority?

    a. Monitoring temperature and reflexes

    b. Providing comfort measures

    c. Have emergency equipment readily available

    d. Providing pain relief as ordered

12. When a local anesthetic is administered in increasing doses, which sensation is lost first?

    a. Touch

    b. Temperature

    c. Proprioception

    d. Skeletal muscle tone

13. A patient is to have an intravenous line inserted, and the nurse prepares to apply a dermal patch to provide local anesthesia to the area. The nurse would apply the patch at which time before initiating intravenous access?

    a. 15 minutes

    b. 30 minutes

    c. 45 minutes

    d. 60 minutes

14. When preparing a patient for the application of a local anesthetic, which of the following would be most important?

    a. Inspecting the application area for intactness

    b. Checking the reflexes in that area

    c. Assessing the peripheral pulses

    d. Determining muscle tone

15. After teaching a group of students about local anesthetic agents, the instructor determines that the teaching was successful when the students identify which of the following as an example of an ester?

    a. Mepivacaine

    b. Lidocaine

    c. Benzocaine

    d. Dibucaine

Copyright © 2011 by Wolters Kluwer Health I Lippincott Williams & Wilkins. *Study Guide for Focus on Nursing Pharmacology.*

Neuromuscular Junction Blocking Agents

LEARNING OBJECTIVES

Upon completion of this chapter, you will be able to:

1. Draw and label a neuromuscular junction.

2. Describe the therapeutic actions, indications, pharmacokinetics, contraindications, most common adverse reactions, and important drug–drug interactions associated with the depolarizing and nondepolarizing neuromuscular junction blockers.

3. Discuss the use of neuromuscular junction blockers across the life span.

4. Compare and contrast the prototype drugs pancuronium and succinylcholine with other neuromuscular junction blockers.

5. Outline the nursing considerations, including important teaching points, for patients receiving a neuromuscular junction blocker.

■ ASSESSING YOUR UNDERSTANDING

FILL IN THE BLANKS

Provide the missing term or terms in the blanks provided.

1. Nerves communicate with muscles at a synapse

   called the _____ _____.

2. The _____, the functional unit of a muscle, is made up of light and dark filaments.

3. The striated appearance of a muscle's functional unit is due to the orderly arrangement of

   _____ and _____ molecules.

4. At the synaptic cleft, the neurotransmitter

   _____ interacts with the nicotinic cholinergic receptors to cause depolarization of the muscle membrane.

5. Drugs that act as antagonists to the neurotransmitter at the neuromuscular

   junction (NMJ) are called _____ NMJ blockers.

6. Succinylcholine is a drug classified as a

   _____ NMJ blocker.

SEQUENCING

Each of the statements below identify an event that occurs with muscle contraction based on the sliding filament theory. Place the number of the statement in the box below based on the order in which they occur.

1. Depolarization allows the release of calcium ions.

2. Acetylcholine is broken down; receptor free.

3. Nerve impulse arrives at motor nerve terminal.

4. Actin and myosin are released from binding sites.

5. Filament becomes shorter.

6. Acetylcholine interacts with nicotinic cholinergic receptors.

7. Calcium binds to troponin.

8. Muscle membrane depolarizes.

9. Actin and myosin repeatedly react with each other.

10. Acetylcholine is released into the synaptic cleft.

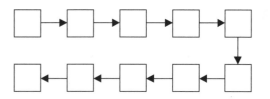

■ APPLYING YOUR KNOWLEDGE

CASE STUDY

An adolescent is brought into the emergency department after being involved in a motor vehicle accident. He has sustained multiple trauma, including a fractured right femur, and is being evaluated for a possible spinal cord injury. The adolescent has a history of asthma. His respiratory status begins to deteriorate, and the decision is made to intubate him and begin mechanical ventilation. The physician administers pancuronium. His parents are at the bedside.

a. What would be the most likely rationale for using pancuronium?

b. What precautions would be necessary related to the use of this drug and the patient's history and current condition?

c. What information would be important to provide to the patient and family about this drug?

PRACTICING FOR NCLEX

Circle the letter that corresponds to the best answer for each question.

1. After reviewing the various NMJ blockers, a group of students demonstrate understanding of the information when they identify which agent as having the longest duration?

   a. Atracurium

   b. Succinylcholine

   c. Vecuronium

   d. Cisatracurium

2. Which agent would be least appropriate to use before anesthesia induction?

   a. Atracurium

   b. Cisatracurium

   c. Pancuronium

   d. Rocuronium

3. A patient is to receive a nondepolarizing NMJ blocker. The patient also takes a calcium channel blocker. Which of the following would most likely occur?

   a. The patient would receive a cholinesterase inhibitor.

   b. The dosage of the NMJ blocker will be less.

   c. A depolarizing NMJ blocker would be used instead.

   d. The dosage of the calcium channel blocker would be increased.

4. After a patient receives succinylcholine, the nurse would assess the patient for which of the following initially?

   a. Muscle pain

   b. Hyperthermia

   c. Hypotension

   d. Respiratory depression

5. Which of the following conditions would predispose a patient to experience a prolonged action of succinylcholine?

   a. Renal failure

   b. Cirrhosis

   c. Heart disease

   d. Inflammatory bowel disease

Copyright © 2011 by Wolters Kluwer Health I Lippincott Williams & Wilkins. *Study Guide for Focus on Nursing Pharmacology.*

6. After reviewing the events associated with the sliding filament theory of muscle contraction, a group students demonstrate a need for additional study when they identify which of the following?

    a. Acetylcholine interacts with muscarnic receptors.

    b. Calcium combines with tropinin.

    c. Actin and myosin, when reacting, shorten the fiber.

    d. Depolarization allows the release of calcium ions.

7. Which of the following statements best reflects the action of NMJ blockers?

    a. They cause muscle paralysis along with total central nervous system depression.

    b. They have relatively few adverse effects.

    c. Most do not affect pain perception and consciousness.

    d. They readily cross the blood–brain barrier.

8. A nurse is monitoring a patient closely for malignant hyperthermia because the patient received which NMJ blocker?

    a. Pancuronium

    b. Vecuronium

    c. Atracurium

    d. Succinylcholine

9. A patient experienced significant muscle pain after receiving an NMJ blocker for a procedure. Which of the following would be most appropriate for the nurse to administer for pain relief?

    a. Dantrolene

    b. Aspirin

    c. Morphine

    d. Naloxone

10. When a depolarizing NMJ agent is used, which of the following occurs?

    a. Prevention of depolarization

    b. Irreversible muscular contraction

    c. Enhancement of repolarization

    d. Continuous sustained muscle contraction

11. Which agent would be associated with increased intraocular pressure?

    a. Succinylcholine

    b. Vecuronium

    c. Rocuronium

    d. Pancuronium

12. A patient is receiving pancuronium. The nurse would expect to see the beginning effects of the drug in which approximate period of time?

    a. 30 to 60 seconds

    b. 1 to 2 minutes

    c. 4 to 6 minutes

    d. 8 to 10 minutes

13. A nurse understands that succinylcholine lasts for approximately how long once it is administered?

    a. 1 to 2 minutes

    b. 4 to 6 minutes

    c. 8 to 12 minutes

    d. 15 to 20 minutes

14. A nurse is reviewing a patient's history for conditions that may contraindicate the use of a nondepolarizing NMJ blocker. Which of the following would be a concern?

    a. Myasthenia gravis

    b. Cirrhosis

    c. Glaucoma

    d. Malnutrition

15. A patient who received a nondepolarizing NMJ blocker is exhibiting signs of excessive neuromuscular blockade. Which of the following would most likely be used?

    a. Peripheral nerve stimulator

    b. Direct-acting skeletal muscle relaxant

    c. Cholinesterase inhibitor

    d. Narcotic antagonist

Copyright © 2011 by Wolters Kluwer Health | Lippincott Williams & Wilkins. *Study Guide for Focus on Nursing Pharmacology.*

CHAPTER 29

Introduction to the Autonomic Nervous System

LEARNING OBJECTIVES

Upon completion of this chapter, you will be able to:

1. Describe how the autonomic nervous system differs anatomically from the rest of the nervous system.

2. Outline a sympathetic response and the clinical manifestation of this response.

3. Describe the alpha- and beta-receptors found within the sympathetic nervous system by sites and actions that follow the stimulation of each kind of receptor.

4. Outline the events that occur with stimulation of the parasympathetic nervous system.

5. Define the terms muscarinic receptor and nicotinic receptor, giving an example of each.

SHORT ANSWER

Supply the information requested.

1. Identify the location of the main nerve centers for the autonomic nervous system.

2. Explain how nerve impulse transmission in the autonomic nervous system is different from that of the central nervous system.

3. State the other name for the sympathetic nervous system.

4. Name the neurotransmitter released by the preganglionic nerves of the sympathetic nervous system.

5. List the four catecholamines.

6. Identify the four classifications of sympathetic nervous system adrenergic receptors.

7. Name the two classifications of parasympathetic nervous system receptors.

8. State the two enzymes involved in terminating a sympathetic nervous system response by metabolizing norepinephrine.

■ ASSESSING YOUR UNDERSTANDING

CROSSWORD

Use the clues to complete the crossword puzzle.

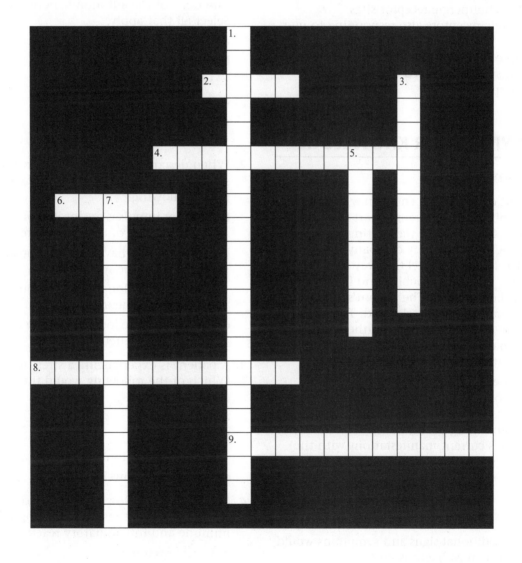

Copyright © 2011 by Wolters Kluwer Health I Lippincott Williams & Wilkins. *Study Guide for Focus on Nursing Pharmacology.*

Across

2. Adrenergic receptor found in the heart and lungs
4. Receptor sites on effects responding to acetylcholine
6. Adrenergic receptors found in smooth muscle
8. Nervous system involved in the fight-or-flight response
9. Receptor sites on effectors responding to norepinephrine

Down

1. Enzyme important for preventing overstimulation of cholinergic receptor sites
3. Cholinergic receptors also responding to muscarine
5. A group of closely packed nerve cell bodies
7. Nervous system involved in the rest-and-digest response

■ APPLYING YOUR KNOWLEDGE

CASE STUDY

A patient comes to the emergency department complaining of a very rapid heart rate and sweating. She states, "I was getting ready to do a presentation for my company, and all of a sudden I started to feel this way. I really don't like to speak in public, and I get really nervous before I do." The patient's heart rate and respiratory rate are elevated. The patient's hands are cool and clammy. Further evaluation reveals that the patient is experiencing an anxiety attack.

a. When evaluating the patient's signs and symptoms, which branch of the autonomic nervous system would the nurse suspect as predominating at this point? Correlate the patient's current manifestations with the system's action.

b. What additional signs and symptoms would the nurse most likely assess?

c. How would the nurse explain to the patient what is happening?

■ PRACTICING FOR NCLEX

Circle the letter that corresponds to the best answer for each question.

1. Which of the following would be considered functions of the autonomic nervous system? Select all that apply.
   a. Control of heart rate
   b. Maintenance of water balance
   c. Level of consciousness
   d. Sensory perception
   e. Muscle movement
   f. Regulation of respiration

2. When describing the sympathetic nervous system, the instructor would include which of the following?
   a. Cells for impulses are located primarily in the sacral area of the spinal cord.
   b. Cells typically have very long preganglionic fibers out to the synapse.
   c. The relatively long postganglionic fibers synapse with neuroeffectors.
   d. The ganglia are located close to the organ or area being affected.

3. A patient is experiencing a stress response. Which of the following would the nurse expect to assess?
   a. Bradycardia
   b. Hypotension
   c. Pupil constriction
   d. Diminished bowel sounds

4. Which of the following is secreted during the fight-or-flight response to suppress the immune and inflammatory reactions?
   a. Corticosteroid
   b. Thyroid hormone
   c. Aldosterone
   d. Glucose

Copyright © 2011 by Wolters Kluwer Health I Lippincott Williams & Wilkins. *Study Guide for Focus on Nursing Pharmacology.*

5. The nurse understands that vasoconstriction that leads to a rise in blood pressure is due to stimulation of which type of receptor?

   a. Alpha-1
   b. Alpha-2
   c. Beta-1
   d. Beta-2

6. A patient is receiving a drug that helps to relax the bladder detrusor muscle. The nurse would understand that this drug is affecting which type of receptor?

   a. Alpha-1
   b. Alpha-2
   c. Beta-1
   d. Beta-2

7. Which of the following would be assessed with parasympathetic nervous system stimulation?

   a. Reduced secretions
   b. Increased gastric motility
   c. Pupillary dilation
   d. Constriction of the rectal sphincter

8. Which neurotransmitter is involved in pre- and postganglionic activity in the parasympathetic nervous system?

   a. Norepinephrine
   b. Epinephrine
   c. Acetylcholine
   d. Dopamine

9. Which of the following would be discussed when describing the parasympathetic nervous system?

   a. Vagus nerve
   b. Adrenergic receptors
   c. Norepinephrine
   d. Monoamine oxidase

10. After teaching a group of students about the differences between the sympathetic nervous system and the parasympathetic nervous system, the instructor determines that the students have understood the information when they state which of the following?

   a. Unlike the sympathetic nervous system, the parasympathetic nervous system ganglia are located in chains along the spinal cord.
   b. The sympathetic nervous system preganglionic fibers are short, while those in the parasympathetic nervous system are long.
   c. The sympathetic nervous system helps the body recuperate from the stress response of the parasympathetic nervous system.
   d. The sympathetic nervous system contains nicotinic receptors that the parasympathetic nervous system does not have.

11. Which of the following would occur if a drug stimulated beta-2 receptors?

   a. Bronchoconstriction
   b. Uterine contraction
   c. Piloerection
   d. Vasodilation

12. Which of the following receptors is found in the beta cells of the pancreas?

   a. Alpha-1
   b. Alpha-2
   c. Beta-1
   d. Beta-2

13. After reviewing the autonomic nervous system and cholinergic neurons, the students demonstrate a need for additional study when they identify which of the following as a location for cholinergic neurons?

   a. Motor nerves on skeletal muscles
   b. All preganglionic nerves
   c. Most postganglionic sympathetic nervous system nerves
   d. Postganglionic parasympathetic nervous system nerves

Copyright © 2011 by Wolters Kluwer Health I Lippincott Williams & Wilkins. *Study Guide for Focus on Nursing Pharmacology.*

14. Muscarinic receptors would be found most likely at which location?

  a. Adrenal medulla

  b. Sweat glands

  c. Neuromuscular junction

  d. Central nervous system

15. Norepinephrine is made by nerve cells using which substance?

  a. Choline

  b. Tyrosine

  c. Decarboxylase

  d. Glycogen

Copyright © 2011 by Wolters Kluwer Health l Lippincott Williams & Wilkins. *Study Guide for Focus on Nursing Pharmacology*.

CHAPTER 30

Adrenergic Agonists

LEARNING OBJECTIVES

Upon completion of this chapter, you will be able to:

1. Describe two ways that sympathomimetic drugs act to produce effects at adrenergic receptors.

2. Describe the therapeutic actions, indications, pharmacokinetics, contraindications, most common adverse reactions, and important drug–drug interactions associated with adrenergic agonists.

3. Discuss the use of adrenergic agents across the life span.

4. Compare and contrast the prototype drugs dopamine, phenylephrine, and isoproterenol with other adrenergic agonists.

5. Outline the nursing considerations, including important teaching points, for patients receiving an adrenergic agent.

■ ASSESSING YOUR UNDERSTANDING

LABELING

Place the name of the drug in the appropriate box under the correct drug class.

Albuterol	Isoproterenol
Clonidine	Phenylephrine
Dobutamine	Terbutaline
Dopamine	

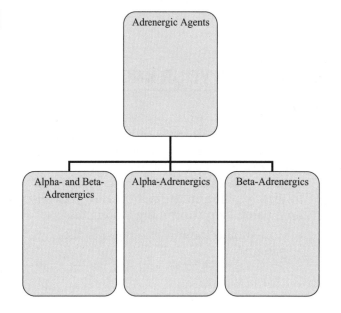

SHORT ANSWER

Supply the information requested.

1. Name the two primary actions of adrenergic agonists.

2. Explain why adrenergic agonists are also referred to as sympathomimetic agents.

3. Name the sympathomimetic drug of choice for the treatment of shock.

4. Describe the rationale for using clonidine to treat hypertension.

5. Explain the result of an interaction between a sympathomimetic agent and an adrenergic antagonist.

6. Identify the reason why adrenergic agonists should be used with caution in patients with vascular problems.

■ APPLYING YOUR KNOWLEDGE

CASE STUDY

A patient is diagnosed with hypertension, and the health care provider prescribes clonidine as a transdermal patch. The patient is concerned because the drug is in patch form instead of pill form. He states, "How will this little patch help control my blood pressure?"

a. How should the nurse respond to the patient?

b. What information would the nurse need to include when teaching the patient about this drug?

■ PRACTICING FOR NCLEX

Circle the letter that corresponds to the best answer for each question.

1. Which of the following would the nurse identify as a naturally occurring catecholamine?
   a. Dobutamine
   b. Dopamine
   c. Ephedrine
   d. Metaraminol

2. Which of the following would a nurse keep in mind about dobutamine when used to treat congestive heart failure?
   a. It has slight preference for beta-1 receptor sites.
   b. It causes a significant increase in the heart rate.
   c. Myocardial oxygen demand is increased.
   d. It rarely interacts with herbal products.

3. Which of the following would the nurse expect to assess in a patient receiving an alpha- and beta-adrenergic agonist?
   a. Hypotension
   b. Dyspnea
   c. Diarrhea
   d. Personality changes

4. A patient is experiencing shock and is extremely hypotensive. Which of the following would the nurse expect as the drug most likely to be given?
   a. Ephedrine
   b. Epinephrine
   c. Dopamine
   d. Dobutamine

5. The nurse is reviewing the medical record of a patient who is taking an alpha- and beta-adrenergic agonist. Which of the following would be of least concern to the nurse?
   a. St. John's wort
   b. Caffeine
   c. Ma huang
   d. Over-the-counter (OTC) cold preparations

Copyright © 2011 by Wolters Kluwer Health | Lippincott Williams & Wilkins. *Study Guide for Focus on Nursing Pharmacology.*

6. The intravenous line of a patient receiving dobutamine infiltrates and the drug extravasates. The nurse would infiltrate the site with which of the following?

a. Lactated Ringer's solution

b. Hyaluronidase

c. Sodium bicarbonate

d. Phentolamine

7. Which of the following adverse effects might a patient receiving clonidine exhibit? Select all that apply.

a. Photophobia

b. Hyperglycemia

c. Pupil constriction

d. Personality changes

e. Difficulty urinating

8. A patient is receiving phenylephrine via intramuscular injection. The nurse would expect the drug to begin acting in approximately which amount of time?

a. 1 to 5 minutes

b. 5 to 10 minutes

c. 10 to 15 minutes

d. 15 to 20 minutes

9. Which assessment finding would indicate to the nurse that the administered isoproterenol is effective?

a. Decreased heart rate

b. Bronchoconstriction

c. Improved cardiac contractility

d. Uterine contraction

10. Which of the following would a nurse expect to administer if a patient who is receiving isoproterenol develops a severe reaction?

a. Beta-adrenergic blockers

b. Sympathomimetic agents

c. Narcotic antagonist

d. Neuromuscular blocking agent

11. A patient is being treated for asthma. Which of the following would the nurse expect to administer?

a. Alpha- and beta-adrenergic agonist

b. Alpha-specific adrenergic agonist

c. Beta-1–specific adrenergic agonist

d. Beta-2–specific adrenergic agonist

12. The nurse is reviewing the history of a patient receiving isoproterenol. Which of the following would the nurse identify as being a contraindication?

a. Pulmonary hypertension

b. Glaucoma

c. Pheochromocytoma

d. Hypovolemia

13. Which of the following agents would the nurse expect to be used to prevent hypotension if dopamine or norepinephrine cannot be used?

a. Dobutamine

b. Ephedrine

c. Metaraminol

d. Epinephrine

14. Which of the following would be most important for the nurse to assess in a patient receiving midodrine?

a. Changes in respiratory rate

b. Positional blood pressure changes

c. Changes in urinary output

d. Appetite changes

15. A patient is taking an OTC allergy product. The nurse would expect to find that this product most likely contains which of the following?

a. Ephedra

b. Phenylephrine

c. Metaraminol

d. Albuterol

CHAPTER 31

Adrenergic Blocking Antagonists

LEARNING OBJECTIVES

Upon completion of this chapter, you will be able to:

1. Describe the effects of adrenergic blocking agents on adrenergic receptors, correlating these effects with their clinical effects.

2. Describe the therapeutic actions, indications, pharmacokinetics, contraindications and cautions, most common adverse reactions, and important drug–drug interactions associated with adrenergic blocking agents.

3. Discuss the use of adrenergic blocking agents across the life span.

4. Compare and contrast the prototype drugs labetalol, phentolamine, doxazosin, propranolol, and atenolol with other adrenergic blocking agents.

5. Outline the nursing considerations, including important teaching points, for patients receiving an adrenergic blocking agent.

■ ASSESSING YOUR UNDERSTANDING

LABELING

Place the name of each drug below in the appropriate column that reflects its selectivity.

Atenolol

Carteolol

Doxazosin

Esmolol

Phentolamine

Pindolol

Propranolol

Terazosin

Timolol

Nonselective Alpha	Alpha-1 Selective	Nonselective Beta	Beta-1 Selective

FILL IN THE BLANKS

Provide the missing term in the blanks provided.

1. Adrenergic blocking agents are also called

   _____ because they block the effects of the sympathetic nervous system.

2. Adrenergic blockers prevent the release of

   _____ from the nerve terminal or from the adrenal medulla.

3. A patient who is receiving a nonselective adrenergic blocker and an antidiabetic agent

   is at risk for _____.

4. Carvedilol is used to treat congestive heart

   failure and _____.

5. Blocking of all receptor sites within the sympathetic nervous system leads to a

   _____ of blood pressure.

6. Alpha-1 selective adrenergic blockers decrease

   blood pressure by blocking the _____ alpha-1 receptor sites.

7. Nonselective beta-adrenergic blockers are used

   primarily to treat _____ problems.

8. An effect associated with nonselective

   beta-adrenergic blockers is _____ exercise tolerance.

9. Adrenergic blocking agents should not be discontinued abruptly but rather should be gradually tapered over a period of

   _____ weeks.

10. The prototype beta-1 selective adrenergic

    blocker is _____.

■ APPLYING YOUR KNOWLEDGE

CASE STUDY

A 58-year-old patient is being seen by his cardiologist for a follow-up visit. The patient has a history of hypertension for which he is receiving carvedilol and furosemide (a diuretic). He is also receiving sotalol as treatment for atrial fibrillation. During the visit, the patient tells the physician that he has been experiencing some light-headedness. "It's mostly when I get up out of bed or when I go to stand up after I've been sitting. I have to stop and hold on for a minute or so and then it passes. I almost stopped taking the drugs because of this."

a. What might the patient be experiencing and why?

b. What information would be important to obtain to help confirm this suspicion?

c. What instructions would be important for this patient?

■ PRACTICING FOR NCLEX

Circle the letter that corresponds to the best answer for each question.

1. Which of the following would be most important to monitor in a patient receiving carvedilol?
   a. Liver function studies
   b. Renal function studies
   c. Complete blood count
   d. Coagulation studies

2. A patient is receiving sotalol. Which instruction would be most important for the nurse to provide to the patient to ensure maximum effectiveness of the drug?
   a. "Take an antacid at the same time you take the drug."
   b. "Be sure to take the drug on an empty stomach."
   c. "Eat a large meal and then take the drug."
   d. "Take the entire daily dose at one time."

3. After reviewing information about nonselective adrenergic blockers, a group of students demonstrate a need for additional teaching when they identify which of the following as an effect of these agents?
   a. Lowered blood pressure
   b. Increased pulse rate
   c. Increased renal perfusion
   d. Decreased renin levels

Copyright © 2011 by Wolters Kluwer Health I Lippincott Williams & Wilkins. *Study Guide for Focus on Nursing Pharmacology.*

4. A patient with diabetes who uses insulin is also receiving labetalol. The nurse would monitor the patient closely for which of the following?

   a. Hypotension

   b. Arrhythmias

   c. Hypoglycemia

   d. Bronchospasm

5. When explaining the use of an alpha-1 selective adrenergic blocker to a patient, which of the following would the nurse need to keep in mind?

   a. Reflex tachycardia may occur.

   b. Bladder relaxation leads to improved urine flow.

   c. The overall vascular tone increases.

   d. Blood pressure decreases due to vasoconstriction.

6. After teaching a group of students about adrenergic blockers that may be used to treat benign prostatic hypertrophy, the instructor determines that the teaching has been successful when the students identify which of the following?

   a. Tamsulosin

   b. Prazosin

   c. Carteolol

   d. Amiodarone

7. A patient experiences diarrhea after receiving a nonselective adrenergic blocking agent. The nurse understands that this effect is most likely due to which of the following?

   a. Drug's effect on liver functioning

   b. Increased parasympathetic dominance

   c. Blockage of norepinephrine in the central nervous system

   d. Loss of vascular tone

8. After administering the oral form of labetalol to a patient, the nurse would monitor the patient for a peak drug effect at which time?

   a. 1 to 2 hours

   b. 2 to 3 hours

   c. 3 to 4 hours

   d. 4 to 5 hours

9. The nurse is preparing a teaching plan for a patient who is to receive a nonselective beta blocker. The nurse would make sure to address safety measures as a priority for the patient receiving which of the following?

   a. Carteolol

   b. Nadolol

   c. Sotalol

   d. Propranolol

10. Which patient statement indicates the need for additional teaching about propranolol?

    a. "I need to get up slowly after sitting or lying down."

    b. "I can stop the drug once my blood pressure is controlled."

    c. "I should space activities throughout the day."

    d. "I need to report if I have any chest pain or problems breathing."

11. A patient has a history of smoking. Which of the following agents would the nurse most likely expect to be ordered?

    a. Timolol

    b. Pindolol

    c. Nadolol

    d. Atenolol

12. Which of the following would a nurse identify as a contraindication for the use of a beta-1 selective blocker?

    a. Diabetes

    b. Thyroid disease

    c. Sinus bradycardia

    d. Chronic obstructive pulmonary disease

13. A patient is experiencing an acute myocardial infarction. The physician orders metoprolol to be given as an intravenous bolus injection. The patient responds, and the physician then orders metoprolol oral therapy. The nurse would expect to administer the first oral dose at which time after the last intravenous bolus dose?

    a. Immediately

    b. 5 minutes

    c. 10 minutes

    d. 15 minutes

14. Which agent would be the most likely drug of choice for an older adult patient with hypertension who requires an adrenergic blocker?

  a. Bisoprolol

  b. Betaxolol

  c. Atenolol

  d. Esmolol

15. A patient is receiving a beta-1 selective blocker after a myocardial infarction to prevent reinfarction. The nurse understands that the rationale for using the drug would be which of the following?

  a. Improve contractility

  b. Enhanced excitability

  c. Decreased cardiac workload

  d. Decreased blood pressure

Copyright © 2011 by Wolters Kluwer Health I Lippincott Williams & Wilkins. *Study Guide for Focus on Nursing Pharmacology.*

CHAPTER 32

Cholinergic Agonists

LEARNING OBJECTIVES

Upon completion of this chapter, you will be able to:

1. Describe the effects of cholinergic receptors, correlating these effects with the clinical effects of cholinergic agonists.

2. Describe the therapeutic actions, indications, pharmacokinetics, contraindications and cautions, most common adverse reactions, and important drug–drug interactions associated with the direct- and indirect-acting cholinergic agonists.

3. Discuss the use of cholinergic agonists across the life span.

4. Compare and contrast the prototype drugs bethanechol, donepezil, and pyridostigmine with other cholinergic agonists.

5. Outline the nursing considerations, including important teaching points, for patients receiving a cholinergic agonist.

■ ASSESSING YOUR UNDERSTANDING

LABELING

Place the name of the following drugs in the appropriate box under the correct drug class.

Bethanechol   Galantamine

Donepezil   Pilocarpine

Edrophonium   Pyridostigmine

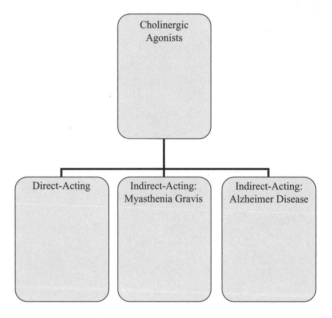

MATCHING

Select the description from column 2 that best describes the term in column 1.

Column 1

_____ 1. Acetylcholinesterase

_____ 2. Parasympathomimetic

_____ 3. Cholinergic

_____ 4. Acetylcholine

_____ 5. Nerve gas

Column 2

a. Another name for cholinergic agonists

b. Irreversible acetylcholinesterase inhibitor

c. Neurotransmitter

d. Enzyme responsible for neurotransmitter breakdown

e. Receptor sites stimulated by acetylcholine

■ APPLYING YOUR KNOWLEDGE

CASE STUDY

A 35-year-old woman is brought to the emergency department by her husband for evaluation. The patient has a history of myasthenia gravis for which she takes pyridostigmine daily. The patient began to have difficulty breathing. Her husband noticed that she was experiencing more problems swallowing and speaking. He also reports that it was difficult to see her eyes because her eyelids were drooping so severely.

a. What might be happening with this patient and why?

b. What would the nurse expect to be done to determine the appropriate plan of treatment?

c. What interventions would be instituted for this patient?

■ PRACTICING FOR NCLEX

Circle the letter that corresponds to the best answer for each question.

1. Which of the following physiologic effects would be related to the use of cholinergic agents?

   a. Pupil dilation

   b. Increased salivation

   c. Increased heart rate

   d. Decreased bladder muscle tone

2. A patient receives pilocarpine eye drops. Which of the following effects would the nurse expect to assess?

   a. Miosis

   b. Mydriasis

   c. Ptosis

   d. Paralysis of eye muscles

3. When assessing a patient for possible adverse effects of direct-acting cholinergic agents, which of the following might the nurse find?

   a. Tachycardia

   b. Hypertension

   c. Constipation

   d. Urinary urgency

4. A patient is experiencing urinary retention after surgery. The nurse would anticipate administering which of the following?

   a. Cevimeline

   b. Pilocarpine

   c. Bethanechol

   d. Carbachol

5. When describing the action of indirect-acting cholinergic agonists to a group of students, which of the following would the instructor include?

   a. Imitation of acetylcholine action at receptor sites

   b. Prevention of acetylcholinesterase action

   c. Reduction in the amount of acetylcholine available

   d. Occupation of acetylcholine receptor sites

6. Which of the following agents would be most appropriate to administer to a patient with Alzheimer's disease?

   a. Pyridostigmine

   b. Neostigmine

   c. Ambenonium

   d. Donepezil

Copyright © 2011 by Wolters Kluwer Health I Lippincott Williams & Wilkins. *Study Guide for Focus on Nursing Pharmacology.*

7. A nurse is preparing a presentation for a local group of emergency first responders about biological and chemical weapons. The nurse is describing the effects of exposure to nerve gas. Which of the following would the nurse include?

   a. Tachycardia

   b. Pupil dilation

   c. Bronchial constriction

   d. Muscle flaccidity

8. A patient is prescribed donepezil. The nurse would expect to administer this drug at which frequency?

   a. Once a day

   b. Twice a day

   c. Three times a day

   d. Four times a day

9. The nurse would be alert for which of the following in a patient who is taking rivastigmine and ibuprofen?

   a. Fecal incontinence

   b. Abdominal cramps

   c. Gastrointestinal bleeding

   d. Diarrhea

10. Which of the following would be most important to have readily available for a patient who is receiving an indirect-acting cholinergic agonist and develops a severe reaction?

    a. Edrophonium

    b. Atropine

    c. Phentolamine

    d. Naloxone

11. A patient with myasthenia gravis is having difficulty swallowing and adhering to a routine schedule. Which agent would be the most appropriate?

    a. Ambenonium

    b. Neostigmine

    c. Pyridostigmine

    d. Rivastigmine

12. A patient is receiving galantamine as treatment for Alzheimer's disease. The nurse would instruct the patient and his family about which of the following as possible adverse effects? Select all that apply.

    a. Urinary urgency

    b. Blurred vision

    c. Constipation

    d. Hypertension

    e. Flushing

13. A patient is receiving tacrine and uses theophylline for chronic bronchospasm. Which of the following would be most important for the nurse to monitor?

    a. Respiratory status

    b. Serum theophylline levels

    c. Blood pressure

    d. Mental status

14. Which of the following would the nurse identify as a contraindication to the use of an anticholinesterase inhibitor?

    a. Asthma

    b. Peptic ulcer disease

    c. Intestinal obstruction

    d. Parkinsonism

15. When describing the action of direct-acting cholinergic agonists, which receptors would the nurse identify as being stimulated?

    a. Muscarinic

    b. Nicotinic

    c. Alpha

    d. Beta

Copyright © 2011 by Wolters Kluwer Health I Lippincott Williams & Wilkins. *Study Guide for Focus on Nursing Pharmacology.*

Anticholinergic Agents

LEARNING OBJECTIVES

Upon completion of the chapter, you will be able to:

1. Define anticholinergic agents.

2. Describe the therapeutic actions, indications, pharmacokinetics, contraindications and cautions, most common adverse reactions, and important drug–drug interactions of anticholinergic agents.

3. Discuss the use of anticholinergic agents across the life span.

4. Compare and contrast the prototype drug atropine with other anticholinergic agents.

5. Outline the nursing considerations, including important teaching points, for patients receiving anticholinergic agents.

■ ASSESSING YOUR UNDERSTANDING

FILL IN THE BLANKS

Provide the missing term in the blanks provided.

1. A plant that contains atropine as an alkaloid,

_____, is used in herbal medicine today.

2. _____ agents are drugs that block the effects of acetylcholine.

3. The most widely used parasympatholytic

agent is _____.

4. Relaxation of the pupil of the eye is called

_____.

5. The adverse effects associated with anticholinergic agents are due to the systemic blockade

of _____ receptors.

6. An antidote for atropine toxicity is

_____.

7. Antihistamines _____ the adverse effects of anticholinergic agents.

8. Blockage of the parasympathetic system leads

to _____ gastrointestinal (GI) activity.

MATCHING

Select the condition in column 2 that would be an indication for the drug listed in column 1.

Column 1

____ 1. Dicyclomine

____ 2. Ipratropium

____ 3. Propantheline

____ 4. Scopolamine

____ 5. Hyoscyamine

Column 2

a. Adjunct therapy for peptic ulcer disease
b. Treatment of irritable bowel
c. Maintenance treatment of bronchospasm
d. Treatment of motion sickness
e. Alleviation of GI spasms

■ APPLYING YOUR KNOWLEDGE

CASE STUDY

A 62-year-old black man comes to the clinic for an eye examination. The patient has a history of depression for which the patient takes a tricyclic antidepressant. The patient is to receive atropine eye drops in preparation for the ophthalmologic examination.

a. What issues would be important for the nurse to consider in this situation?

b. Would the nurse expect the patient to exhibit adverse effects? Why or why not?

■ PRACTICING FOR NCLEX

Circle the letter that corresponds to the best answer for each question.

1. A nurse suspects that a patient may be experiencing atropine toxicity. Which of the following would the nurse assess?
  a. Diaphoresis
  b. Excess salivation
  c. Slight cardiac slowing
  d. Cough

2. Which of the following statements best reflects the action of scopolamine?
  a. It blocks the nicotinic receptors in the parasympathetic nervous system.
  b. It exerts a major effect on the neuromuscular junction.
  c. It competes with acetylcholine at muscarinic effector sites.
  d. It acts specifically on the smooth muscles of the urinary tract.

3. Which agent would a nurse expect to administer transdermally?
  a. Atropine
  b. Scopolamine

  c. Dicyclomine
  d. Propantheline

4. A patient is prescribed propantheline. The nurse would administer this drug by which route?
  a. Oral
  b. Subcutaneous
  c. Intramuscular
  d. Intravenous

5. A patient with hypertension is to receive an anticholinergic agent. The nurse would be especially alert for which of the following?
  a. Bladder obstruction
  b. Paralytic ileus
  c. Increased intraocular pressure
  d. Increased blood pressure

6. A patient is experiencing urgency, nocturia, and frequency secondary to cystitis. Which of the following might the health care provider prescribe?
  a. Flavoxate
  b. Dicyclomine
  c. Glycopyrrolate
  d. Methscopolamine

7. An older patient is taking an anticholinergic agent. After teaching the patient about the drug, which patient statement indicates the need for additional teaching?
  a. "I should make sure that I drink plenty of fluids."
  b. "I need to exercise frequently outside in the warm weather."
  c. "I should avoid driving if I feel light-headed or dizzy."
  d. "I should eat plenty of fiber to prevent constipation."

8. A patient is diagnosed with atropine toxicity that resulted from the ingestion of herbal therapies. Which of the following would be done first?
  a. Administration of physostigmine
  b. Gastric lavage
  c. Administration of diazepam
  d. Cool sponge baths

Copyright © 2011 by Wolters Kluwer Health l Lippincott Williams & Wilkins. *Study Guide for Focus on Nursing Pharmacology.*

9. Which of the following agents would be least likely to cause increased adverse effects if given with an anticholinergic agent?
   a. Antihistamines
   b. Antiparkinson agents
   c. Monoamine oxidase inhibitors
   d. Nonsteroidal anti-inflammatory drugs

10. The nurse administers atropine intramuscularly at 9:00 AM. At which time would the nurse expect the drug's peak effects to occur?
    a. 9:15 AM
    b. 9:30 AM
    c. 9:45 AM
    d. 10:00 AM

11. A patient is prescribed glycopyrrolate. The nurse understands that this drug may be administered by which route? Select all that apply.
    a. Oral
    b. Intramuscular
    c. Subcutaneous
    d. Transdermal
    e. Intravenous

12. Which of the following would the nurse expect to assess in a patient who has been given propantheline?
    a. Pupil constriction
    b. Diarrhea
    c. Bradycardia
    d. Excitement

13. A patient is using a transdermal application of scopolamine. Which of the following instructions would the nurse include when teaching the patient how to use this drug?
    a. "Shave the area where you are planning to apply the patch."
    b. "Place your fingers on the adhesive side of the patch to apply it."
    c. "Make sure the area you are using is clean, dry, and free from cuts."
    d. "Apply a new patch before you remove the old one."

14. Which agent would the nurse identify as acting specifically on the receptors in the GI tract?
    a. Ipratropium
    b. Tiotropium
    c. Trospium
    d. Hyoscyamine

15. A patient is using a scopolamine patch for treatment of motion sickness. The nurse would instruct the patient to change the patch at which frequency?
    a. Every day
    b. Every 3 days
    c. Every 5 days
    d. Every 7 days

Copyright © 2011 by Wolters Kluwer Health l Lippincott Williams & Wilkins. *Study Guide for Focus on Nursing Pharmacology.*

34

Introduction to the Endocrine System

Upon completion of this chapter, you will be able to:

1. Label a diagram showing the glands of the traditional endocrine system and list the hormones produced by each.

2. Describe two theories of hormone action.

3. Discuss the role of the hypothalamus as the master gland of the endocrine system, including influences on the actions of the hypothalamus.

4. Outline a negative feedback system within the endocrine system and explain the ways that this system controls hormone levels in the body.

5. Describe the hypothalamic-pituitary axis and what would happen if a hormone level were altered within the hypothalamic-pituitary axis.

■ ASSESSING YOUR UNDERSTANDING

LABELING

Place the name of the hormone in the appropriate column.

Adrenocorticotropic hormone (ACTH)

Antidiuretic hormone

Follicle-stimulating hormone

Gonadotropin-releasing hormone

Growth hormone

Luteinizing hormone

Melanocyte-stimulating hormone

Oxytocin

Prolactin

Somatostatin

Thyroid-releasing hormone

Thyroid-stimulating hormone

Hypothalamus	Anterior Pituitary	Posterior Pituitary

MATCHING

Select the hormone produced from column 2 that is secreted by the gland in column 1.

Column 1

___ **1.** Adrenal cortex

___ **2.** Ovaries

___ **3.** Pancreas

___ **4.** Kidney

___ **5.** Stomach

___ **6.** Testes

___ **7.** Thyroid

___ **8.** Pineal gland

Column 2

a. Erythropoietin

b. Melatonin

c. Gastrin

d. Aldosterone

e. Progesterone

f. Glucagon

g. Calcitonin

h. Testosterone

■ APPLYING YOUR KNOWLEDGE

CASE STUDY

A patient is diagnosed with a brain tumor. Diagnostic studies reveal that the tumor is located at the very back of the cerebrum (the forebrain), extending into the area between the cerebrum and the brain stem, in an area termed the *diencephalon*. The tumor is pressing on a small portion of the hypothalamus. The patient is to undergo radiation therapy to help shrink the tumor in the hopes that the tumor can then be surgically removed.

a. How might the patient's hormonal balance be affected by this condition?

b. What other effects might occur as a result of the tumor's location?

■ PRACTICING FOR NCLEX

Circle the letter that corresponds to the best answer for each question.

1. Which of the following best reflects hormones?

  a. Produced in large quantities

  b. Secreted directly into the bloodstream

  c. Require time to be broken down

  d. Travel via ducts to receptor sites

2. After reviewing the structures of the endocrine system, the students demonstrate understanding when they identify which of the following as the master gland?

  a. Thyroid

  b. Pituitary

  c. Hypothalamus

  d. Pancreas

3. A hormone that takes a while to produce an effect is most likely reacting in which manner?

  a. With a receptor on the cell membrane

  b. With a cell as it travels through the bloodstream

  c. In a specialized target area of the body

  d. Inside the cell receptor site to change messenger RNA

4. Which of the following would the nurse identify as being secreted by the hypothalamus?

  a. Somatostatin

  b. ACTH

  c. Luteinizing hormone

  d. Prolactin

5. Which of the following would be delivered by the neurologic network from the hypothalamus to the pituitary?

  a. Growth hormone-releasing hormone

  b. Gonadotropin-releasing hormone

  c. Corticotropin-releasing hormone

  d. Oxytocin

Copyright © 2011 by Wolters Kluwer Health I Lippincott Williams & Wilkins. *Study Guide for Focus on Nursing Pharmacology.*

6. After teaching a group of students about the factors that affect the release of hormones from the anterior pituitary gland, the instructor determines that the students need additional teaching when they identify which of the following as a factor?
   a. Central nervous system activity
   b. Hypothalamic hormones
   c. Drugs
   d. Plasma osmolality

7. Which of the following would a nurse identify as being released from the intermediate lobe of the pituitary gland?
   a. Oxytocin
   b. Endorphins
   c. Antidiuretic hormone
   d. Melanocyte-stimulating hormone

8. Which hormone would a nurse identify as being involved in diurnal rhythm?
   a. Corticotropin-releasing factor
   b. Thyroid-stimulating hormone
   c. Growth hormone release-inhibiting factor
   d. Luteinizing hormone

9. Which hormone would be responsible for the letdown reflex in lactating women?
   a. Prolactin
   b. Follicle-stimulating hormone
   c. Oxytocin
   d. Luteinizing hormone

10. After teaching a group of students about the negative feedback system, the instructor determines that the students have understood the information when they identify which hormone as not being regulated by this mechanism?
    a. Prolactin
    b. Thyroid hormone
    c. Follicle-stimulating hormone
    d. ACTH

11. Which of the following regulates the release of parathormone?
    a. Acid in the gastrointestinal tract
    b. Calcium levels
    c. Blood pressure
    d. Blood glucose levels

12. Which hormone is released by activation of the sympathetic nervous system?
    a. Aldosterone
    b. Prostaglandin
    c. ACTH
    d. Calcitonin

13. When describing the hypothalamic-pituitary axis, which event would occur first?
    a. Anterior pituitary release of stimulating hormones
    b. Hypothalamus secretion of releasing factor
    c. Hormone secretion by the endocrine gland
    d. Rising levels of secreted hormone

14. Which of the following is a primary effect of aldosterone secretion?
    a. Increased glucose levels
    b. Increased red blood cell production
    c. Increased sodium levels
    d. Increased potassium levels

15. Stimulation of which of the following would result from thyroid hormone secretion?
    a. Stomach acid production
    b. Basal metabolic rate
    c. Male secondary sex characteristics
    d. Pancreatic juice secretion

Copyright © 2011 by Wolters Kluwer Health | Lippincott Williams & Wilkins. *Study Guide for Focus on Nursing Pharmacology.*

CHAPTER 35

Hypothalamic and Pituitary Agents

LEARNING OBJECTIVES

Upon completion of this chapter, you will be able to:

1. Describe the anatomic and physiologic relationship between the hypothalamus and the pituitary gland and list the hormones produced by each.

2. Describe the therapeutic actions, indications, pharmacokinetics, contraindications, most common adverse reactions, and important drug–drug interactions associated with the hypothalamic and pituitary agents.

3. Discuss the use of hypothalamic and pituitary agents across the life span.

4. Compare and contrast the prototype drugs leuprolide, somatropin, bromocriptine mesylate, and desmopressin with other hypothalamic and pituitary agents.

5. Outline the nursing considerations, including important teaching points, for patients receiving a hypothalamic or pituitary agent.

■ ASSESSING YOUR UNDERSTANDING

CROSSWORD

Use the clues to solve the crossword puzzle.

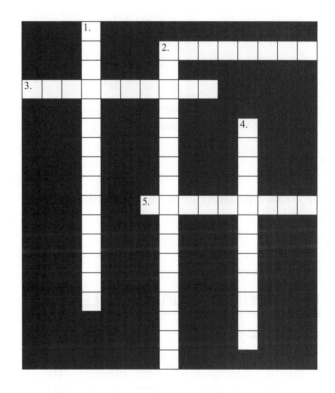

Across

2. Small stature; lack of growth hormone in children
3. Thickening of bony surfaces due to excess growth hormone after closure of the epiphyseal plates
5. Excess levels of growth hormone before closure of the epiphyseal plates

Down

1. Lack of adequate pituitary function
2. Lack of antidiuretic hormone
4. Master gland

SHORT ANSWER

Supply the information requested.

1. Describe the primary uses for hypothalamic hormones.

2. Explain the difference between gigantism and acromegaly.

3. Identify the prototype growth hormone antagonist.

4. List three signs of water intoxication that can occur with desmopressin.

5. Name two growth hormone antagonists.

■ APPLYING YOUR KNOWLEDGE

CASE STUDY

A child is to receive growth hormone therapy due to a deficiency of growth hormone. The plan is to administer somatropin, which is a synthetic human growth hormone. The child has undergone numerous screening procedures and testing. During a recent visit, he says to the nurse, "I can't wait until I start growing. I'm so tired of being the shortest one in my class."

a. How should the nurse respond to this child?

b. What psychosocial issues might arise with this therapy?

■ PRACTICING FOR NCLEX

Circle the letter that corresponds to the best answer for each question.

1. A patient is to receive nafarelin. The nurse would instruct the patient in administering this drug by which route?
   a. Oral
   b. Intranasal
   c. Intramuscular
   d. Subcutaneous

2. Which of the following would the nurse assess in a patient receiving a hypothalamic agonist?
   a. Dehydration
   b. Decreased glucose levels
   c. Impaired healing
   d. Loss of energy

3. After teaching a patient about the adverse effects of leuprolide, the nurse determines that additional teaching is needed when the patient identifies which of the following as an adverse effect?
   a. Hematuria
   b. Chills
   c. Peripheral edema
   d. Constipation

4. Which agent would the nurse expect to be used to diagnosis Cushing's disease?
   a. Corticotropin-releasing hormone
   b. Gonadorelin
   c. Goserelin
   d. Sermorelin

5. Which agent would the nurse identify as a growth hormone agonist?
   a. Bromocriptine
   b. Octreotide
   c. Somatropin
   d. Pegvisomant

Copyright © 2011 by Wolters Kluwer Health I Lippincott Williams & Wilkins. *Study Guide for Focus on Nursing Pharmacology.*

6. The nurse is assessing a child who is receiving growth hormone therapy. Which of the following would the nurse identify as suggesting glucose intolerance?

   a. Injection site pain

   b. Fatigue

   c. Thirst

   d. Cold intolerance

7. The nurse is preparing to administer octreotide. The nurse expects to administer this drug by which route?

   a. Oral

   b. Subcutaneous

   c. Intramuscular

   d. Intranasal

8. A patient is receiving pegvisomant as treatment for acromegaly. Which of the following might the nurse assess as a possible adverse effect?

   a. Gastrointestinal upset

   b. Drowsiness

   c. Postural hypotension

   d. Infection

9. A patient who is receiving a growth hormone antagonist develops acute cholecystitis. Which agent would the patient most likely be receiving?

   a. Bromocriptine

   b. Pegvisomant

   c. Somatropin

   d. Octreotide

10. A patient is to undergo fertility treatment and is to receive an agent that induces ovulation because her ovaries are functioning. Which agent would this most likely be?

    a. Chorionic gonadotropin

    b. Corticotropin

    c. Cosyntropin

    d. Thyrotropin alfa

11. The nurse would administer which of the following to a patient is in labor to improve her uterine contractions?

    a. Desmopressin

    b. Oxytocin

    c. Menotropins

    d. Chorionic gonadotropin alfa

12. When describing desmopressin to a group of students, the instructor explains that it is a synthetic form of which of the following?

    a. Oxytocin

    b. Adrenocorticotropic hormone

    c. Thyroid hormone

    d. Antidiuretic hormone

13. A patient receives desmopressin intravenously at 10:00 AM. The nurse would expect the drug to begin working at which time?

    a. 10:15 AM

    b. 10:30 AM

    c. 10:45 AM

    d. 11:00 AM

14. A patient is undergoing testing for Cushing's disease and is to receive corticotropin-releasing hormone. The nurse would prepare to administer this drug as which of the following?

    a. Intravenous bolus injection

    b. Intramuscular injection

    c. Intravenous infusion

    d. Depot injection

15. After reviewing agents that act as gonadotropin-releasing hormone antagonists, the students demonstrate a need for additional study when they identify which of the following as an example?

    a. Leuprolide

    b. Ganirelix

    c. Goserelin

    d. Abarelix

Copyright © 2011 by Wolters Kluwer Health | Lippincott Williams & Wilkins. *Study Guide for Focus on Nursing Pharmacology.*

36

Adrenocortical Agents

LEARNING OBJECTIVES

Upon completion of this chapter, you will be able to:

1. Explain the control of the synthesis and secretion and the physiologic effects of the adrenocortical agents.

2. Describe the therapeutic actions, indications, pharmacokinetics, contraindications, most common adverse reactions, and important drug–drug interactions associated with the adrenocortical agents.

3. Discuss the use of adrenocortical agents across the life span.

4. Compare and contrast the prototype drugs prednisone and fludrocortisone with other adrenocortical agents.

5. Outline the nursing considerations, including important teaching points, for patients receiving an adrenocortical agent.

■ ASSESSING YOUR UNDERSTANDING

LABELING

Place the name of the following drugs in the appropriate box under the correct drug class.

Beclomethasone   Hydrocortisone

Budesonide   Prednisone

Cortisone   Triamcinolone

Dexamethasone

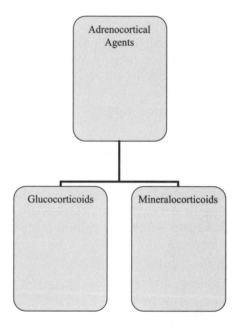

SHORT ANSWER

Supply the information requested.

1. Explain diurnal rhythm as it relates to hormonal secretion.

2. Describe the chemicals that are released by the adrenal medulla.

3. List the three types of corticosteroids produced by the adrenal cortex.

4. Explain how an adrenal crisis occurs.

5. Describe what happens with the prolonged use of corticosteroids.

6. Identify the functions of glucocorticoids in the body.

■ APPLYING YOUR KNOWLEDGE

CASE STUDY

A 9-year-old child is admitted to the facility after experiencing a severe asthmatic attack that responds to bronchodilator therapy (systemic and inhaled) and large doses of corticosteroids. The child was diagnosed with asthma at age 2½ years and has had repeated asthmatic attacks for which he was hospitalized frequently before the age of 6 years. Since that time, the child has had two previous attacks that required hospitalization. Each time, bronchodilator and corticosteroid therapy was used as treatment. Currently, the child, who has been receiving intravenous corticosteroids, is being switched to oral therapy. The child is talking with the nurse about his condition and states, "I hate to take these steroids. My face gets all round, and I get so fat. My friends started to call me "mega Jon." Maybe I won't have to take them when I go home."

a. What effects might the child be experiencing related to his prescribed therapy?

b. How should the nurse respond to the child's statement about not taking the drugs at home?

■ PRACTICING FOR NCLEX

Circle the letter that corresponds to the best answer for each question.

1. Which of the following would a nurse identify as being secreted by the adrenal medulla?
  a. Androgens
  b. Neurotransmitters
  c. Glucocorticoids
  d. Mineralocorticoids

2. At which time would a nurse expect peak levels of adrenocorticotropic hormone to occur?
  a. 10 PM to 12 AM
  b. 1 AM to 3 AM
  c. 6 AM to 9 AM
  d. 12 PM to 3 PM

3. Which corticosteroid would a nurse identify as having the greatest glucocorticoid effects?
  a. Prednisone
  b. Cortisone
  c. Dexamethasone
  d. Triamcinolone

4. A child is to receive a topical corticosteroid agent. Which statement by the parents indicates a need for additional teaching?
  a. "We'll apply the cream in a thin layer over the area, using a small amount."
  b. "We need to cover the area snugly with plastic wrap to prevent scratching."
  c. "We'll keep the cream away from any open areas that might develop."
  d. "We'll avoid putting the cream on any areas where the skin is abraded."

5. The nurse is preparing to administer prednisone. The nurse would expect to administer this agent by which route?
  a. Oral
  b. Intralesional
  c. Inhalation
  d. Intravenous

Copyright © 2011 by Wolters Kluwer Health | Lippincott Williams & Wilkins. *Study Guide for Focus on Nursing Pharmacology.*

6. The nurse is monitoring a child who has been receiving long-term therapy with systemic corticosteroids. Which of the following would be most important for the nurse to assess?

   a. Weight changes

   b. Rectal bleeding

   c. Epistaxis

   d. Growth pattern

7. A patient receives prednisone at 7:00 AM. The nurse would expect to assess for the drug's peak effectiveness at which time after administration?

   a. 7:30 AM

   b. 8:30 AM

   c. 9:30 AM

   d. 10:30 AM

8. The nurse is teaching a patient who is receiving a glucocorticoid about the drug. Which of the following would the nurse instruct the patient to report immediately?

   a. Weight gain

   b. Abdominal distention

   c. Fever

   d. Increased appetite

9. A nurse would instruct a patient to take an oral glucocorticoid at which time?

   a. In the morning

   b. Around lunchtime

   c. Before dinner

   d. At bedtime

10. A nurse is reviewing the history of a patient who is to receive glucocorticoid therapy. Which of the following would the nurse identify as a contraindication to the drug's use?

    a. Diabetes

    b. Peptic ulcer disease

    c. Allergic disorder

    d. Acute infection

11. Which glucocorticoid also exerts some mineralocorticoid effects?

    a. Triamcinolone

    b. Prednisolone

    c. Dexamethasone

    d. Betamethasone

12. After teaching a group of students about the effects of mineralocorticoids, the instructor determines that additional teaching is needed when the students identify which of the following as an effect?

    a. Increased sodium reabsorption

    b. Water retention

    c. Increased calcium retention

    d. Increased potassium excretion

13. When monitoring a patient who is receiving mineralocorticoid therapy, the nurse would report which assessment finding?

    a. Shortness of breath

    b. Headache

    c. Weakness

    d. Slight pedal edema

14. When reviewing the serum potassium levels of a patient receiving fludrocortisone, which of the following would be a concern?

    a. 2.8 mEq/L

    b. 3.1 mEq/L

    c. 3.5 mEq/L

    d. 4.2 mEq/L

15. A group of students are reviewing material about the action of the adrenal glands and the stress response. The students demonstrate understanding of the material when they identify which of the following as a result of adrenocortical hormones?

    a. Decreased blood volume

    b. Glucose release for energy

    c. Increased protein production

    d. Stimulation of the inflammatory response

Copyright © 2011 by Wolters Kluwer Health l Lippincott Williams & Wilkins. *Study Guide for Focus on Nursing Pharmacology.*

Thyroid and Parathyroid Agents

LEARNING OBJECTIVES

Upon completion of this chapter, you will be able to:

1. Explain the control of the synthesis and secretion of thyroid hormones and parathyroid hormones, applying this to alterations in the control process (e.g., using thyroid hormones to treat obesity, Paget's disease, etc.).

2. Describe the therapeutic actions, indications, pharmacokinetics, contraindications, most common adverse reactions, and important drug–drug interactions associated with thyroid and parathyroid agents.

3. Discuss the use of thyroid and parathyroid drugs across the life span.

4. Compare and contrast thyroid and parathyroid prototype drugs with agents in their class.

5. Outline nursing considerations, including important teaching points, for patients receiving drugs used to affect thyroid or parathyroid function.

■ ASSESSING YOUR UNDERSTANDING

CROSSWORD

Use the clues to complete the crossword puzzle.

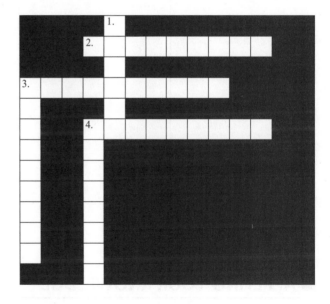

Across

2. Cells circularly arranged that form the structural unit of the thyroid gland
3. Hormone produced to counteract the effects of parathyroid hormone
4. Rate at which cells burn energy

Down

1. Dietary element used to produce thyroid hormone
3. Thyroid hormone deficiency in an infant
4. Lack of thyroid hormone in adults

LABELING

Place the following signs or symptoms in the appropriate column as indicating a deficiency or excess of thyroid hormones.

Coarse, dry skin

Tachycardia

Lethargy

Diffuse goiter

Fine, soft hair

Emotional dullness

Intolerance to heat

Weight gain

Thyroid Hormone Deficiency	Thyroid Hormone Excess

■ APPLYING YOUR KNOWLEDGE

CASE STUDY

A woman has undergone surgery to remove most of her thyroid gland as treatment for hyperthyroidism. Initially, drug therapy with methimazole was tried, but it was not effective. The patient is preparing to go home. She asks the nurse, "First I was on medicine to control my thyroid, then I had it removed. Now I have to take medicine. Now I have to take more medicine. I thought I was done with all of this!"

a. What information would be important for the nurse to address with this patient?

b. What instructions would be important to include when teaching the patient about this drug?

■ PRACTICING FOR NCLEX

Circle the letter that corresponds to the best answer for each question.

1. Which agent would a nurse expect to administer to a patient with hypothyroidism?
   a. Levothyroxine
   b. Methimazole
   c. Propylthiouracil
   d. Calcitriol

2. Which of the following would a nurse expect to assess in a patient experiencing hyperthyroidism?
   a. Slow and deep tendon reflexes
   b. Bradycardia
   c. Flushed, warm skin
   d. Intolerance to cold

3. When describing the parafollicular cells to a group of students, which hormone would the instructor identify as being produced by these cells?
   a. Parathormone
   b. Calcitonin
   c. Levothyroxine
   d. Liothyronine

4. Which of the following would be the initial substance responsible for thyroid hormone regulation?
   a. Iodine intake
   b. Thyrotropin-releasing hormone
   c. Thyroid-stimulating hormone
   d. Levothyroxine

5. A patient is prescribed levothyroxine. The nurse understands that this drug contains which of the following?

   a. T3

   b. Iodine

   c. T4

   d. Vitamin D

6. A patient is receiving propylthiouracil. The nurse anticipates a reduction in the patient's dosage based on assessment of which of the following?

   a. Nervousness

   b. Tachycardia

   c. Weight loss

   d. Decreased appetite

7. A group of students are reviewing hypo- and hypercalcemia. The students demonstrate a need for additional review when they identify which of the following as indicating hypercalcemia?

   a. Lethargy

   b. Tetany

   c. Muscle weakness

   d. Personality changes

8. A patient is prescribed calcitriol. Which instruction would be most important for the nurse to include in the teaching plan?

   a. "Take the drug with a magnesium antacid."

   b. "Limit your intake of dairy products."

   c. "Have your calcium levels check periodically."

   d. "Take the drug with food if gastrointestinal upset occurs."

9. After teaching a group of students about bisphosphonates, the students demonstrate understanding of the information when they identify which drug as an example?

   a. Teriparatide

   b. Calcitonin-salmon

   c. Dihydrotachysterol

   d. Pamidronate

10. A patient is prescribed ibandronate. The nurse instructs the patient to take the drug at which frequency?

    a. Once a week

    b. Once every 2 weeks

    c. Once a month

    d. Once every 3 months

11. While reviewing the medication history of a patient receiving alendronate, the nurse notes that the patient also takes a multivitamin. Which instruction would be most appropriate?

    a. "Stop taking the multivitamin at once."

    b. "Take the multivitamin just before the alendronate."

    c. "Take the alendronate with an antacid before the multivitamin."

    d. "Separate taking the two drugs by about a half hour."

12. A patient is prescribed calcitonin. The nurse would teach the patient to administer the drug by which route?

    a. Oral

    b. Subcutaneous

    c. Sublingual

    d. Topical

13. Which of the following would lead a nurse to suspect that a patient receiving bisphosphonate therapy is experiencing hypercalcemia?

    a. Lethargy

    b. Paresthesias

    c. Muscle cramps

    d. Carpopedal spasms

Copyright © 2011 by Wolters Kluwer Health | Lippincott Williams & Wilkins. *Study Guide for Focus on Nursing Pharmacology.*

14. A patient who is receiving a strong iodide solution, potassium iodide, develops iodism. Which of the following would the nurse expect to find?

   a. Sweet taste in the mouth

   b. Constipation

   c. Sore teeth

   d. Rash

15. A patient is to receive teriparatide. The nurse would instruct the patient in which of the following?

   a. Oral administration

   b. Subcutaneous injection

   c. Intranasal spray administration

   d. Transdermal application

Copyright © 2011 by Wolters Kluwer Health | Lippincott Williams & Wilkins. *Study Guide for Focus on Nursing Pharmacology.*

Agents to Control Blood Glucose Levels

LEARNING OBJECTIVES

Upon completion of this chapter, you will be able to:

1. Describe the pathophysiology of diabetes mellitus, including alterations in metabolic pathways and changes to basement membranes.

2. Describe the therapeutic actions, indications, pharmacokinetics, contraindications, most common adverse reactions, and important drug–drug interactions associated with insulin and other antidiabetic and glucose-elevating agents.

3. Discuss the use of antidiabetic and glucose-elevating agents across the life span.

4. Compare and contrast the prototype drugs insulin, chlorpropamide, glyburide, and metformin with other antidiabetic agents in their class.

5. Outline the nursing considerations, including important teaching points, for patients receiving an antidiabetic or glucose-elevating agent.

■ ASSESSING YOUR UNDERSTANDING

MATCHING

Select the description from column 2 that best describes the term in column 1.

Column 1

___ **1.** Glycosuria

___ **2.** Insulin

___ **3.** Ketosis

___ **4.** Polyphagia

___ **5.** Polydipsia

___ **6.** Adiponectin

___ **7.** Glycogen

___ **8.** Incretins

Column 2

a. Increased thirst

b. Breakdown of fats for energy

c. Glucose in the urine

d. Hormone that increases insulin sensitivity

e. Peptides produced in the gastrointestinal (GI) tract

f. Hormone of the pancreatic beta cells

g. Increased hunger

h. Storage form of glucose

SHORT ANSWER

Supply the information requested.

1. Explain the role of the pancreas as an endocrine and exocrine gland.

2. Describe the action of glucagonlike polypeptide-1.

3. List four disorders that may occur as a result of diabetes.

4. Identify the test that is used to evaluate overall blood glucose level control.

5. Name the condition in which the pancreatic beta cells are no longer functioning.

6. List three manifestations of hyperglycemia.

■ APPLYING YOUR KNOWLEDGE

CASE STUDY

A 12-year-old boy is newly diagnosed with diabetes. The child is to receive insulin twice a day via subcutaneous injection. The patient also is actively involved in soccer and swimming, competing competitively and practicing four to five times a week. The parents and child are concerned about how the diabetes will affect his ability to participate in these activities.

a. How might the nurse address the child and parents' concerns related to sports?

b. What other issues might occur based on the child's developmental stage?

■ PRACTICING FOR NCLEX

Circle the letter that corresponds to the best answer for each question.

1. Which of the following would a nurse identify as an example of a sulfonylurea?
   a. Glyburide
   b. Metformin
   c. Acarbose
   d. Miglitol

2. Which agent would a nurse expect to administer as a single oral dose in the morning?
   a. Repaglinide
   b. Rosiglitazone
   c. Exenatide
   d. Miglitol

3. Which of the following would alert the nurse to suspect that a patient is developing ketoacidosis?
   a. Fluid retention
   b. Blurred vision
   c. Hunger
   d. Fruity breath odor

4. After teaching a group of students about the various insulin preparations, the instructor determines that the teaching was successful when the students identify that which type of insulin cannot be mixed with other types?
   a. Regular
   b. Lente
   c. Detemir
   d. Lispro

Copyright © 2011 by Wolters Kluwer Health | Lippincott Williams & Wilkins. *Study Guide for Focus on Nursing Pharmacology.*

5. A patient receives regular insulin at 8:00 AM. The nurse would be alert for signs and symptoms of hypoglycemia at which time?

   a. Between 10:00 AM and 12:00 PM

   b. Between 8:30 AM and 9:30 AM

   c. Between 2:00 PM and 4:00 PM

   d. Between 12:00 PM and 8:00 PM

6. Which of the following would be least appropriate when administering insulin by subcutaneous injection?

   a. Using a 25 gauge ½ -inch needle

   b. Inserting the needle at a 45-degree angle

   c. Injecting the insulin slowly

   d. Massaging the site after removing the needle

7. A nurse is preparing a syringe that contains regular and NPH insulin. To ensure effectiveness, the nurse would administer the insulins within which time frame?

   a. 10 minutes

   b. 15 minutes

   c. 30 minutes

   d. 60 minutes

8. A patient is receiving glipizide as treatment for his type 2 diabetes. The nurse understands that this drug acts by which of the following?

   a. Binding to potassium channels on pancreatic beta cells

   b. Inhibiting alpha-glucosidase to delay glucose absorption

   c. Increasing the uptake of glucose

   d. Decreasing insulin resistance

9. A patient is taking metformin as part of his treatment for diabetes. The nurse would warn the patient that he may experience signs and symptoms of hypoglycemia within approximately which time frame?

   a. 1 hour

   b. 2 hours

   c. 3 hours

   d. 4 hours

10. A patient newly diagnosed with type 1 diabetes asks the nurse why he cannot just take a pill. The nurse would incorporate knowledge of which of the following when responding to this patient?

    a. Insulin is needed because the beta cells of the pancreas are no longer functioning.

    b. The insulin is more effective in establishing control of blood glucose levels initially.

    c. More insulin is needed than that which the patient can produce naturally.

    d. The patient most likely does not exercise enough to control his glucose levels.

11. When describing the effects of incretins on blood glucose control to a group of students, which of the following would an instructor include?

    a. Increases glucagon release

    b. Increases GI emptying

    c. Increases insulin release

    d. Increases protein building

12. A nurse is preparing an in-service presentation for a group of staff members on diabetes. Which of the following would the nurse include as the primary delivery system for insulin?

    a. Jet injector

    b. Insulin pen

    c. External pump

    d. Subcutaneous injection

13. A man is brought to the emergency department. He is nonresponsive, and his blood glucose level is 32 mg/dL. Which of the following would the nurse expect to be ordered?

    a. Insulin lispro

    b. Glucagon

    c. Diazoxide

    d. Regular insulin

Copyright © 2011 by Wolters Kluwer Health I Lippincott Williams & Wilkins. *Study Guide for Focus on Nursing Pharmacology.*

14. When reviewing sites for insulin administration with a patient, which site, if stated by the patient as an appropriate site, indicates the need for additional teaching?

a. Upper arm

b. Abdomen

c. Buttocks

d. Upper thigh

15. The nurse is instructing a patient how to take his prescribed pramlintide. Which of the following would be most appropriate?

a. "Give it by subcutaneous injection immediately before your major meals."

b. "Take the drug orally once a day, preferably in the morning."

c. "Give yourself an injection 1 hour before you eat breakfast and dinner."

d. "Take the drug orally with the first bite of each meal."

Copyright © 2011 by Wolters Kluwer Health I Lippincott Williams & Wilkins. *Study Guide for Focus on Nursing Pharmacology.*

Introduction to the Reproductive System

LEARNING OBJECTIVES

Upon completion of this chapter, you will be able to:

1. Label a diagram depicting the structures of the female ovaries and male testes as part of the reproductive systems and explain the function of each structure.

2. Outline the control mechanisms involved with the male and female reproductive systems, using this outline to explain the negative feedback systems involved with each system.

3. List five effects for each of these sex hormones: Estrogen, progesterone, and testosterone.

4. Describe the changes that occur to the female body during pregnancy.

5. Describe the phases of the human sexual response and briefly describe the clinical presentation of each stage.

■ ASSESSING YOUR UNDERSTANDING

LABELING

Place the name of the structure at the appropriate location on the illustration below.

    Bladder
    Fallopian tube
    Labia
    Ovary
    Uterus
    Vagina
    Rectum

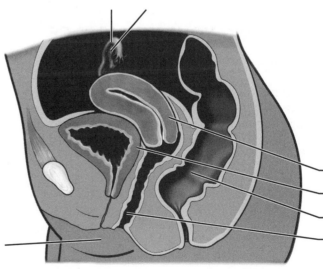

LABELING

Place the name of the structure at the appropriate location on the illustration below.

Corpus cavernosum
Corpus spongiosum
Epididymis
Glans penis
Prostate
Pubic symphysis

Rectum
Scrotum
Seminal vesicle
Testis
Ureter
Urethra
Urinary bladder
Vas deferens

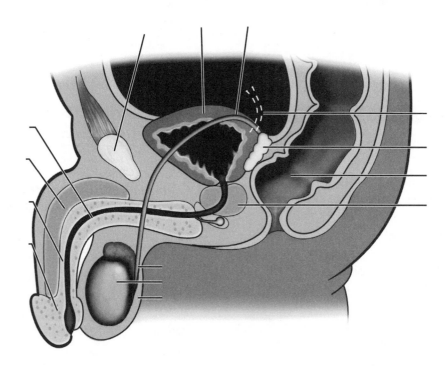

■ APPLYING YOUR KNOWLEDGE

CASE STUDY

A nurse has been invited to teach a health class to a group of freshmen girls at a local high school on the topic of female reproduction. The girls are between the ages of 13 and 14 years.

a. What topics would be most important for the nurse to address?

b. How might the age of the girls in the class influence the nurse's methods for teaching?

Copyright © 2011 by Wolters Kluwer Health I Lippincott Williams & Wilkins. *Study Guide for Focus on Nursing Pharmacology.*

■ PRACTICING FOR NCLEX

Circle the letter that corresponds to the best answer for each question.

1. Which hormone would be initially responsible for hormone secretion from the ovaries and testes?
   a. Follicle-stimulating hormone
   b. Luteinizing hormone
   c. Gonadotropin-releasing hormone
   d. Interstitial cell-stimulating hormone

2. Which of the following statements about the female reproductive system structures is most accurate?
   a. A female produces ova continuously, starting from the time of birth.
   b. An ovum contains one-half of the genetic material to produce a whole cell.
   c. The fallopian tube is a muscular tube connected directly to the ovary.
   d. The uterus is responsible for producing estrogen and progesterone.

3. Which hormone is involved if a couple engages in the rhythm method of birth control?
   a. Estradiol
   b. Estrone
   c. Estriol
   d. Progesterone

4. Which of the following would a nurse attribute to estrogen?
   a. Breast growth
   b. Thickened cervical mucus
   c. Increased body temperature
   d. Increased appetite

5. After teaching a group of students about female reproductive hormones, the instructor determines that the teaching was successful when the students identify which hormone as being primarily responsible for maintaining pregnancy?
   a. Estrogen
   b. Progesterone
   c. Follicle-stimulating hormone
   d. Luteinizing hormone

6. Which hormone is responsible for ovulation?
   a. Estrogen
   b. Progesterone
   c. Follicle-stimulating hormone
   d. Luteinizing hormone

7. If an ovum is fertilized and implants into the uterine wall, which of the following would occur next?
   a. Development of the placenta
   b. Increasing production of estrogen
   c. Production of human chorionic gonadotropin
   d. Formation of corpus albicans

8. Which of the following is associated with an increase in gonadotropin-releasing hormone secretion?
   a. Stress
   b. Starvation
   c. Extreme exercise
   d. Increased light exposure

9. A group of students are reviewing information about the menstrual cycle. The students demonstrate understanding when they identify which of the following as the onset of the menstrual cycle?
   a. Puberty
   b. Menarche
   c. Andropause
   d. Menopause

10. A patient complains of menstrual cramps. The nurse understands that this is due to which of the following?
    a. High levels of plasminogen
    b. Lowered estrogen levels
    c. Prostaglandins
    d. Follicle-stimulating hormone

11. During pregnancy, which of the following becomes a massive endocrine gland?
    a. Umbilical cord
    b. Placenta
    c. Embryo
    d. Uterus

Copyright © 2011 by Wolters Kluwer Health | Lippincott Williams & Wilkins. *Study Guide for Focus on Nursing Pharmacology.*

12. Which structure is responsible for producing sperm?

    a. Seminiferous tubules

    b. Leydig cells

    c. Vas deferens

    d. Prostate gland

13. Which of the following would a nurse attribute to the effect of testosterone? Select all that apply.

    a. Increased high-density lipoprotein levels

    b. Vocal cord thickening

    c. Increased hematocrit

    d. Facial hair growth

    e. Increased skin elasticity

14. When describing the human sexual response cycle, which of the following would a nurse include as occurring first?

    a. Recovery

    b. Climax

    c. Stimulation

    d. Plateau

15. Which of the following occurs during andropause?

    a. Atrophy of the seminiferous tubules

    b. Development of the interstitial cells

    c. Decreased release of follicle-stimulating hormone

    d. Increased inhibin levels

Copyright © 2011 by Wolters Kluwer Health l Lippincott Williams & Wilkins. *Study Guide for Focus on Nursing Pharmacology.*

CHAPTER 40

Drugs Affecting the Female Reproductive System

LEARNING OBJECTIVES

Upon completion of this chapter, you will be able to:

1. Integrate knowledge of the effects of sex hormones on the female body to explain the therapeutic and adverse effects of these agents when used clinically.

2. Describe the therapeutic actions, indications, pharmacokinetics, contraindications, most common adverse reactions, and important drug–drug interactions associated with drugs that affect the female reproductive system.

3. Discuss the use of drugs that affect the female reproductive system across the life span.

4. Compare and contrast the prototype drugs estradiol, raloxifene, norethindrone, clomiphene, oxytocin, and dinoprostone with other agents in their class.

5. Outline the nursing considerations, including important teaching points to stress, for patients receiving drugs that affect the female reproductive system.

■ ASSESSING YOUR UNDERSTANDING

FILL IN THE BLANKS

Provide the missing term in the blanks provided.

1. Female sex hormones include estrogens and

   _____.

2. Drugs such as norethindrone acetate transform the proliferative endometrium

   into a _____ endometrium.

3. The combination of estrogens with

   _____ increases the risk for development of thrombi and emboli.

4. Two estrogen receptor modulators are

   _____ and toremifene.

5. The prototype fertility agent is _____.

6. _____ are a group of drugs that stimulate uterine contraction.

SHORT ANSWER

Supply the information requested.

1. Explain the two major indications for using female sex hormones.

2. Describe the characteristics of a woman who may be a candidate for the use of fertility drugs.

3. Name the drug that may be used to stimulate spermatogenesis in a male.

4. Describe the effect that may occur if a woman with ovarian cysts uses fertility drugs.

5. Identify the uterine motility agent that can be used intranasally to stimulate the letdown reflex in a lactating woman.

■ APPLYING YOUR KNOWLEDGE

CASE STUDY

A 45-year-old woman comes to the clinic for an evaluation. The woman is experiencing menopausal symptoms, complaining of extreme moodiness and hot flashes, especially during the nighttime hours and sleep. She is visibly upset about these changes. "Sometimes my hot flashes are so bad that I find myself having to change my pajamas because they get so wet. And sometimes I just feel like I want to burst into tears for no reason. I just don't know what to do. My friend said to try hormone therapy, but I'm afraid. I've heard so many stories about the side effects."

a. How should the nurse respond to this patient?

b. What information would the nurse and patient need to discuss related to the patient's current complaints and concerns?

■ PRACTICING FOR NCLEX

Circle the letter that corresponds to the best answer for each question.

1. A patient is prescribed estradiol in a vaginal ring form. The nurse would instruct the patient to insert a new vaginal ring at which frequency?
   a. Daily
   b. Weekly
   c. Monthly
   d. Every 3 months

2. When reviewing the history of a patient, which of the following would the nurse identify as a contraindication for the use of progestins?
   a. Migraine headaches
   b. Asthma
   c. Pelvic inflammatory disease
   d. Epilepsy

3. A patient is using an oral contraceptive combination that include drospirenone. The nurse would assess the patient for which of the following?
   a. Irritation
   b. Headache
   c. Abdominal pain
   d. Hyperkalemia

4. After teaching a woman who is receiving estrogen hormonal therapy about substances to avoid, the nurse determines that additional teaching is needed when the patient cites which of the following?
   a. St. John's wort
   b. Orange juice
   c. Smoking
   d. Grapefruit juice

Copyright © 2011 by Wolters Kluwer Health I Lippincott Williams & Wilkins. *Study Guide for Focus on Nursing Pharmacology.*

5. A postmenopausal woman is receiving raloxifene as part of a treatment plan for osteoporosis. The nurse would instruct the patient that this drug is administered by which route?

   a. Oral

   b. Transdermal

   c. Intravaginal

   d. Intramuscular

6. A group of students are reviewing the various fertility drugs that are available. The students demonstrate understanding when they identify which drug as being administered orally?

   a. Cetrorelix

   b. Follitropin alfa

   c. Clomiphene

   d. Ganirelix

7. Which agent would a nurse expect to be ordered for a patient who experiences preterm labor?

   a. Ergonovine

   b. Oxytocin

   c. Dinoprostone

   d. Terbutaline

8. The nurse monitors a patient receiving oxytocin for water intoxication based on the understanding that this condition is the result of which of the following?

   a. Stimulation of the neuroreceptor sites

   b. Release of antidiuretic hormone

   c. Effects secondary to ergotism

   d. Blockage of estrogen receptor sites

9. A patient is beginning therapy with a combined oral contraceptive. The nurse would instruct the patient to take the first pill on which of the following?

   a. First day of menstrual bleeding

   b. Fifth day of the cycle

   c. Fourteenth day of the usual cycle

   d. First day of the next month

10. A patient who is taking oral contraceptives develops an upper respiratory infection for which a tetracycline is ordered. Which instruction would be most important for the nurse to include?

    a. Taking the tetracycline 2 hours after taking the oral contraceptive

    b. Using an alternative means of contraception while taking the tetracycline

    c. Reducing the oral contraceptive to every other day

    d. Monitoring for increased adverse effects of the oral contraceptive

11. A patient is receiving estrogen therapy. Which of the following would the nurse instruct the patient to report immediately?

    a. Abdominal bloating

    b. Weight gain

    c. Dizziness

    d. Shortness of breath

12. Which of the following would a nurse identify as a gonadotropin-releasing hormone antagonist?

    a. Cetrorelix

    b. Chorionic gonadotropin

    c. Follitropin alfa

    d. Menotropins

13. A patient is to receive lutropin alfa. The nurse would expect to administer this agent by which route?

    a. Oral

    b. Subcutaneous

    c. Intramuscular

    d. Intravaginal

14. A patient is to receive dinoprostone at 4:00 PM. The nurse would expect the patient to begin to experience uterine contractions at which time?

    a. 4:10 PM

    b. 4:15 PM

    c. 6:00 PM

    d. 7:00 PM

15. A patient who has come to the emergency department after being raped is given a dose of emergency contraception at 12 AM. The nurse would instruct the patient to take another dose of the drug at which time?

    a. 4 AM

    b. 6 AM

    c. 10 AM

    d. 12 PM

Copyright © 2011 by Wolters Kluwer Health I Lippincott Williams & Wilkins. *Study Guide for Focus on Nursing Pharmacology.*

CHAPTER 41

Drugs Affecting the Male Reproductive System

LEARNING OBJECTIVES

Upon completion of this chapter, you will be able to:

1. Discuss the effects of testosterone and androgens on the male body and use this information to explain the therapeutic and adverse effects of these agents when used clinically.

2. Describe the therapeutic actions, indications, pharmacokinetics, contraindications, most common adverse reactions, and important drug–drug interactions associated with drugs affecting the male reproductive system.

3. Discuss the use of drugs that affect the male reproductive system across the life span.

4. Compare and contrast the prototype drugs testosterone, oxandrolone, and sildenafil with other agents in their class.

5. Outline the nursing considerations, including important teaching points, for patients receiving drugs used to affect the male reproductive system.

■ ASSESSING YOUR UNDERSTANDING

FILL IN THE BLANKS

Provide the missing term in the blanks provided.

1. Male sex hormones, or _____, are produced in the testes and adrenal glands.

2. Underdevelopment of the testes in males is called _____.

3. Testosterone is considered class _____ controlled substances.

4. Patients taking testosterone can experience _____ or increased hair distribution.

5. Anabolic steroids are known to be used illegally for the enhancement of _____ performance.

SHORT ANSWER

Supply the information requested.

1. Explain how anabolic steroids work.

2. Identify the hormones that are considered androgens.

3. List three androgenic effects associated with testosterone administration.

4. Describe the action of alprostadil.

5. Name two dietary factors that could affect the action of PDE5 inhibitors.

■ APPLYING YOUR KNOWLEDGE

CASE STUDY

A 55-year-old man comes to the clinic for a routine physical examination. During the examination, the patient mentions that he has noticed a change in his sexual activity ability. He mentions that it has been taking longer to achieve an erection and that the erection does not last as long. He also mentions that he has had several episodes where an erection did not occur. He states, "It's really embarrassing. I guess this is what it means to get old. Maybe I should try that "viva Viagra" stuff like I've seen on TV."

a. How would the nurse respond to the patient?

b. What information would be important for the nurse to gather about the patient's current condition to determine if the medication would be appropriate for this patient?

■ PRACTICING FOR NCLEX

Circle the letter that corresponds to the best answer for each question.

1. A patient is receiving a medication that has androgenic effects. Which of the following would the nurse expect to assess?
   a. Flushing
   b. Sweating
   c. Oily skin
   d. Nervousness

2. After reviewing the various methods for administering testosterone to patient, the nurse indicates a need for additional review when the nurse identifies which route as appropriate?
   a. Depot injection
   b. Transdermal patch
   c. Intramuscular injection
   d. Oral

3. The nurse is reviewing the history of a patient who is to receive testosterone. Which of the following would alert the nurse to the need for close monitoring of the patient?
   a. Prostate cancer
   b. Breast cancer
   c. Cardiovascular disease
   d. Penile implant

4. A patient has been receiving long-term testosterone therapy. The nurse would expect to monitor which of the following?
   a. Renal function studies
   b. Liver function studies
   c. Complete blood count
   d. Coagulation studies

5. A patient is using a transdermal system for androgen administration. Which drug would the patient most likely be using?
   a. Fluoxymesterone
   b. Danazol
   c. Testosterone
   d. Methyltestosterone

Copyright © 2011 by Wolters Kluwer Health I Lippincott Williams & Wilkins. *Study Guide for Focus on Nursing Pharmacology.*

6. Which of the following would a nurse expect to occur with the administration of anabolic steroids?

   a. Increased catabolism

   b. Decreased hemoglobin

   c. Reduced tissue building

   d. Increased red blood cell mass

7. A 30-year-old debilitated patient is receiving anabolic steroids. Which of the following might the patient experience?

   a. Breast size reduction

   b. Priapism

   c. Testicular enlargement

   d. Excessive hair growth

8. A patient is receiving androgen therapy. Which of the following would cause the nurse the greatest concern?

   a. Decreased thyroid function

   b. Elevated liver enzyme levels

   c. Increased creatinine level

   d. Increased creatinine clearance

9. When teaching a group of high school students about using anabolic steroids, the nurse would include information that these drugs are classified as which class of controlled substances?

   a. I

   b. II

   c. III

   d. IV

10. A group of students are reviewing the drugs available for treating penile erectile dysfunction. The students demonstrate understanding when they identify which drug as a PDE5 inhibitor?

    a. Alprostadil

    b. Sildenafil

    c. Oxandrolone

    d. Danazol

11. Which agent would a patient most likely be prescribed for penile erectile dysfunction if the patient is very sexually active and the timing of sexual stimulation is not known?

    a. Sildenafil

    b. Tadalafil

    c. Vardenafil

    d. Alprostadil

12. Sildenafil may be used in women to treat which of the following?

    a. Pulmonary hypertension

    b. Sexual dysfunction

    c. Coronary artery disease

    d. Peptic ulcer disease

13. A nurse is reviewing the medication history of a patient. The nurse understands that a PDE5 inhibitor would be inappropriate for a patient taking which of the following?

    a. Ketoconazole

    b. Indinavir

    c. Nitroglycerin

    d. Erythromycin

14. A nurse is instructing a patient about vardenafil. The nurse would instruct the patient to take the drug how many minutes before sexual stimulation?

    a. 15 minutes

    b. 30 minutes

    c. 45 minutes

    d. 60 minutes

15. The nurse would instruct a patient who is using a transdermal system for testosterone administration to apply a new patch at which frequency?

    a. Every 12 hours

    b. Every day

    c. Every 3 days

    d. Every 7 days

Copyright © 2011 by Wolters Kluwer Health I Lippincott Williams & Wilkins. *Study Guide for Focus on Nursing Pharmacology.*

CHAPTER 42

Introduction to the Cardiovascular System

Upon completion of this chapter, you will be able to:

1. Label a diagram of the heart, including all chambers, valves, great vessels, coronary vessels, and the conduction system.

2. Describe the flow of blood during the cardiac cycle, including flow to the cardiac muscle.

3. Outline the conduction system of the heart, correlating the normal electrocardiogram pattern with the underlying electrical activity in the heart.

4. Discuss four normal controls of blood pressure.

5. Describe the capillary fluid shift, including factors that influence the movement of fluid in clinical situations.

■ ASSESSING YOUR UNDERSTANDING

LABELING

Place the name of the structures listed below in the appropriate location on the illustration.

Aorta
Inferior vena cava
Left atrium

Left ventricle
Mitral valve
Pulmonary arteries
Pulmonary veins
Pulmonic valve
Right atrium
Right ventricle
Superior vena cava
Triscupid valve

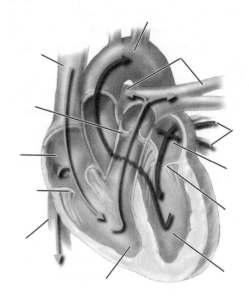

SEQUENCING

Place the number of the statement in the box based on the correct sequence of events for conduction through the heart.

1. Impulse travels via the bundle branches

2. Atrial bundles carry impulses

3. Ventricular cells are stimulated

4. Impulse reaches the atrioventricular (AV) node

5. Purkinje fibers carry the impulse

6. Sinoatrial (SA) node fires

7. Impulse travels via the bundle of His

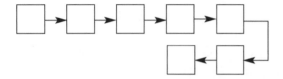

■ APPLYING YOUR KNOWLEDGE

CASE STUDY

It has been several days since a patient with a history of hypertension was admitted to the health care facility with an acute myocardial infarction. The patient has responded well to treatment and will be discharged the next day. The nurse is talking with the patient about his condition, the medications that are being prescribed, and instructions for activity and exercise. "I was taking my blood pressure medicine pretty regularly, but then I forgot to get them refilled. And when I remembered to call, I didn't pick them up right away."

a. How might the patient's history of hypertension have played a role in his myocardial infarction?

b. What would the nurse teach the patient about activity and oxygen consumption?

■ PRACTICING FOR NCLEX

Circle the letter that corresponds to the best answer for each question.

1. When describing Starling's law of the heart, the instructor compares this to which of the following?

    a. Moving up and down on a staircase

    b. Stretching of a rubber band

    c. Pushing and pulling of a rope

    d. Flowing of water through a pipe

2. Which of the following would the nurse explain as the pacemaker of the heart?

    a. SA node

    b. AV node

    c. Bundle of His

    d. Purkinje fibers

3. An instructor is describing the unique characteristic of cells of the conducting system, explaining that these cells can generate action potentials without outside stimulation. The instructor is describing which of the following?

    a. Conductivity

    b. Contractility

    c. Automaticity

    d. Capacitancy

4. Sodium ion concentrations are equal inside and outside the cell during which phase of the action potential of the cardiac muscle?

    a. Phase 0

    b. Phase 1

    c. Phase 2

    d. Phase 3

5. When explaining the contraction of the heart muscle, the instructor describes the basic unit as which of the following?

    a. Actin

    b. Myosin

    c. Troponin

    d. Sarcomere

Copyright © 2011 by Wolters Kluwer Health | Lippincott Williams & Wilkins. *Study Guide for Focus on Nursing Pharmacology.*

6. After explaining an electrocardiogram to a patient, which statement indicates that the patient understands this test?

   a. "It will show the chambers of my heart in different views."

   b. "It will measure the amount of blood being pumped."

   c. "It will show how impulses are moving through my heart."

   d. "It will help to identify how my heart is working mechanically."

7. A nurse is reviewing a patient's electrocardiogram. Which of the following would the nurse identify as indicating depolarization of the bundle of His and ventricles?

   a. P wave

   b. QRS complex

   c. T wave

   d. PR interval

8. The nurse is reviewing a patient's electrocardiogram and notes that the P waves are saw-toothed in shape and there are three P waves for every QRS complex. The nurse would interpret this as suggesting which of the following?

   a. Sinus bradycardia

   b. Paroxysmal atrial tachycardia

   c. Atrial fibrillation

   d. Atrial flutter

9. When describing circulation, which of the following would a nurse include?

   a. Low to high pressure system

   b. One course of blood flow

   c. A closed system

   d. Primarily a resistance system

10. Fluid moves into the arterial end of a capillary due to which of the following?

    a. Hydrostatic pressure

    b. Fluid needs of the cells

    c. Oncotic pressure

    d. Loose endothelial cells

11. Which area of the heart is supplied by the right coronary artery?

    a. Left ventricle

    b. Right side of the heart

    c. Cardiac septum

    d. Conduction system

12. Which of the following is released initially when blood flow to the kidneys is decreased?

    a. Renin

    b. Angiotensin I

    c. Angiotensin II

    d. Aldosterone

13. Blood returning to the heart arrives at the right ventricle by way of which of the following?

    a. Aorta

    b. Pulmonary vein

    c. Vena cava

    d. Triscupid valve

14. Which of the following is responsible for transmitting the nerve impulse to the ventricular cells?

    a. AV node

    b. Bundle of His

    c. Bundle branches

    d. Purkinje fibers

15. At which area is the conduction velocity the slowest?

    a. Bundle of His

    b. AV node

    c. Purkinje fibers

    d. Bundle branches

Copyright © 2011 by Wolters Kluwer Health I Lippincott Williams & Wilkins. *Study Guide for Focus on Nursing Pharmacology.*

Drugs Affecting Blood Pressure

LEARNING OBJECTIVES

Upon completion of this chapter, you will be able to:

1. Outline the normal controls of blood pressure and explain how the various drugs used to treat hypertension or hypotension affect these controls.

2. Describe the therapeutic actions, indications, pharmacokinetics, contraindications, most common adverse reactions, and important drug–drug interactions associated with drugs affecting blood pressure.

3. Discuss the use of drugs that affect blood pressure across the life span.

4. Compare and contrast the prototype drugs captopril, losartan, diltiazem, nitroprusside, mecamylamine, and midodrine with other agents in their class and with other agents used to affect blood pressure.

5. Outline the nursing considerations, including important teaching points, for patients receiving drugs used to affect blood pressure.

■ ASSESSING YOUR UNDERSTANDING

LABELING

Place the name of the following drugs in the correct box for the drug class.

Captopril	Losartan
Diltiazem	Quinapril
Enalaprilat	Valsartan
Felodipine	Verapamil

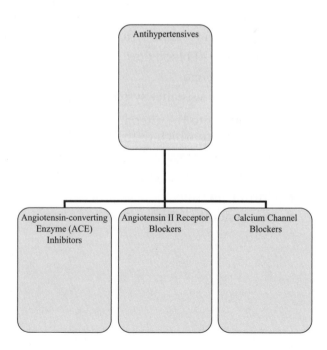

SHORT ANSWER

Supply the information requested.

1. Identify the three elements that determine pressure in the cardiovascular system.

2. Name the two areas where baroreceptors are located.

3. Describe two dangers associated with hypertension.

4. List four factors that are known to increase blood pressure.

5. Explain the focus of treatment for hypertension.

6. Identify the drugs of choice for treating stage 1 hypertension in a patient who does not have any complicating conditions.

7. Describe the lifestyle modifications that are indicated as part of step 1 treatment for hypertension.

■ APPLYING YOUR KNOWLEDGE

CASE STUDY

A 58-year-old man has been diagnosed with hypertension and has been receiving carvedilol. The patient also has a history of left ventricular hypertrophy. The patient's blood pressure on the last few visits has remained somewhat elevated. The physician has decided to add quinapril to the patient's regimen. The nurse is talking with the patient about his drug therapy when the patient states, "It always seems that my pressure is much higher when I come here. I started checking my blood pressure at the local drug store, and it is usually lower than the readings here."

a. How might the nurse interpret the patient's statement? What would the nurse need to consider when responding to the patient?

b. What would the nurse need to address when teaching the patient about the new drug?

■ PRACTICING FOR NCLEX

Circle the letter that corresponds to the best answer for each question.

1. When describing the pressures in the cardiovascular system, the nurse would identify which of the following as the area of highest pressure?
   a. Right atrium
   b. Right ventricle
   c. Left atrium
   d. Left ventricle

2. Which of the following would be considered the most important factor in determining peripheral resistance?
   a. Arterioles
   b. Capillaries
   c. Arteries
   d. Veins

3. Which of the following functions continually maintain blood pressure within a predetermined range of normal?
   a. Cardiovascular center
   b. Medulla
   c. Baroreceptors
   d. Carotid arteries

Copyright © 2011 by Wolters Kluwer Health | Lippincott Williams & Wilkins. *Study Guide for Focus on Nursing Pharmacology.*

4. A patient develops a severe elevation in blood pressure. The physician orders an ACE inhibitor to be given intravenously. Which agent would be most likely?

   a. Captopril
   b. Enalapril
   c. Lisinopril
   d. Enalaprilat

5. A patient receiving an ACE inhibitor reports a problem with coughing. The nurse would ask the patient if he is receiving which of the following?

   a. Ramipril
   b. Benazepril
   c. Lisinopril
   d. Quinapril

6. A patient is receiving captopril. Which of the following would be most important for the nurse to monitor?

   a. Electrocardiogram
   b. Nutritional status
   c. Complete blood count
   d. Liver function studies

7. A group of students are reviewing the various antihypertensive agents. The students demonstrate understanding of the information when they identify which of the following as an example of an angiotensin II receptor blocker?

   a. Moexipril
   b. Losartan
   c. Minoxidil
   d. Amlodipine

8. When describing the action of calcium channel blockers, which of the following would be an expected effect?

   a. Increased contractility
   b. Arterial contraction
   c. Increased venous return
   d. Slowed impulse formation

9. The nurse is teaching a patient how to take his diltiazem. Which instruction would be most appropriate?

   a. "Cut the tablet in half to make it easier to swallow."

   b. "Mix the crushed tablet with applesauce to improve the taste."
   c. "Swallow the drug whole with a large glass of water."
   d. "Chew the tablet thoroughly before swallowing."

10. A patient who has been receiving verapamil for several months comes to the clinic reporting significant dizziness, lightheadedness, and fatigue. He also reports frequent episodes of nausea and swelling of his ankles. Drug toxicity is suspected. Which question would be critical to ask the patient?

    a. "Are you taking any over-the-counter pain relievers like ibuprofen?"
    b. "Have you been drinking any grapefruit juice lately?"
    c. "Are your splitting or crushing your pills?"
    d. "When did you take the last dose of the drug?"

11. A patient is receiving nitroprusside. The nurse suspects that the patient is experiencing cyanide toxicity based on assessment of which of the following?

    a. Increased hair growth
    b. Absent reflexes
    c. Pupil constriction
    d. Chest pain

12. Which of the following agents would be used to treat hypertension by blocking the postsynaptic alpha-1 receptor sites?

    a. Prazosin
    b. Labetalol
    c. Guanabenz
    d. Nadolol

13. A patient is experiencing orthostatic hypotension that is affecting his ability to function. Which of the following would be most appropriate?

    a. Dopamine
    b. Methyldopa
    c. Midodrine
    d. Clonidine

14. A patient is receiving a diuretic as the first-line treatment of mild hypertension. The nurse monitors the patient for signs and symptoms of hypokalemia with which agent?

    a. Amiloride

    b. Spironolactone

    c. Triamterene

    d. Hydrochlorothiazide

15. A group of students are reviewing the various antihypertensive agents available. The students demonstrate understanding of the information when they identify which agent as an example of a renin inhibitor?

    a. Mecamylamine

    b. Aliskiren

    c. Candesartan

    d. Captopril

44

Cardiotonic Agents

LEARNING OBJECTIVES

Upon completion of this chapter, you will be able to:

1. Describe the pathophysiologic process of heart failure and the resultant clinical signs.

2. Explain the body's compensatory mechanisms that occur in response to heart failure.

3. Describe the therapeutic actions, indications, pharmacokinetics, contraindications and cautions, most common adverse reactions, and important drug–drug interactions associated with the cardiotonic agents.

4. Discuss the use of cardiotonic agents across the life span.

5. Compare and contrast the prototype drugs digoxin and inamrinone as well as digoxin immune Fab.

6. Outline the nursing considerations, including important teaching points, for patients receiving cardiotonic agents.

■ ASSESSING YOUR UNDERSTANDING

MATCHING

Select the description from column 2 that best describes the term in column 1.

Column 1

___ 1. Cardiomegaly

___ 2. Heart failure

___ 3. Dyspnea

___ 4. Cardiomyopathy

___ 5. Hemoptysis

___ 6. Nocturia

___ 7. Orthopnea

___ 8. Positive inotropic

Column 2

a. Getting up to void at night

b. Effect resulting in an increased contraction force

c. Enlargement of the heart

d. Discomfort with respirations

e. Disease of the heart muscle

f. Inability of the heart to pump adequately

g. Blood-tinged sputum

h. Difficulty breathing when lying down

FILL IN THE BLANKS

Provide the missing term or terms in the blanks provided.

1. _____ redrugs are used to increase the contractility of the heart muscle in patients experiencing heart failure.

2. Severe heart failure causing the left ventricle to pump inefficiently can lead to

   _____ _____ manifested by rales and wheezes.

3. In heart failure, the heart rate

   will be _____ secondary to sympathetic stimulation.

4. In left-sided heart failure, rales indicate the presence of _____ in the lung tissue.

5. In right-sided heart failure, venous return to the heart is _____ because the pressure on the right side of the heart is increased.

6. Increased _____ venous pressure is manifested by distended neck veins.

7. With right-sided heart failure, increased blood flow to the kidneys can lead to increased urination and _____.

8. Cardiotonic drugs are also called _____ drugs.

■ APPLYING YOUR KNOWLEDGE

CASE STUDY

A patient has a history of atrial fibrillation for which he takes amiodarone and hypertension for which he takes a thiazide diuretic. The patient comes to the office for a checkup. During the visit, the nurse notes that the patient has slight pitting edema of both lower extremities and jugular vein distention. The patient is tachypneic. Auscultation reveals rales and a third heart sound. The patient states, "Over the last week, I've noticed that I've had to sleep with two pillows instead of one. And I've been getting up at night to urinate." The physician decides to order digoxin 0.125 mg daily for the patient.

a. Based on the patient's assessment findings, what type of heart failure would this patient be experiencing?

b. What information would be crucial for the nurse to cover when teaching the patient about the newly prescribed drug?

■ PRACTICING FOR NCLEX

Circle the letter that corresponds to the best answer for each question.

1. A nurse suspects that a patient is experiencing left-sided heart failure. Which of the following would the nurse assess? Select all that apply.
   a. Tachypnea
   b. Hemoptysis
   c. Peripheral edema
   d. Hepatomegaly
   e. Orthopnea
   f. Polyuria

2. When describing how vasodilators help alleviate heart failure, which of the following would the nurse include?
   a. Increase cardiac workload
   b. Decrease afterload
   c. Increase preload
   d. Decrease blood volume

3. Which of the following would be considered a therapeutic effect of digoxin?
   a. Decreased cardiac output
   b. Increased heart rate
   c. Increased force of contraction
   d. Decreased renal perfusion

4. Which serum digoxin level would the nurse interpret as indicating digoxin toxicity?
   a. 0.6 ng/mL
   b. 1.4 ng/mL
   c. 1.8 ng/mL
   d. 2.3 ng/mL

5. A nurse is administering digoxin intravenously as ordered. The nurse would administer the drug over which time frame?
   a. 2 minutes
   b. 3 minutes
   c. 4 minutes
   d. 5 minutes

Copyright © 2011 by Wolters Kluwer Health I Lippincott Williams & Wilkins. *Study Guide for Focus on Nursing Pharmacology.*

6. A patient who is prescribed digoxin asks the nurse how he should take the drug. Which instruction would be most appropriate?

   a. "Take the medicine with an antacid at any time of the day."

   b. "Take the drug after eating your breakfast."

   c. "Eat a small snack just before taking the drug."

   d. "Take the drug on an empty stomach at the same time each day."

7. A patient takes his pulse rate before taking his regular daily dose of digoxin and finds his pulse to be 52 beats/min. Which of the following would the patient do next?

   a. Take the drug as ordered and note the pulse rate in a log

   b. Hold the dose and retake the pulse in 1 hour

   c. Withhold the drug and call the doctor immediately

   d. Go the nearest emergency care facility for evaluation

8. A nurse is preparing to administer inamrinone. The nurse would administer this drug most likely by which route?

   a. Oral

   b. Subcutaneous

   c. Intramuscular

   d. Intravenous

9. A patient is receiving inamrinone. Which of the following would be most important for the nurse to monitor?

   a. Pulmonary function studies

   b. Platelet count

   c. White blood cell count

   d. Renal function studies

10. A patient received an intravenous bolus of inamrinone. The nurse would anticipate repeating the dose at which time if needed?

    a. 10 minutes

    b. 20 minutes

    c. 30 minutes

    d. 40 minutes

11. After teaching a class of students about heart failure and drug therapy, the instructor determines that the teaching has been successful when the students identify which drug as most often used as treatment?

    a. Digoxin

    b. Human B-type natriuretic peptide

    c. Nitrate

    d. Furosemide

12. Which of the following conditions would least likely contribute to the development of heart failure?

    a. Coronary artery disease

    b. Renal failure

    c. Valvular disease

    d. Hypertension

13. A patient who is taking digoxin would withhold the drug if his pulse rate were which of the following?

    a. 78 beats/minute

    b. 70 beats/minute

    c. 64 beats/minute

    d. 56 beats/minute

14. Which of the following would the nurse identify as a cardiac glycoside?

    a. Inamrinone

    b. Milrinone

    c. Digoxin

    d. Captopril

15. Which of the following would a nurse expect to assess if a patient is experiencing right-sided heart failure?

    a. Wheezing

    b. Peripheral edema

    c. Hemoptysis

    d. Dyspnea

Copyright © 2011 by Wolters Kluwer Health | Lippincott Williams & Wilkins. *Study Guide for Focus on Nursing Pharmacology.*

CHAPTER 45

Antiarrhythmic Agents

LEARNING OBJECTIVES

Upon completion of this chapter, you will be able to:

1. Describe the cardiac action potential and its phases to explain the changes made by each class of antiarrhythmic agent.

2. Describe the therapeutic actions, indications, pharmacokinetics, contraindications and cautions, most common adverse reactions, and important drug–drug interactions associated with antiarrhythmic agents.

3. Discuss the use of antiarrhythmic agents across the life span.

4. Compare and contrast the prototype antiarrhythmic drugs lidocaine, propranolol, sotalol, and diltiazem with other agents in their class and with other classes of antiarrhythmics.

5. Outline the nursing considerations, including important teaching points, for patients receiving antiarrhythmic agents.

■ ASSESSING YOUR UNDERSTANDING

LABELING

Place the name of the drugs listed below in the proper column identifying the antiarrhythmic class.

Acebutolol

Amiodarone

Diltiazem

Disopyramide

Flecainide

Lidocaine

Mexiletine

Propafenone

Propranolol

Quinidine

Sotalol

Verapamil

Class I	Class II	Class III	Class IV

SEQUENCING

Each of the following statements describes an event in the phases of the action potential of the cardiac muscle cell. Place the number of the statement in the box based on the order in which the events occur.

1. Cell comes to rest; restoration of the resting membrane potential

2. Cells becomes stimulated and sodium gates open, allowing sodium to rush into the cell

3. Rapid repolarization occurs with sodium gates closing and potassium flowing out of the cell

4. Sodium ion concentration equalizes inside and outside the cell

5. Plateau stage with the cell membrane becoming less permeable to sodium and calcium slowly entering and potassium beginning to leave the cell

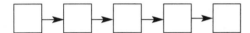

■ APPLYING YOUR KNOWLEDGE

CASE STUDY

A patient goes to see his primary care provider because he has been "feeling strange" lately. He is complaining of fatigue and lack of energy for about the past 2 weeks. "It seems like all I do is sleep. At first, I thought I had the flu or had just overdone things. But I should be rested with all the sleep I've had." Examination reveals an irregular pulse. An electrocardiogram reveals atrial fibrillation. The patient is sent to the emergency department of the local hospital for admission. Intravenous heparin is started, and sotalol is ordered. After 3 days, the sotalol is discontinued due to lack of effectiveness, and the patient is started on amiodarone. Warfarin therapy and heparin are discontinued once the patient has achieved the desired level of anticoagulation. The patient remains in atrial fibrillation and is discharged home on amiodarone and warfarin.

a. What would be the most likely reason for the use of warfarin and heparin for this patient?

b. What monitoring would be essential for this patient?

■ PRACTICING FOR NCLEX

Circle the letter that corresponds to the best answer for each question.

1. When describing the action of antiarrhythmics, which effect would most likely be included?
   a. Reduction of peripheral resistance
   b. Enhancement of automaticity
   c. Alteration in conductivity
   d. Reduction in cardiac output

2. Which arrhythmia would the nurse identify as being related to an alteration in conduction through the heart muscle?
   a. Premature atrial contraction
   b. Atrial flutter
   c. Ventricular fibrillation
   d. Heart block

3. Which of the following agents would be classified as a class Ia antiarrhythmic?
   a. Lidocaine
   b. Procainamide
   c. Mexiletine
   d. Flecainide

4. Which phase of the cardiac muscle action potential is affected by class I antiarrhythmics?
   a. Phase 0
   b. Phase 1
   c. Phase 2
   d. Phase 3

5. A patient is prescribed disopyramide. The nurse would expect to administer this drug by which route?
   a. Oral
   b. Intramuscular
   c. Subcutaneous
   d. Intravenous

Copyright © 2011 by Wolters Kluwer Health I Lippincott Williams & Wilkins. *Study Guide for Focus on Nursing Pharmacology.*

6. The health care provider orders quinidine for a patient who is receiving digoxin. The nurse would monitor this patient for which of the following?
   a. Increased quinidine effect
   b. Digoxin toxicity
   c. Bleeding
   d. Renal dysfunction

7. The nurse is teaching a patient who is receiving quinidine about foods to avoid. The patient demonstrates the need for additional teaching when he identifies the need to avoid which of the following?
   a. Citrus juices
   b. Antacids
   c. Milk
   d. Apple juice

8. A patient receives lidocaine by intramuscular injection. The nurse would expect the drug to begin to exert its therapeutic effects within which time frame?
   a. 5 to 10 minutes
   b. 10 to 20 minutes
   c. 20 to 30 minutes
   d. 30 to 40 minutes

9. When describing the action of class II antiarrhythmics, which of the following would the nurse include?
   a. Membrane stabilization with depression of phase 0 action potential
   b. Blockage of beta receptors in the heart and kidneys
   c. Blockage of potassium channels during phase 3 action potential
   d. Interference with calcium ion movement across the membrane

10. A patient is to receive esmolol. The nurse would expect to administer this agent by which route?
    a. Oral
    b. Intramuscular
    c. Intravenous
    d. Subcutaneous

11. Which of the following would be a contraindication for the use of a class II antiarrhythmic?
    a. Sinus bradycardia
    b. Diabetes
    c. Thyroid dysfunction
    d. Hepatic dysfunction

12. The nurse would instruct a patient receiving acebutolol about which of the following adverse effects?
    a. Hypertension
    b. Increased libido
    c. Improved exercise tolerance
    d. Bronchospasm

13. When describing the action of dofetilide, the nurse understands that the drug affects which phase of the action potential?
    a. Phase 0
    b. Phase 1
    c. Phase 2
    d. Phase 3

14. A patient is prescribed sotalol. Which instruction would be most important?
    a. "Sit up for at least 30 minutes after taking the drug."
    b. "Be sure to take the drug on an empty stomach."
    c. "Try using an antacid along with this drug."
    d. "Hold the drug if your pulse rate is less than 60 beats per minute."

15. A patient is receiving adenosine for treatment of supraventricular tachycardia. The nurse understands that this drug results in which of the following?
    a. Increased conduction through the atrioventricular node
    b. Prolonged refractory period
    c. Increased automaticity in the atrioventricular node
    d. Slowed release of calcium leaving the cell

Copyright © 2011 by Wolters Kluwer Health I Lippincott Williams & Wilkins. *Study Guide for Focus on Nursing Pharmacology.*

CHAPTER 46

Antianginal Agents

LEARNING OBJECTIVES

Upon completion of this chapter, you will be able to:

1. Describe coronary artery disease, including identified risk factors and clinical presentation.

2. Describe the therapeutic actions, indications, pharmacokinetics, contraindications and cautions, most common adverse reactions, and important drug–drug interactions associated with the nitrates, beta-blockers, and calcium channel blockers used to treat angina.

3. Discuss the use of antianginal agents across the life span.

4. Compare and contrast the prototype drugs nitroglycerin, metoprolol, and diltiazem with other agents used to treat angina.

5. Outline the nursing considerations, including important teaching points, for patients receiving drugs used to treat angina.

■ ASSESSING YOUR UNDERSTANDING

MATCHING

Select the description from column 2 that best describes the term in column 1.

Column 1

____ **1.** Atheroma

____ **2.** Atherosclerosis

____ **3.** Angina pectoris

____ **4.** Prinzmetal's angina

____ **5.** Myocardial infarction

____ **6.** Stable angina

____ **7.** Coronary artery disease

____ **8.** Unstable angina

Column 2

a. Episode of myocardial ischemia with pain due to an imbalance of myocardial oxygen supply and demand when a person is at rest

b. Drop in blood flow through coronary arteries due to vasospasm

c. Disorder involving progressive narrowing of arteries supplying the myocardium

d. Suffocation of the chest

e. Narrowing of the arteries resulting in a loss of elasticity

f. Pain due to imbalance of myocardial oxygen supply and demand that is relieved by rest

g. Plaque in the endothelial lining of the arteries

h. End result of vessel blockage leading to ischemia and then necrosis

SHORT ANSWER

Supply the information requested.

1. Identify the leading cause of death in the Western world.

2. Explain the difference in how the heart muscle receives its blood supply when compared with other tissues.

3. Describe what happens when a person with atherosclerosis experiences an increased demand on the heart.

4. List two ways that antianginal agents work to improve blood delivery to the heart.

5. Describe the action of nitrates.

■ APPLYING YOUR KNOWLEDGE

CASE STUDY

A patient comes to the clinic for an evaluation. The patient has a history of stable angina for which he has used nitroglycerin sublingually. The patient tells the nurse that he has not had any complaints of chest pain for the past 6 months or so. As the nurse is reviewing the patient's medications, the patient removes a small plastic bag from his back pants pocket that contains his nitroglycerin. He says, "See, I still have all the pills. I haven't used any for quite a while."

a. What problem would the nurse need to address with the patient?

b. What actions by the nurse would be appropriate?

■ PRACTICING FOR NCLEX

Circle the letter that corresponds to the best answer for each question.

1. When describing angina to a group of patients, which of the following would be most accurate?

   a. Pain due to lack of oxygen in the heart muscle

   b. Chest pain that occurs with exercise

   c. Damage to the heart muscle

   d. Spasm of the blood vessels

2. A patient experiences pain in the chest that radiates to the jaw, occurring when the patient is at rest. The nurse would interpret this as which of the following?

   a. Stable angina

   b. Unstable angina

   c. Prinzmetal's angina

   d. Myocardial infarction

3. When describing the effects of a myocardial infarction, the nurse understands that the majority of deaths related to this condition result from which of the following?

   a. Shock

   b. Arrhythmias

   c. Heart failure

   d. Stroke

4. Which of the following would a nurse identify as a nitrate?

   a. Metoprolol

   b. Amlodipine

   c. Nicardipine

   d. Isosorbide

5. A group of students are reviewing information about isosorbide dinitrate. The students demonstrate the need for additional study when they identify that this drug is available in which form?

   a. Oral

   b. Sublingual

   c. Intravenous

   d. Chewable tablet

Copyright © 2011 by Wolters Kluwer Health I Lippincott Williams & Wilkins. *Study Guide for Focus on Nursing Pharmacology.*

6. Which of the following would contraindicate the use of nitrates?
   a. Cardiac tamponade
   b. Hypotension
   c. Cerebral hemorrhage
   d. Hepatic disease

7. A patient is using nitroglycerin in sublingual spray form. The nurse would inform the patient that the drug would begin working within which time frame?
   a. 1 minute
   b. 2 minutes
   c. 3 minutes
   d. 4 minutes

8. Which of the following indicates that a patient understands how to use sublingual nitroglycerin?
   a. "I should feel a fizzing or burning sensation."
   b. "I should put the pill between my tongue and cheek."
   c. "I need to avoid taking any sips of water before using the drug."
   d. "I can chew the tablet once it starts dissolving."

9. The nurse instructs the patient that he can repeat the dose of nitroglycerin every 5 minutes up to a maximum total of how many doses?
   a. Two
   b. Three
   c. Four
   d. Five

10. Which of the following drugs should be avoided by a patient taking nitrates?
    a. Phosphodiesterase 5 inhibitors
    b. Beta-blockers
    c. Nonsteroidal anti-inflammatory drugs
    d. Cardiac glycosides

11. After teaching a group of students about drugs used as antianginal agents, the instructor determines that the teaching was successful when the students identify which of the following as a beta-blocker antianginal agent?
    a. Amlodipine
    b. Nadolol
    c. Verapamil
    d. Ranolazine

12. A patient has had a myocardial infarction and is to receive propranolol. The nurse understands that this drug is being used to achieve which of the following?
    a. Reduce the risk for recurrent anginal attacks
    b. Control the risk for vasospasm
    c. Prevent reinfarction
    d. Prevent the development of hypertension

13. Which of the following agents would be most appropriate for a patient with Prinzmetal's angina?
    a. Nitroglycerin
    b. Metoprolol
    c. Nadolol
    d. Amlodipine

14. When describing the action of ranolazine, which of the following would be most appropriate?
    a. Shortens the QT interval
    b. Decreases myocardial workload
    c. Decreases heart rate
    d. Decreases blood pressure

15. A patient is using transdermal nitroglycerin. The nurse would instruct the patient to apply a new patch at which frequency?
    a. Each time he has chest pain
    b. Before activities that may cause chest pain
    c. Every day
    d. Every week

Copyright © 2011 by Wolters Kluwer Health l Lippincott Williams & Wilkins. *Study Guide for Focus on Nursing Pharmacology.*

CHAPTER 47

Lipid-Lowering Agents

LEARNING OBJECTIVES

Upon completion of this chapter, you will be able to:

1. Outline the mechanisms of fat metabolism in the body and discuss the role of hyperlipidemia as a risk factor for coronary artery disease.

2. Describe the therapeutic actions, indications, pharmacokinetics, contraindications and cautions, most common adverse reactions, and important drug–drug interactions associated with the bile acid sequestrants, HMG-CoA inhibitors, cholesterol absorption inhibitors, and other agents used to lower lipid levels.

3. Discuss the use of drugs that lower lipid levels across the life span.

4. Compare and contrast the various drugs used to lower lipid levels.

5. Outline the nursing considerations, including important teaching points, for patients receiving drugs used to lower lipid levels.

■ ASSESSING YOUR UNDERSTANDING

LABELING

Place the name of the following drugs in the appropriate box under the correct drug class.

Cholestyramine   Simvastatin

Colestipol   Ezetimibe

Fluvastatin

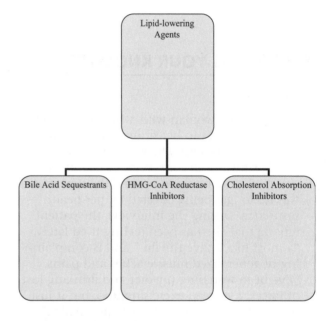

SHORT ANSWER

Supply the information requested.

1. List the six characteristics associated with metabolic syndrome.

2. Name the three nonmodifiable risk factors for coronary artery disease.

3. Explain how gout is a risk factor for coronary artery disease.

4. Describe the variations in lipoprotein levels of black Americans as compared with white Americans.

5. Identify three ways to modify risk factors for coronary artery disease.

6. Name the substance that carries micelles for absorption.

■ APPLYING YOUR KNOWLEDGE

CASE STUDY

A 55-year-old woman with a history of hyper-lipidemia comes to her primary care provider's office for a checkup. The woman had been taking simvastatin for several years but was switched to atorvastatin because the simvastatin was no longer being covered by her health insurance. During the interview, the patient reports that she has been feeling tired lately, "almost like I have the flu," and is complaining of generalized muscle aches and pains. "I've been watching my diet and drinking lost of juices. I've been exercising, too, but it just seems like my muscles are getting smaller."

a. What information would be important for the nurse to obtain about the patient's diet?

b. What might the patient be experiencing, and what testing would be indicated for the patient based on her complaints?

■ PRACTICING FOR NCLEX

Circle the letter that corresponds to the best answer for each question.

1. An instructor is describing the characteristics associated with metabolic syndrome. Which of the following would the instructor include in the description? Select all that apply.
   a. Fasting blood glucose less than 110 mg/dL
   b. Waist measurement over 40 inches in men
   c. Triglyceride levels greater than 150 mg/dL
   d. Blood pressure less than 130/85 mm Hg
   e. Decreased levels of plasminogen activator

2. The nurse is reviewing the results of a patient's lipid profile. Which of the following would the nurse identify as borderline high?
   a. Total cholesterol 160 mg/dL
   b. Low-density lipoprotein (LDL) cholesterol 110 mg/dL
   c. High-density lipoprotein (HDL) cholesterol 45 mg/dL
   d. Triglycerides 180 mg/dL

3. Which substance would a group of students identify as being responsible for breaking up dietary fasts into smaller units?
   a. Bile acids
   b. Cholesterol
   c. Chylomicrons
   d. Micelles

4. After reviewing information about lipo-proteins, a group of students demonstrate understanding of the information when they identify which of the following as being loosely packed?
   a. LDLs
   b. HDLs
   c. Triglycerides
   d. Lipids

5. Which of the following would be classified as a bile acid sequestrant?
   a. Lovastatin
   b. Ezetimibe
   c. Cholestyramine
   d. Gemfibrozil

Copyright © 2011 by Wolters Kluwer Health I Lippincott Williams & Wilkins. *Study Guide for Focus on Nursing Pharmacology.*

6. A patient who is receiving colestipol is also taking a thiazide diuretic. Which instruction would be most appropriate for the nurse to give?

   a. "Take the colestipol at the same time as the thiazide diuretic."

   b. "Take the thiazide diuretic about 4 hours before the colestipol."

   c. "Take the colestipol first and then take the diuretic a half hour later."

   d. "Take the thiazide diuretic about 1 hour before the colestipol."

7. A nurse would caution a patient receiving cholestyramine to avoid mixing the drug with which of the following?

   a. Soups

   b. Carbonated beverages

   c. Fruit juices

   d. Cereals

8. The nurse instructs a patient to take the prescribed pravastatin at bedtime based on the understanding about which of the following?

   a. Adverse effects are less likely during the night.

   b. Compliance is enhanced with nighttime administration.

   c. Greater drug effectiveness is achieved at this time.

   d. Lack of dietary intake during sleep increases absorption.

9. Which of the following best reflects the action of ezetimibe?

   a. Blocks the enzyme involved in cholesterol synthesis

   b. Binds with bile acids to form an insoluble complex for excretion

   c. Stimulates the breakdown of lipoproteins from tissues

   d. Decreases the absorption of dietary cholesterol from the small intestine

10. A patient with atrial fibrillation who is receiving oral anticoagulant therapy is receiving atorvastatin. The nurse would monitor this patient for which of the following?

    a. Abdominal pain

    b. Cataract development

    c. Liver failure

    d. Bleeding

11. A patient is being prescribed fluvastatin. The nurse reviews the patient's medical record to ensure that the patient has attempted lifestyle changes for at least a minimum of which amount of time?

    a. 2 weeks

    b. 4 weeks

    c. 8 weeks

    d. 12 weeks

12. A patient is receiving niacin as part of therapy for hyperlipoproteinemia. The nurse would explain that the lipid levels will usually begin to drop in approximately which amount of time?

    a. 3 to 5 days

    b. 5 to 7 days

    c. 7 to 10 days

    d. 10 to 14 days

13. Which agent would the nurse identify as inhibiting the release of free fatty acids from adipose tissue?

    a. Niacin

    b. Fenofibrate

    c. Gemfibrozil

    d. Fenofibric acid

14. A patient who is receiving a bile acid sequestrant is being prescribed an additional agent to lower lipid levels. Which agent would the nurse most likely expect the provider to order?

    a. Statin

    b. Fibrate

    c. Bile acid sequestrant

    d. Cholesterol absorption inhibitor

15. After teaching a group of students about fats and biotransformation, the instructor determines that the teaching was successful when the students identify which of the following as the storage location of bile acids?

    a. Liver

    b. Gallbladder

    c. Small intestine

    d. Stomach

Copyright © 2011 by Wolters Kluwer Health l Lippincott Williams & Wilkins. *Study Guide for Focus on Nursing Pharmacology.*

CHAPTER 48

Drugs Affecting Blood Coagulation

LEARNING OBJECTIVES

Upon completion of this chapter, you will be able to:

1. Outline the mechanisms by which blood clots dissolve in the body, correlating this information with the actions of drugs used to affect blood clotting.

2. Describe the therapeutic actions, indications, pharmacokinetics, contraindications, most common adverse reactions, and important drug–drug interactions associated with drugs affecting blood coagulation.

3. Discuss the use of drugs that affect blood coagulation across the life span.

4. Compare and contrast the prototype drugs aspirin, heparin, urokinase, antihemophilic factor, and aminocaproic acid with other agents used to affect blood coagulation.

5. Outline the nursing considerations, including important teaching points, for patients receiving drugs used to affect blood coagulation.

■ ASSESSING YOUR UNDERSTANDING

MATCHING

Select the description in column 2 that best describes the term in column 1.

Column 1

____ **1.** Plasminogen

____ **2.** Clotting factors

____ **3.** Hageman factor

____ **4.** Platelet aggregation

____ **5.** Thrombolytic agents

____ **6.** Anticoagulants

____ **7.** Hemostatic agents

____ **8.** Extrinsic pathway

____ **9.** Intrinsic pathway

____ **10.** Coagulation

Column 2

a. Drugs that stop blood loss

b. Clumping together to plug an injury to the vascular system

c. Clotting factors leading to clot formation within an injured vessel

d. Drugs that prevent or slow clot formation

e. Natural clot-dissolving substance

f. First substance activated with blood vessel or cell injury

g. Clotting factors forming a clot on the outside of the injured vessel

h. Substances formed in the liver, many of which require vitamin K

i. Drugs that lyse a formed clot

j. Blood changing from a fluid state to a solid state to plug vascular system injuries

LABELING

Place the name of the following drugs in the appropriate box under the correct drug class.

Abciximab   Heparin

Alteplase   Streptokinase

Clopidogrel   Ticlopidine

Desirudin   Warfarin

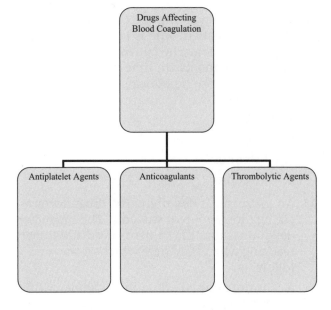

■ APPLYING YOUR KNOWLEDGE

CASE STUDY

A patient is brought to the emergency department with complaints of severe, sharp chest pain that is accompanied by diaphoresis, hemoptysis, and tachycardia. The patient has a history of deep vein thrombosis. Further assessment reveals a pulmonary embolism. The patient receives alteplase, which is followed by anticoagulant therapy with a heparin infusion. The patient improves and is started on warfarin while continuing to

receive the heparin infusion. The heparin infusion is discontinued, and the patient is being discharged on warfarin therapy.

a. What was the rationale for using alteplase?

b. Why was the patient receiving heparin and warfarin at the same time?

c. What instructions are important to include in the discharge teaching plan for this patient?

■ PRACTICING FOR NCLEX

Circle the letter that corresponds to the best answer for each question.

1. Which of the following would be considered a topical hemostatic agent?

   a. Thrombin

   b. Protamine sulfate

   c. Pentoxifylline

   d. Urokinase

2. When describing the clotting process, which step would the nurse identify as the first reaction to occur with injury to a blood vessel?

   a. Platelet aggregation

   b. Vasoconstriction

   c. Release of factor XI

   d. Thrombin formation

3. A patient is to receive clopidogrel. The nurse would expect to administer this agent by which route?

   a. Oral

   b. Intravenous

   c. Intramuscular

   d. Subcutaneous

Copyright © 2011 by Wolters Kluwer Health l Lippincott Williams & Wilkins. *Study Guide for Focus on Nursing Pharmacology.*

4. The nurse would monitor the platelet levels closely for a patient receiving which of the following?

   a. Aspirin

   b. Abciximab

   c. Anagrelide

   d. Dipyridamole

5. A patient is receiving warfarin. The nurse would expect to administer this drug by which route?

   a. Oral

   b. Subcutaneous

   c. Intravenous

   d. Intramuscular

6. A patient is receiving heparin. Which of the following would the nurse use to monitor the effects of the drug?

   a. Partial thromboplastin time

   b. International normalized ratio

   c. Prothrombin time

   d. Vitamin K level

7. Which of the following would a nurse identify as inhibiting factor Xa?

   a. Heparin

   b. Warfarin

   c. Argatroban

   d. Fondaparinux

8. A patient exhibits signs and symptoms of heparin overdose. The nurse would anticipate administering which of the following?

   a. Vitamin K

   b. Protamine sulfate

   c. Urokinase

   d. Drotrecogin alfa

9. After reviewing the drugs that may interfere with warfarin, the students indicate that they need additional study when they identify which of the following as requiring a dosage increase in the warfarin?

   a. Clofibrate

   b. Quinidine

   c. Phenytoin

   d. Cefoxitin

10. A patient who is experiencing the signs and symptoms of an acute myocardial infarction says that his symptoms started at 10:00 AM this morning. It is now 11:15 AM. The nurse understands that the latest time that the patient could receive a thrombolytic agent would be which of the following?

    a. 1:00 PM

    b. 2:00 PM

    c. 3:00 PM

    d. 4:00 PM

11. A patient is started on enoxaparin immediately after hip surgery. The nurse would explain to the patient that this drug will be continued for how long?

    a. 1 to 3 days

    b. 3 to 7 days

    c. 7 to 10 days

    d. 10 to 14 days

12. The nurse is reviewing the coagulation studies of a patient who is receiving a heparin infusion. The patient's baseline partial thromboplastin time is 32 seconds. Which result would indicate therapeutic effectiveness?

    a. 32 seconds

    b. 40 seconds

    c. 64 seconds

    d. 96 seconds

13. An instructor is describing the drug drotrecogin alfa to a group of students. The instructor determines that the students need additional teaching when they state which of the following?

    a. The drug is used primarily for adults with severe sepsis.

    b. The drug is administered by intravenous infusion for a total of 4 days.

    c. The drug is fairly expensive, possibly limiting its used.

    d. The drug is associated with a high risk for embolism.

Copyright © 2011 by Wolters Kluwer Health I Lippincott Williams & Wilkins. *Study Guide for Focus on Nursing Pharmacology.*

14. A patient is receiving antihemophilic factor. The nurse understands that this drug is which factor?

    a. VIII
    b. VIIa
    c. IX
    d. X

15. Which of the following would a nurse identify as a systemic hemostatic agent?

    a. Absorbable gelatin
    b. Aminocaproic acid
    c. Human fibrin sealant
    d. Thrombin

Copyright © 2011 by Wolters Kluwer Health I Lippincott Williams & Wilkins. *Study Guide for Focus on Nursing Pharmacology*.

Drugs Used to Treat Anemias

●

LEARNING OBJECTIVES

Upon completion of this chapter, you will be able to:

1. Explain the process of erythropoiesis and its correlation to the development of three types of anemias.

2. Describe the therapeutic actions, indications, pharmacokinetics, contraindications and cautions, most common adverse reactions, and important drug–drug interactions associated with drugs used to treat anemias.

3. Discuss the use of drugs used to treat anemias across the life span.

4. Compare and contrast the prototype drugs epoetin alfa, ferrous sulfate, folic acid, and hydroxocobalamin with other agents in their class.

5. Outline the nursing considerations, including important teaching points, for patients receiving drugs used to treat anemias.

■ ASSESSING YOUR UNDERSTANDING

MATCHING

Select the description in column 2 that best describes the term in column 1.

Column 1

___ **1.** Anemia

___ **2.** Plasma

___ **3.** Erythrocytes

___ **4.** Erythropoiesis

___ **5.** Erythropoietin

___ **6.** Reticulocyte

Column 2

a. Liquid portion of the blood

b. Control of the rate of red blood cell production in the bone marrow

c. Immature nonnucleated red blood cell

d. Cell responsible for carrying oxygen to the tissues

e. Disorder of too few or ineffective red blood cells

f. Production and life cycle of red blood cells

SHORT ANSWER

Supply the information requested.

1. Describe how erythropoietin produces a red blood cell.

2. Identify the average life span of a red blood cell.

3. List three important elements in the bone marrow needed to produce healthy red blood cells.

4. Describe the three major types of anemia.

5. Name the type of anemia that occurs when the gastric mucosa cannot produce intrinsic factor.

■ APPLYING YOUR KNOWLEDGE

CASE STUDY

A patient has been undergoing cancer chemotherapy and has developed anemia. The patient has been prescribed ferrous sulfate 100 mg three times a day. He has been taking the medication for approximately 4 months, but he continues to exhibit signs and symptoms of anemia. Blood tests confirm this. The health care provider orders epoetin alfa.

a. What would be the rationale for using epoetin alfa?

b. What areas would require close monitoring of the patient receiving this drug?

■ PRACTICING FOR NCLEX

Circle the letter that corresponds to the best answer for each question.

1. Which of the following would a nurse identify as the primary issue associated with anemias?
   a. Defective white blood cells
   b. Increased plasma proteins
   c. Ineffective red blood cells
   d. Lack of vitamin B_{12}

2. After reviewing the major types of anemia, students demonstrate understanding of the information when they identify which of the following as an example of a hemolytic anemia?
   a. Iron deficiency anemia
   b. Pernicious anemia
   c. Folic acid deficiency anemia
   d. Sickle cell anemia

3. Which of the following would the nurse encourage a patient to consume to prevent folic acid anemia? Select all that apply.
   a. Fruits
   b. Fish
   c. Broccoli
   d. Milk
   e. Liver

4. A patient is receiving hydroxocobalamin for treatment of pernicious anemia. The nurse would administer this agent by which route?
   a. Oral
   b. Subcutaneous
   c. Intramuscular
   d. Intravenous

5. A patient is diagnosed with sickle cell anemia. Which agent would the nurse expect to be ordered?
   a. Hydroxyurea
   b. Epoetin alfa
   c. Ferrous sulfate
   d. Iron dextran

Copyright © 2011 by Wolters Kluwer Health l Lippincott Williams & Wilkins. *Study Guide for Focus on Nursing Pharmacology.*

6. A patient is receiving darbepoetin alfa. The nurse would inform the patient that he will be receiving this drug at which frequency?

   a. Once a week

   b. Two to three times/week

   c. Every other week

   d. Monthly

7. A patient is prescribed iron therapy using iron dextran. The nurse would administer this drug by which route?

   a. Oral

   b. Subcutaneous

   c. Intramuscular

   d. Intravenous

8. A patient is receiving ferrous sulfate as treatment for iron deficiency anemia. After teaching the patient, which statement indicates the need for additional teaching?

   a. "I need to take an antacid with the pill to prevent an upset stomach."

   b. "I need to make sure that I eat enough foods containing iron."

   c. "It might take several months before my iron levels get back to normal."

   d. "I need to avoid taking the drug with coffee or tea."

9. Which of the following would be appropriate for a patient who is receiving iron therapy?

   a. Ensuring that the patient consumes three large meals per day

   b. Cautioning the patient that stool may be dark or green

   c. Encouraging the patient to take the drug on an empty stomach

   d. Advising the patient to limit the amount of fiber in his diet

10. When describing the function of vitamin B_{12}, which of the following would be appropriate to include?

    a. Maintenance of myelin sheath

    b. Prevention of neural tube defects

    c. Important role in cell division

    d. Oxygen transport to the tissues

11. Which of the following would be least important in producing healthy, efficient red blood cells? Select all that apply.

    a. Iron

    b. Carbohydrates

    c. White blood cells

    d. Amino acids

    e. Plasma

12. A patient is receiving epoetin alfa. The nurse understands that this drug's duration of effect would be which amount of time?

    a. 12 hours

    b. 24 hours

    c. 36 hours

    d. 48 hours

13. A patient is experiencing iron toxicity. Which agent would the nurse expect to be given?

    a. Dimercaprol

    b. Succimer

    c. Deferoxamine

    d. Edetate calcium disodium

14. Which of the following would the nurse expect the health care provider to prescribe for a patient receiving methotrexate?

    a. Cyanocobalamin

    b. Leucovorin

    c. Hydroxyurea

    d. Iron sucrose

15. A patient is prescribed oral ferrous sulfate solution. Which statement by the patient indicates that he understands how to take the drug?

    a. "I'll mix the dose with orange juice to make it easier to swallow."

    b. "I should drink a big glass of water after swallowing the solution."

    c. "I can mix the dose with a small amount of yogurt to make it taste better."

    d. "I should drink the solution through a straw so my teeth don't get stained."

Copyright © 2011 by Wolters Kluwer Health | Lippincott Williams & Wilkins. *Study Guide for Focus on Nursing Pharmacology.*

CHAPTER 50

Introduction to the Renal System

LEARNING OBJECTIVES

Upon completion of this chapter, you will be able to:

1. Review the anatomy of the kidney, including the structure of the nephron.

2. Explain the basic processes of the kidney and where these processes occur.

3. Explain the control of calcium, sodium, potassium, and chloride in the nephron.

4. Discuss the countercurrent mechanism and the control of urine concentration and dilution, applying these effects to various clinical scenarios.

5. Describe the renin-angiotensin-aldosterone system, including controls and clinical situations where this system is active.

6. Discuss the roles of the kidney with acid-base balance, calcium regulation, and red blood cell production, integrating this information to explain the clinical manifestations of renal failure.

■ ASSESSING YOUR UNDERSTANDING

MATCHING

Select the description from column 2 that best describes the term in column 1.

Column 1

_____ 1. Aldosterone

_____ 2. Antidiuretic hormone

_____ 3. Carbonic anhydrase

_____ 4. Filtration

_____ 5. Reabsorption

_____ 6. Secretion

_____ 7. Countercurrent mechanism

_____ 8. Nephron

Column 2

a. Movement of substances from the renal tubule back into vascular system

b. Catalyst that speeds up the reaction combining water and carbon dioxide

c. Hormone produced by the adrenal gland

d. Functional unit of the kidney

e. Active movement of substances from the blood into the renal tubule

f. Hormone produced by the hypothalamus

g. Passage of fluid and small components through the glomerulus into the tubule

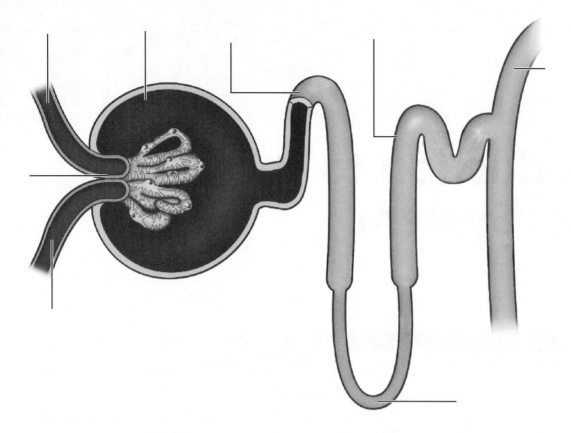

h. Process used by medullary nephrons to concentrate or dilute urine

LABELING

Place the name of the structure in the appropriate location on the illustration above.

Afferent arteriole

Bowman's capsule

Collecting duct

Distal convoluted tubule

Efferent arteriole

Glomerulus

Loop of Henle

Proximal convoluted tubule

■ APPLYING YOUR KNOWLEDGE

CASE STUDY

As part of a class assignment, a group of students are to role-play the processes that occur in the nephron. In addition, the students are to depict how the nephron

maintains the volume and composition of body fluids.

a. What processes would the student need to demonstrate, and how might they accomplish this task?

b. What key electrolytes would the students act out?

■ PRACTICING FOR NCLEX

Circle the letter that corresponds to the best answer for each question.

1. Which of the following statements best reflects information about the renal system?

   a. The kidneys consist of two protective layers.

   b. The system includes the kidneys and urinary tract.

Copyright © 2011 by Wolters Kluwer Health I Lippincott Williams & Wilkins. *Study Guide for Focus on Nursing Pharmacology*.

c. The system is primarily involved with regulating blood pressure.

d. Most of the fluid filtered by the kidneys is excreted.

2. After reviewing the structure of the kidneys, the students demonstrate understanding of the information when they identify which of the following?

a. The renal medulla drains the urine into the ureters.

b. The renal arteries come directly off the iliac artery.

c. The medullary nephrons are able to concentrate or dilute urine.

d. Erythropoietin is produced in the glomerulus.

3. The kidneys receive approximately what percentage of the cardiac output?

a. 5%

b. 15%

c. 25%

d. 40%

4. When describing the signs and symptoms associated with renal failure, which of the following would be most important for a nurse to keep in mind?

a. A small number of nephrons usually are affected when manifestations develop.

b. Most signs and symptoms are unrelated to nephron damage.

c. Renal failure reflects injury to the protective layers of the kidneys.

d. Renal failure suggests that extensive kidney damage has already occurred.

5. An instructor is reviewing the process of tubular secretion. Which of the following would the nurse include?

a. Movement of fluid and small components through the glomerulus into the tubule

b. Active movement of substances from the blood into the renal tubule

c. Movement of substances from the tubule back into the vascular system

d. Activity to create a more concentrated or diluted urine

6. The amount of fluid excreted as urine each day averages approximately less than how many liters?

a. 1 L

b. 2 L

c. 3 L

d. 4 L

7. Which of the following substances are moved from the glomerulus into the tubule due to hydrostatic pressure?

a. Lipids

b. Proteins

c. Blood cells

d. Water

8. Sodium ions are actively reabsorbed in which location?

a. Proximal convoluted tubule

b. Loop of Henle

c. Ascending loop of Henle

d. Distal convoluted tubule

9. Which of the following would lead to a release of aldosterone?

a. Low potassium levels

b. Parasympathetic stimulation

c. Angiotensin III

d. Natriuretic hormone

10. When describing the fluid in the ascending loop of Henle, which of the following would be most accurate?

a. Highly concentrated

b. Hypotonic

c. Hypertonic

d. Osmotically balanced

11. Where is the majority of potassium that is filtered at the glomerulus reabsorbed?

a. Bowman's capsule

b. Descending loop of Henle

c. Ascending loop of Henle

d. Distal convoluted tubule

12. Which substance stimulates the reabsorption of calcium in the distal convoluted tubule?

a. Aldosterone

b. Antidiuretic hormone

c. Vitamin D

d. Parathyroid hormone

13. Which of the following is released in response to a decrease in blood flow to the nephron?

   a. Calcium

   b. Renin

   c. Angiotensinogen

   d. Aldosterone

14. The nurse is describing the need to maintain the acidity of urine based on the understanding that this is necessary for which of the following?

   a. Maintain fluid balance

   b. Destroy any bacteria that may enter

   c. Prevent loss of sphincter control

   d. Maintain peristaltic movement

15. A nurse is describing the reasons why more women than men are affected by cystitis. Which of the following would the nurse identify as a major reason?

   a. "A woman's urine has a tendency to be more alkaline."

   b. "The urethra doesn't have the protection of the prostate gland."

   c. "The urethra exits into an area rich in gram-negative bacteria."

   d. "A woman's bladder stretches to accommodate more urine."

Copyright © 2011 by Wolters Kluwer Health I Lippincott Williams & Wilkins. *Study Guide for Focus on Nursing Pharmacology.*

CHAPTER 51

Diuretic Agents

LEARNING OBJECTIVES

Upon completion of this chapter, you will be able to:

1. Define the term *diuretic* and list four types of diuretic drugs.

2. Describe the therapeutic actions, indications, pharmacokinetics, contraindications and cautions, most common adverse reactions, and important drug–drug interactions associated with the various classes of diuretic drugs.

3. Discuss the use of diuretic agents across the life span.

4. Compare and contrast the prototype drugs of each class of diuretic drugs with other agents in their class.

5. Outline the nursing considerations, including important teaching points, for patients receiving diuretic agents.

■ ASSESSING YOUR UNDERSTANDING

LABELING

Place the name of the following drugs in the appropriate box under the correct drug class.

Amiloride	Mannitol
Bumetanide	Spironolactone
Ethacrynic acid	Triamterene
Furosemide	Urea

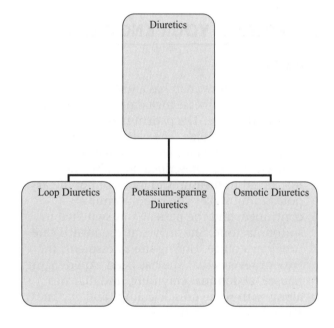

SHORT ANSWER

Supply the information requested.

1. Explain the clinical significance of the action of diuretics.

2. Describe what is meant by fluid rebound.

3. Explain how heart failure can cause edema.

4. Identify how thiazide and thiazidelike diuretics act.

5. Name the prototype loop diuretic.

6. Identify the most common use for carbonic anhydrase inhibitors.

■ APPLYING YOUR KNOWLEDGE

CASE STUDY

An older adult woman has a history of cardiovascular disease including hypertension and heart failure. The patient had been receiving furosemide. The patient developed mild hypokalemia for which a potassium supplement was prescribed. She also was instructed in measures to increase her dietary potassium intake. The hypokalemia continued, and the patient was switched to spironolactone. She arrives at the health care provider's office. During the assessment, the patient reveals that she has been experiencing nausea, abdominal cramping, and diarrhea along with some muscle cramps and weakness. Hyperkalemia is suspected.

a. What information would be most important for the nurse to obtain?

b. What should the nurse emphasize in the teaching plan for this patient?

■ PRACTICING FOR NCLEX

Circle the letter that corresponds to the best answer for each question.

1. A patient is receiving a diuretic and tells the nurse that he has decreased his fluid intake so that he does not have to make so many trips to the bathroom. The nurse interprets this information, realizing that this patient is at risk for which of the following?
   a. Hypokalemia
   b. Fluid rebound
   c. Weight loss
   d. Dehydration

2. After reviewing the different classes of diuretics available, a student demonstrates understanding when he identifies which of the following as an example of a thiazidelike diuretic?
   a. Metolazone
   b. Chlorothiazide
   c. Furosemide
   d. Triamterene

3. A patient is receiving hydrocholorothiazide. The nurse would expect to administer this drug by which route?
   a. Oral
   b. Subcutaneous
   c. Intramuscular
   d. Intravenous

4. Which of the following would contraindicate the use of indapamide?
   a. Diabetes
   b. Systemic lupus erythematosus
   c. Hypokalemia
   d. Gout

5. The nurse is monitoring the results of laboratory testing for a patient receiving chlorthalidone. Which of the following would be a cause for concern?
   a. Decreased uric acid levels
   b. Hypercalcemia
   c. Hyperkalemia
   d. Anemia

Copyright © 2011 by Wolters Kluwer Health l Lippincott Williams & Wilkins. *Study Guide for Focus on Nursing Pharmacology.*

6. A patient is receiving hydrochlorothiazide. The nurse would expect this drug to begin acting within which time frame?
   a. 1 hour
   b. 2 hours
   c. 3 hours
   d. 4 hours

7. When describing where bumetanide acts, which of the following would the nurse include?
   a. Proximal convoluted tubule
   b. Loop of Henle
   c. Collecting tubule
   d. Glomerulus

8. The nurse assesses a patient receiving furosemide for which of the following?
   a. Acidosis
   b. Hypercalcemia
   c. Hypotension
   d. Hypoglycemia

9. A patient receives a dose of furosemide intravenously at 8:00 AM. The nurse would expect this drug to exert is peak effects at which time?
   a. 8:15 AM
   b. 8:30 AM
   c. 8:45 AM
   d. 9:00 AM

10. After teaching a group of students about loop diuretics, the instructor determines that the teaching has been successful when the students identify which agent as the safest for use in the home?
    a. Furosemide
    b. Ethacrynic acid
    c. Bumetanide
    d. Torsemide

11. Which of the following would the nurse expect to find in a patient receiving acetazolamide?
    a. Metabolic alkalosis
    b. Metabolic acidosis
    c. Respiratory acidosis
    d. Respiratory alkalosis

12. When describing the action of spironolactone, the nurse would explain that this drug acts by which of the following?
    a. Blocking potassium secretion through the tubule
    b. Slowing the movement of hydrogen ions
    c. Blocking the chloride pump
    d. Blocking aldosterone in the distal tubule

13. A patient is receiving triamterene. The nurse instructs the patient to avoid which of the following? Select all that apply.
    a. Bananas
    b. Prunes
    c. Lettuce
    d. Broccoli
    e. Apples

14. Which of the following instructions would be most appropriate for a patient who is taking a diuretic?
    a. "Take the daily dose around dinnertime."
    b. "It's okay to take it with food."
    c. "Lie down after taking the drug."
    d. "Limit the amount of fluids you drink."

15. A patient is diagnosed with increased intracranial pressure. Which of the following would the nurse expect to be ordered?
    a. Mannitol
    b. Furosemide
    c. Amiloride
    d. Bumetanide

Copyright © 2011 by Wolters Kluwer Health | Lippincott Williams & Wilkins. *Study Guide for Focus on Nursing Pharmacology.*

52

Drugs Affecting the Urinary Tract and the Bladder

LEARNING OBJECTIVES

Upon completion of this chapter, you will be able to:

1. Describe four common problems associated with the urinary tract, including the clinical manifestations of these problems.

2. Describe the therapeutic actions, indications, pharmacokinetics, contraindications and cautions, most common adverse reactions, and important drug–drug interactions associated with urinary tract anti-infectives, antispasmodics, and analgesics, bladder protectants, and drugs used to treat benign prostatic hyperplasia.

3. Discuss the use of drugs affecting the urinary tract and bladder across the life span.

4. Compare and contrast the prototype drugs norfloxacin, oxybutynin, and doxazosin with other agents in their class.

5. Outline the nursing considerations, including important teaching points, for patients receiving drugs affecting the urinary tract and bladder.

■ ASSESSING YOUR UNDERSTANDING

MATCHING

Select the description from column 2 that best describes the term in column 1.

Column 1

_____ **1.** Cystitis

_____ **2.** Dysuria

_____ **3.** Nocturia

_____ **4.** Urgency

_____ **5.** Frequency

Column 2

a. Feeling of the need to void often

b. Inflammation of the bladder

c. Getting up to void at night

d. Painful urination

e. Feeling of needing to void immediately

SHORT ANSWER

Supply the information requested.

1. Describe the difference between cystitis and pyelonephritis.

2. List the two types of urinary tract anti-infectives.

3. Explain how urinary tract antispasmodics act.

4. Identify the indication for use of pentosan polysulfate sodium.

5. Describe the two types of drugs used to treat benign prostatic hyperplasia (BPH).

6. Name the herbal therapy that may be used to relieve the symptoms of BPH.

■ APPLYING YOUR KNOWLEDGE

CASE STUDY

A 42-year-old woman comes to the clinic for an evaluation. The woman reports urgency and frequency and some stress incontinence but denies any pain or burning on urination. She states, "There are times when I literally have to run to the bathroom because I have to go so badly. It's really embarrassing. It doesn't matter how much I've had to drink. In fact, whenever I go anywhere, I find where the restrooms are first, just in case. There have been several times when I almost didn't make it to the bathroom." Further assessment and a urine culture rule out a urinary tract

infection. The health care provider prescribes trospium.

a. When explaining the action of this drug, what information would the nurse need to address?

b. What information would the nurse need to include when teaching the patient about using this drug?

■ PRACTICING FOR NCLEX

Circle the letter that corresponds to the best answer for each question.

1. A group of students are reviewing the agents used as urinary tract anti-infectives. The students demonstrate understanding of the material when they cite which of the following as an example?
   a. Flavoxate
   b. Phenazopyridine
   c. Doxazosin
   d. Nitrofurantoin

2. When describing a urinary tract anti-infective, which of the following would a nurse identify as one that acidifies the urine?
   a. Cinoxacin
   b. Fosfomycin
   c. Methenamine
   d. Co-trimoxazole

3. A patient has a history of renal dysfunction. Which agent would the nurse expect to administer as the usual dosage?
   a. Cinoxacin
   b. Nitrofurantoin
   c. Norfloxacin
   d. Co-trimoxazole

4. A patient with cystitis is receiving fosfomycin. Which statement indicates that the patient has understood the instructions?
   a. "I need to drink lots of citrus juices."
   b. "I mix one packet in water to take the drug."

Copyright © 2011 by Wolters Kluwer Health I Lippincott Williams & Wilkins. *Study Guide for Focus on Nursing Pharmacology.*

c. "I can drink milk with the drug if my stomach is upset."

d. "I have to take the drug for no less than 7 days."

5. A physician prescribes a urinary antispasmodic as a transdermal patch. The nurse identifies this as drug as which of the following?

   a. Oxybutynin

   b. Flavoxate

   c. Tolterodine

   d. Darifenacin

6. A patient who takes digoxin for heart failure is also prescribed trospium. The nurse would monitor the patient closely for which of the following?

   a. Increased central nervous system effects

   b. Signs of digoxin toxicity

   c. Excess anticholinergic effects

   d. Changes in urine color

7. A patient is receiving phenazopyridine. The nurse would inform the patient that this drug may cause the urine to become which color?

   a. Brown

   b. Dark yellow

   c. Blue-green

   d. Reddish-orange

8. A patient is prescribed oxybutynin as a transdermal patch. The nurse would instruct the patient to change the patch at which frequency?

   a. Every day

   b. Every other day

   c. Every 4 days

   d. Every 7 days

9. The nurse is reviewing the medical record of a patient who is to receive pentosan. Which of the following would alert the nurse to the need for close monitoring?

   a. Splenic dysfunction

   b. Use of anticoagulants

   c. Thrombocytopenia

   d. Recent surgery

10. When explaining the action of dutasteride as treatment for BPH, the nurse would explain that the drug acts to achieve which of the following?

    a. Blockage of alpha-1 adrenergic receptors

    b. Inhibition of testosterone conversion

    c. Buffering to control cell wall permeability

    d. Interference with DNA replication

11. A patient is prescribed tamsulosin. The nurse would instruct the patient to take the drug in which manner?

    a. At night before going to bed

    b. An hour before the same meal each day

    c. One-half hour before the same meals daily

    d. At a consistent time each day

12. The nurse would inform the patient about which of the following when dutasteride is prescribed?

    a. Hypertension

    b. Bradycardia

    c. Increased libido

    d. Impotence

13. Which of the following would be most important to monitor in a patient receiving an agent for BPH?

    a. Complete blood count

    b. Serum electrolyte levels

    c. Renal function studies

    d. Prostate-specific antigen level

14. Which of the following would lead a nurse to suspect that a patient most likely has pyelonephritis?

    a. Urinary frequency

    b. Flank pain

    c. Dysuria

    d. Urgency

15. A patient is experiencing signs and symptoms of an overactive bladder. Which agent would the nurse expect the health care provider to prescribe?

    a. Nalidixic acid

    b. Methylene blue

    c. Tolterodine

    d. Terazosin

Copyright © 2011 by Wolters Kluwer Health I Lippincott Williams & Wilkins. *Study Guide for Focus on Nursing Pharmacology.*

CHAPTER 53

Introduction to the Respiratory System

LEARNING OBJECTIVES

Upon completion of this chapter, you will be able to:

1. Describe the major structures of the respiratory system, including the role of each in respiration.

2. Describe the process of respiration, with clinical examples of problems that can arise with alterations in the respiratory membrane.

3. Differentiate between the common conditions that affect the upper respiratory system.

4. Identify three conditions involving the lower respiratory tract, including the clinical presentations of these conditions.

5. Discuss the process involved in obstructive respiratory diseases, correlating this to the signs and symptoms of these diseases.

■ ASSESSING YOUR UNDERSTANDING

LABELING

Place the name of the structure in the proper location of the respiratory tract.

Alveoli

Bronchiole

Bronchus

Larynx

Lung

Mouth

Nose

Pharynx

Sinuses

Trachea

Upper Respiratory Tract	Lower Respiratory Tract

MATCHING

Select the description from column 2 that best describes the term in column 1.

Column 1

_____ **1.** Asthma

_____ **2.** Chronic obstructive pulmonary disease (COPD)

___ **3.** Atelectasis

___ **4.** Common cold

___ **5.** Cystic fibrosis

___ **6.** Pneumonia

___ **7.** Pneumothorax

___ **8.** Respiratory distress syndrome

___ **9.** Seasonal rhinitis

___ **10.** Sinusitis

Column 2

a. Hay fever

b. Bacterial or viral inflammation of the lungs

c. Hereditary disease involving copious thick secretions in the lungs

d. Viral upper respiratory tract infection

e. Disorder involving recurrent episodes of bronchospasm

f. Collapse of once-expanded alveoli

g. Condition involving the destruction of respiratory defense mechanisms

h. Disorder of premature neonates related to surfactant deficiency

i. Inflammation of the epithelial lining of the air-filled passages of the skull

j. Air in the pleural space exerting high pressure against the air sacs

■ APPLYING YOUR KNOWLEDGE

CASE STUDY

The nurse is assessing a patient who had abdominal surgery 36 hours ago. Assessment reveals crackles on auscultation and diminished breath sounds at the bases. His respirations are also somewhat shallow. Oxygen saturation levels via pulse oximetry are slightly decreased. The patient is complaining of abdominal pain. The patient states that he is trying not to cough or move because it hurts too much. The patient is receiving morphine for pain.

a. What might the patient be experiencing based on his status and assessment findings and why?

b. What measures might be helpful to promote the patient's respiratory function?

■ PRACTICING FOR NCLEX

Circle the letter that corresponds to the best answer for each question.

1. Which of the following would the nurse identify as being involved with asthma?

a. Acute infection

b. Hyperactive airways

c. Alveolar collapse

d. Progressive loss of lung compliance

2. Which term would be used to describe the movement of air in and out of the body?

a. Perfusion

b. Respiration

c. Ventilation

d. Gas exchange

3. An instructor is describing the respiratory membrane at the alveolar level. Which of the following would the instructor include as a component?

a. Cilia

b. Goblet cells

c. Mast cells

d. Capillary endothelium

4. Sympathetic nervous system stimulation of the respiratory tract would result in which of the following?

a. Diaphragmatic contraction

b. Bronchoconstriction

c. Increased respiratory rate

d. Inspiratory movement

5. A nurse is describing the events associated with a common cold to a local community group. Which of the following would the nurse include?

a. Release of epinephrine

b. Shrinkage of the mucous membranes

c. Increased activity of the goblet cells

d. Invasion by a bacterium

Copyright © 2011 by Wolters Kluwer Health I Lippincott Williams & Wilkins. *Study Guide for Focus on Nursing Pharmacology.*

6. A group of students are reviewing the common conditions associated with the upper respiratory tract. The students demonstrate understanding of the material when they identify which of the following as a response to a specific antigen?

   a. Asthma

   b. Seasonal rhinitis

   c. Sinusitis

   d. Pharyngitis

7. When describing the structure of the lungs, the nurse would identify the left lung as consisting of how many lobes?

   a. Two

   b. Three

   c. Four

   d. Five

8. Which mechanism is involved in the movement of oxygen and carbon dioxide at the alveolar level?

   a. Active transport

   b. Diffusion

   c. Facilitated diffusion

   d. Osmosis

9. Which of the following disorders would alter the ability to move gases in and out of the lungs? Select all that apply.

   a. Atelectasis

   b. Common cold

   c. Bronchitis

   d. Respiratory distress syndrome

   e. Sinusitis

   f. Cystic fibrosis

10. With bronchitis, proteins leak into the area due to which of the following?

    a. Swelling

    b. Increased blood flow

    c. Changes in capillary permeability

    d. Inflammatory reaction

11. With which condition are the bronchial epithelial cells replaced by a fibrous scar tissue?

    a. Asthma

    b. Bronchiectasis

    c. Bronchitis

    d. Pneumonia

12. A neonate develops respiratory distress syndrome. Which of the following would be used?

    a. Anti-infective agents

    b. Bronchodilators

    c. Surfactant replacements

    d. Antihistamines

13. After reviewing information about respiratory tract disorders, a group of students demonstrate understanding of the material when they identify which of the following as the most common cause of COPD?

    a. Infection

    b. Allergen exposure

    c. Genetic inheritance

    d. Cigarette smoking

14. A patient experiences bronchospasm with asthma. The nurse understands that this is due to which of the following?

    a. Cytokines

    b. Histamine

    c. Norepinephrine

    d. Serotonin

15. When describing the mast cells to a group of students, an instructor would include which of the following as being released by these cells? Select all that apply.

    a. Histamine

    b. Serotonin

    c. Adenosine triphosphate

    d. Epinephrine

    e. Dopamine

Copyright © 2011 by Wolters Kluwer Health I Lippincott Williams & Wilkins. *Study Guide for Focus on Nursing Pharmacology.*

CHAPTER 54

Drugs Acting on the Upper Respiratory Tract

LEARNING OBJECTIVES

Upon completion of this chapter, you will be able to:

1. Outline the underlying physiologic events that occur with upper respiratory disorders.

2. Describe the therapeutic actions, indications, pharmacokinetics, contraindications, most common adverse reactions, and important drug–drug interactions associated with drugs acting on the upper respiratory tract.

3. Discuss the use of drugs that act on the upper respiratory tract across the life span.

4. Compare and contrast the prototype drugs with other agents in their class and with other classes of drugs that act on the upper respiratory tract.

5. Outline the nursing considerations, including important teaching points, for patients receiving drugs acting on the upper respiratory tract.

■ ASSESSING YOUR UNDERSTANDING

LABELING

Place the name of the following drugs in the appropriate box under the correct classification.

Azelastine   Diphenhydramine

Benzonatate   Fexofenadine

Buclizine   Hydrocodone

Chlorpheniramine   Hydroxyzine

Dextromethorphan   Loratadine

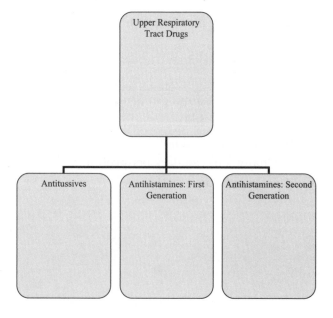

MATCHING

Select the description from column 2 that best describes the term in column 1.

Column 1

___ **1.** Antihistamine

___ **2.** Antitussive

___ **3.** Expectorant

___ **4.** Mucolytic

Column 2

a. Drug that blocks the cough reflex

b. Drug that increases a productive cough

c. Drug that blocks the action of a chemical released during inflammation

d. Drug that liquefies secretions

■ APPLYING YOUR KNOWLEDGE

CASE STUDY

A 20-year-old student comes to the campus health center. Over the past several days, he has developed nasal congestion, sneezing, and itchy and watery eyes. He had been participating in a service project in which they were cleaning up abandoned homes. The student says, "I often get this way when I'm exposed to dust. I wore a mask, but there really was a huge amount of dust flying around." The patient has a prescription for fexofenadine, which has been effective but has not been taking it lately. The nurse practitioner instructs the patient to start taking his fexofenadine and recommends the use of oxymetazoline for his nasal congestion.

a. What might be a reason why the nurse practitioner did not prescribe a nasal steroid?

b. What information would be important for the nurse to address when teaching the patient about the drug?

■ PRACTICING FOR NCLEX

Circle the letter that corresponds to the best answer for each question.

1. Which agent acts directly on the medullary cough center?

   a. Benzonatate

   b. Codeine

   c. Ephedrine

   d. Tetrahydrozoline

2. A nurse administers an antitussive agent cautiously to a patient with asthma for which reason?

   a. The airway needs to be maintained.

   b. The drug can lead to addiction.

   c. A loss of respiratory reserve can occur.

   d. The patient may experience increased sedation.

3. After teaching a patient who is receiving an antitussive about the drug, which statement indicates the need for additional teaching?

   a. "I'll get a humidifier for my bedroom."

   b. "I'll keep the room warm and toasty."

   c. "I can use some lozenges for comfort."

   d. "I need to increase the amount of fluids I drink."

4. Which agent would the nurse instruct a patient to use orally?

   a. Pseudoephedrine

   b. Phenylephrine

   c. Tetrahydrozoline

   d. Xylometazoline

5. An instructor is describing topical decongestants as belonging to which class?

   a. Adrenergics

   b. Anticholinergics

   c. Antihistamines

   d. Sympathomimetics

6. After teaching a group of parents about the use of over-the-counter cough and cold products with their children, which statement indicates the need for additional teaching?

   a. "We can use over-the-counter products for our 5-year-old but not for our 18-month-old."

b. "We need to read the label carefully to see how often and how much to give."

c. "We can use the adult brand, but we just have to decrease the amount."

d. "We should use the cup that comes with the drug to measure it out."

7. A patient is taking pseudoephedrine. The nurse would assess the patient for which of the following adverse effects?

a. Anxiety

b. Lethargy

c. Hypotension

d. Dry skin

8. The nurse instructs a patient who is prescribed a nasal steroid that it may take up to how long before effects may be noted?

a. 2 days

b. 4 days

c. 7 days

d. 21 days

9. A group of students are reviewing information about antihistamines. The students demonstrate understanding of the information when they identify which agent as a second-generation antihistamine?

a. Brompheniramine

b. Promethazine

c. Meclizine

d. Loratadine

10. When describing the effects of second-generation antihistamines, which of the following would the nurse address as being decreased?

a. Hypersensitivity

b. Dry mouth

c. Gastrointestinal upset

d. Sedation

11. A patient receives diphenhydramine orally. The nurse would expect this drug to begin acting within which time frame?

a. 15 to 30 minutes

b. 30 to 45 minutes

c. 45 to 60 minutes

d. 60 to 75 minutes

12. The health care provider suggests that a patient use guaifenesin to help his cough. The nurse instructs the patient to call the health care provider if he continues to have a productive cough after which amount of time?

a. 5 days

b. 1 week

c. 2 weeks

d. 3 weeks

13. Which agent would a nurse expect the health care provider to prescribe for a patient experiencing motion sickness?

a. Clemastine

b. Meclizine

c. Cyproheptadine

d. Hydroxyzine

14. When describing the action of acetylcysteine in treating cystic fibrosis, which of the following would the nurse need to keep in mind about the drug?

a. It binds with a heptatoxic metabolite.

b. It separates extracellular DNA from protein in the mucus.

c. It splits the disulfide bonds that hold mucus together.

d. It liquefies secretions to decrease viscosity.

15. A patient is receiving dornase alfa at home. Which of the following would the nurse instruct the patient to do?

a. "Store the drug at room temperature."

b. "Mix the drug with tap water."

c. "Protect the drug from light."

d. "Take the drug orally with meals."

Copyright © 2011 by Wolters Kluwer Health I Lippincott Williams & Wilkins. *Study Guide for Focus on Nursing Pharmacology.*

55

Drugs Acting on the Lower Respiratory Tract

LEARNING OBJECTIVES

Upon completion of this chapter, you will be able to:

1. Describe the underlying pathophysiology involved in obstructive pulmonary disease and correlate this information with the presenting signs and symptoms.

2. Describe the therapeutic actions, indications, pharmacokinetics, contraindications, most common adverse reactions, and important drug–drug interactions associated with drugs used to treat lower respiratory tract disorders.

3. Discuss the use of drugs used to treat obstructive pulmonary disorders across the life span.

4. Compare and contrast the prototype drugs used to treat obstructive pulmonary disorders with other agents in their class and with other classes of drugs used to treat obstructive pulmonary disorders.

5. Outline the nursing considerations, including important teaching points, for patients receiving drugs used to treat obstructive pulmonary disorders.

■ ASSESSING YOUR UNDERSTANDING

LABELING

Place the name of the following drugs in the appropriate box under the correct drug class.

Albuterol   Salmeterol

Aminophylline   Terbutaline

Epinephrine   Theophylline

Ipratropium   Tiotropium

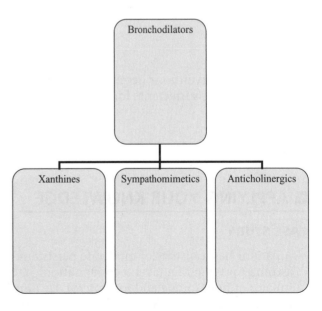

SHORT ANSWER

Supply the information requested.

1. Describe the first step in treatment for pulmonary obstructive diseases.

2. Explain the role of surfactant in the treatment of respiratory distress syndrome in a neonate.

3. Describe why xanthines are no longer considered first-line agents for asthma and bronchospasm.

4. Identify the receptor affected by sympathomimetic agents used as bronchodilators.

5. Explain the action of anticholinergics used as bronchodilators.

6. Define what is meant by the term *mast cell stabilizer*.

7. List three interventions necessary for administration of lung surfactants for an infant.

■ APPLYING YOUR KNOWLEDGE

CASE STUDY

A patient has a history of moderate persistent asthma for which he takes a combination inhaler of budesonide and formoterol. He also takes montelukast daily. His asthma has been fairly well controlled with these medications. The patient calls the health care provider's office to report that he is experiencing some difficulty breathing and feels congested in his chest. He also reports that he is wheezing. He asks if he should use his rescue inhaler of albuterol.

a. How would the albuterol help in this situation?

b. What information would be important to include when talking with the patient?

■ PRACTICING FOR NCLEX

Circle the letter that corresponds to the best answer for each question.

1. When describing the action of mast cell stabilizers, which of the following would the nurse include as being inhibited?
   a. Epinephrine
   b. Intracellular calcium
   c. Prostaglandins
   d. Slow-reacting substance of anaphylaxis

2. After teaching a group of students about drugs as bronchodilators, the instructor determines that the teaching has been successful when the students identify which group of drugs as once being first-line agents?
   a. Mast cell stabilizers
   b. Leukotriene receptor antagonists
   c. Xanthines
   d. Sympathomimetics

3. A patient is receiving theophylline intravenously. The nurse reviews the results of his serum drug levels and notifies the physician for which result?
   a. 10 mcg/mL
   b. 15 mcg/mL
   c. 20 mcg/mL
   d. 25 mcg/mL

Copyright © 2011 by Wolters Kluwer Health I Lippincott Williams & Wilkins. *Study Guide for Focus on Nursing Pharmacology.*

4. A nurse would expect to increase the dosage of theophylline if the patient has a current history of which of the following?

   a. Hyperthyroidism

   b. Cigarette smoking

   c. Gastrointestinal upset

   d. Alcohol intake

5. A nurse is administering levalbuterol to a patient. The nurse would administer this drug by which route?

   a. Oral

   b. Intravenous

   c. Inhalation

   d. Intramuscular

6. A patient is using an inhaled bronchodilator as treatment for exercise-induced asthma. The nurse would instruct the patient to use the inhaler at which time?

   a. Immediately after beginning to exercise

   b. 15 minutes before engaging in exercise

   c. Right before and after exercising

   d. Midway during the exercise routine

7. A patient who is experiencing anaphylaxis with severe wheezing receives a dose of epinephrine intravenously. The nurse would expect the drug to exert it full effects within which time frame?

   a. 5 minutes

   b. 10 minutes

   c. 15 minutes

   d. 20 minutes

8. An 8-year-old child with an acute asthmatic attack is receiving metaproterenol via nebulizer. Which of the following would be most appropriate?

   a. Have the child lie flat.

   b. Mix the drug with saline.

   c. Encourage rapid shallow breaths.

   d. Turn the device off when the mist slows.

9. While reviewing a patient's history, an allergy to which of the following would alert the nurse to a possible problem with the use of ipratropium?

   a. Eggs

   b. Dairy

   c. Peanuts

   d. Shellfish

10. Which statement by a patient who is prescribed triamcinolone indicates the need for additional teaching?

    a. "I should see some results in about 3 to 4 days."

    b. "I can't use this drug if I have an acute attack."

    c. "I might notice some hoarseness with the drug."

    d. "I should rinse my mouth after using the drug."

11. A patient is receiving ipratropium as maintenance therapy for chronic obstructive pulmonary disease. The nurse would caution the patient that up to how many inhalations may be used in 24 hours if needed?

    a. 4

    b. 8

    c. 12

    d. 16

12. Which of the following effects would result from the action of montelukast?

    a. Increased neutrophil aggregation

    b. Decreased eosinophil migration

    c. Decreased capillary permeability

    d. Increased smooth muscle contraction

13. A patient is experiencing an acute asthmatic attack. Which agent would be most effective?

    a. Inhaled steroid

    b. Leukotriene receptor antagonist

    c. Mast cell stabilizer

    d. Beta-2 selective adrenergic agonist

14. Which of the following would a nurse identify as a surfactant?

    a. Cromolyn

    b. Beractant

    c. Zileuton

    d. Theophylline

15. Which of the following would be most important to assess before administering calfactant? Select all that apply.

    a. Endotracheal tube placement

    b. Bowel sounds

    c. Lung sounds

    d. Abdominal girth

    e. Oxygen saturation levels

Copyright © 2011 by Wolters Kluwer Health I Lippincott Williams & Wilkins. *Study Guide for Focus on Nursing Pharmacology.*

CHAPTER 56

Introduction to the Gastrointestinal System

LEARNING OBJECTIVES

Upon completion of this chapter, you will be able to:

1. Label the parts of the gastrointestinal tract on a diagram, describing the secretions, absorption, digestion, and type of motility that occurs in each part.

2. Discuss the nervous system control of the gastrointestinal tract, including influences of the autonomic nervous system on gastrointestinal activity.

3. List three of the local gastrointestinal reflexes and describe the clinical application of each.

4. Describe the steps involved in swallowing, including two factors that can influence this reflex.

5. Discuss the vomiting reflex, addressing three factors that can stimulate the reflex.

■ ASSESSING YOUR UNDERSTANDING

LABELING

Place the name of the structure in its correct location on the diagram.

Duodenum

Epiglottis

Esophagus

Gallbladder

Large intestine

Liver

Pancreas

Parotid gland

Pharynx

Rectum

Salivary glands

Small intestine

Stomach

Tongue

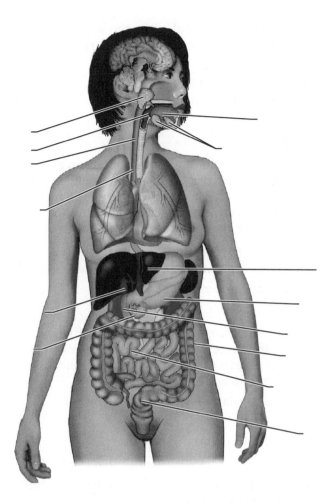

c. Fluid stored in the gallbladder

d. Fluid produced in the mouth in response to tactile stimuli and cerebral stimulation

e. Stomach contents containing ingested food and secreted enzymes, water, and mucus

f. Movement with contraction of one portion of small intestine while the next portion is relaxed

g. Substance secreted by the stomach in response to many stimuli

h. Complex reflex response to a bolus of food in the back of the throat

■ APPLYING YOUR KNOWLEDGE

CASE STUDY

A 45-year-old woman comes to the clinic complaining of right upper quadrant pain that sometimes radiates to the shoulder. She states that it seems to increase after she has eaten a heavy meal. The woman reports that her mother and sister have had gallstones, and she asks if this is what is happening.

a. Based on the nurse's understanding of the gallbladder, what information would be important to assess with this patient?

b. What might be happening that would lead to the patient's complaint of pain?

MATCHING

Select the description from column 2 that best describes the term in column 1.

Column 1

____ **1.** Chyme

____ **2.** Bile

____ **3.** Gastrin

____ **4.** Hydrochloric acid

____ **5.** Peristalsis

____ **6.** Saliva

____ **7.** Segmentation

____ **8.** Swallowing

Column 2

a. Action that moves a food bolus forward via progressive waves of muscular contraction

b. Substance released by parietal cells of the stomach

■ PRACTICING FOR NCLEX

Circle the letter that corresponds to the best answer for each question.

1. Which of the following would the nurse identify as being secreted by the exocrine pancreas?

   a. Insulin

   b. Pancreatin

   c. Gastrin

   d. Hydrochloric acid

Copyright © 2011 by Wolters Kluwer Health I Lippincott Williams & Wilkins. *Study Guide for Focus on Nursing Pharmacology.*

2. Which substance is responsible for making the food bolus slippery?

   a. Saliva

   b. Bile

   c. Chyme

   d. Pancrelipase

3. Which structure would a nurse identify as being responsible for the mechanical breakdown of food?

   a. Mouth

   b. Stomach

   c. Small intestine

   d. Pancreas

4. Which layer of the gastrointestinal tract is innermost?

   a. Mucosal layer

   b. Muscularis layer

   c. Nerve plexus layer

   d. Adventitia

5. Which substance is secreted by the chief cells of the stomach?

   a. Gastrin

   b. Hydrochloric acid

   c. Pepsin

   d. Bile

6. After reviewing the process of secretion, a group of students demonstrate understanding when they identify which pancreatic enzyme as being secreted to break down sugars?

   a. Chymotrypsin

   b. Trypsin

   c. Sodium bicarbonate

   d. Amylase

7. Which process is used by the small intestine for motility?

   a. Peristalsis

   b. Churning

   c. Segmentation

   d. Mass movement

8. After teaching a group of students about the reflexes involved in the gastrointestinal tract, the instructor determines that the teaching has been successful when the students identify which of the following as a central reflex?

   a. Gastroenteric

   b. Somatointestinal

   c. Vomiting

   d. Ileogastric

9. When auscultating bowel sounds on a patient who has had abdominal surgery, the nurse finds that they are absent. The nurse interprets this as indicating a disruption in which of the following?

   a. Ileogastric reflex

   b. Intestinointestinal reflex

   c. Gastroenteric reflex

   d. Gastrocolic reflex

10. Which of the following occurs first when pressure receptors in the back of the throat and pharynx send impulses to the medulla to stimulate nerves?

    a. Soft palate elevates

    b. Larynx rises

    c. Glottis closes

    d. Pharyngeal constrictor muscles contract

11. Which of the following would facilitate the swallowing reflex?

    a. Applying heat to the tongue

    b. Turning the head to one side

    c. Using different textured foods

    d. Providing foods of similar temperature

12. Upon stimulation of the chemotrigger receptor zone, which of the following occurs next?

    a. Increased production of mucus

    b. Increased salivation

    c. Decreased acid production

    d. Increased sweating

13. Which of the following best reflects the gastrointestinal system?

    a. It is one of only a few body systems open to the external environment.

    b. It plays a major role in waste excretion.

    c. It is comprised of one continuous, long tube.

    d. It is subject to high levels of friction with movement.

Copyright © 2011 by Wolters Kluwer Health | Lippincott Williams & Wilkins. *Study Guide for Focus on Nursing Pharmacology.*

14. Which of the following would be least likely to increase gastrin secretion?

   a. Alcohol

   b. Caffeine

   c. Proteins

   d. High acid levels

15. Which substances are primarily absorbed by the large intestine? Select all that apply.

   a. Alcohol

   b. Drugs

   c. Water

   d. Sodium

   e. Vitamins

Copyright © 2011 by Wolters Kluwer Health I Lippincott Williams & Wilkins. *Study Guide for Focus on Nursing Pharmacology.*

Drugs Affecting Gastrointestinal Secretions

■ LEARNING OBJECTIVES

Upon completion of this chapter, you will be able to:

1. Describe the current theories on the pathophysiologic process responsible for the signs and symptoms of peptic ulcer disease.

2. Describe the therapeutic actions, indications, pharmacokinetics, contraindications and cautions, most common adverse reactions, and important drug–drug interactions associated with drugs used to affect gastrointestinal secretions.

3. Discuss the drugs used to affect gastrointestinal secretions across the life span.

4. Compare and contrast the prototype drugs used to affect gastrointestinal secretions with other agents in their class and with other classes of drugs used to affect gastrointestinal secretions.

5. Outline the nursing considerations, including important teaching points, for patients receiving drugs used to affect gastrointestinal secretions.

■ ASSESSING YOUR UNDERSTANDING

LABELING

Place the name of the following drugs in the box corresponding to the correct drug class.

Cimetidine	Omeprazole
Esomeprazole	Ranitidine
Nizatidine	Sucralfate

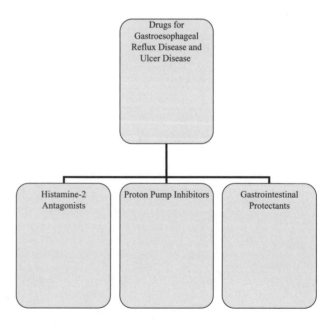

Drugs for Gastroesophageal Reflux Disease and Ulcer Disease

Histamine-2 Antagonists

Proton Pump Inhibitors

Gastrointestinal Protectants

FILL IN THE BLANKS

Provide the missing term or terms in the blanks provided.

1. Histamine-2 receptor antagonists block the

   release of _____ _____ in response
   to gastrin.

2. _____ ulcers are often seen in situations
   such as trauma, burns, or prolonged illness.

3. The only histamine-2 receptor antagonist

   approved for use in children is _____.

4. The reflex response of the stomach to lower

   more than normal acid levels is called
   acid _____ .

5. Antacids _____ stomach acid.

6. An antacid of calcium carbonate often causes

   _____ and acid rebound; magnesium salt

   antacids often cause _____.

7. Proton pump inhibitors are typically

   administered _____ meals.

8. The only gastrointestinal protectant currently

   available is _____.

■ APPLYING YOUR KNOWLEDGE

CASE STUDY

A 62-year-old man comes to the clinic
complaining of heartburn. The patient tells
the nurse that he has acid, frequently experiencing a sour taste in his mouth. He states, "I
was using Tums and chewing them almost all
the time. Then I started taking a liquid
antacid like every 2 hours, but nothing seems
to be helping." The patient is to be evaluated
by the health care provider.

a. What might be happening with this patient
   and why?

b. For which adverse effects would the nurse
   be especially alert?

c. What teaching would be important for this
   patient?

■ PRACTICING FOR NCLEX

Circle the letter that corresponds to the best answer for each question.

1. Which agent would a nurse identify as
   inhibiting the secretion of gastrin?
   a. Histamine-2 receptor antagonist
   b. Proton pump inhibitor
   c. Antacid
   d. Prostaglandin

2. Which agent would a nurse identify as the
   prototype histamine-2 receptor antagonist?
   a. Cimetidine
   b. Ranitidine
   c. Famotidine
   d. Nizatidine

3. A nurse is reviewing information about proton pump inhibitors. The nurse recognizes
   that which of the following is available as an
   over-the-counter agent?
   a. Lansoprazole
   b. Omeprazole
   c. Rabeprazole
   d. Esomeprazole

4. Which of the following would a nurse expect
   as most likely to be used in combination
   with antibiotics for treatment of *Helicobacter
   pylori* infection?
   a. Famotidine
   b. Calcium carbonate
   c. Omeprazole
   d. Sucralfate

5. A patient is taking an antacid that contains
   aluminum salts. The nurse would monitor
   the patient for which of the following?
   a. Diarrhea
   b. Hypercalcemia
   c. Acid rebound
   d. Hypophosphatemia

Copyright © 2011 by Wolters Kluwer Health I Lippincott Williams & Wilkins. *Study Guide for Focus on Nursing Pharmacology.*

6. Which of the following would a nurse expect to administer intravenously?
   a. Esomeprazole
   b. Omeprazole
   c. Rabeprazole
   d. Dexlansoprazole

7. Which instruction would be most important to give to a patient who is receiving omeprazole?
   a. "Chew the tablet thoroughly before swallowing."
   b. "Open the capsule and sprinkle it on applesauce."
   c. "Swallow the tablet whole with a large glass of water."
   d. "Take an antacid immediately before taking the drug."

8. After teaching a patient who is receiving sucralfate about the drug, which statement indicates that the teaching has been successful?
   a. "I need to limit my fluid intake."
   b. "I should eat a high-fiber diet."
   c. "I may need something to control diarrhea."
   d. "I need to avoid sugarless lozenges."

9. A patient is receiving pancrelipase. The nurse would expect to administer this drug at which time?
   a. 1 hour before meals
   b. With meals and snacks
   c. At bedtime
   d. First thing on arising

10. Which of the following best reflects the rationale for using histamine-2 receptor antagonists for stress ulcer prophylaxis?
    a. Reduces the overall acid level, promoting healing and comfort
    b. Blocks the overproduction of hydrochloric acid
    c. Decreases the acid being regurgitated into the esophagus
    d. Protects the stomach lining via acid blockage

11. Which agent is associated with antiandrogenic effects?
    a. Ranitidine
    b. Famotidine
    c. Cimetidine
    d. Nizatidine

12. A patient has a history of liver dysfunction. Which histamine-2 receptor antagonist would the nurse expect to be prescribed?
    a. Cimetidine
    b. Famotidine
    c. Ranitidine
    d. Nizatidine

13. A patient is receiving sodium bicarbonate orally. Which of the following would lead the nurse to suspect that the patient is developing systemic alkalosis? Select all that apply.
    a. Headache
    b. Constipation
    c. Confusion
    d. Irritability
    e. Tetany

14. When describing the possible adverse effects associated with omeprazole therapy, which of the following would the nurse identify as least common?
    a. Dizziness
    b. Headache
    c. Alopecia
    d. Cough

15. A patient is receiving sucralfate. The nurse understands that this drug would begin to act within which time frame?
    a. 15 minutes
    b. 30 minutes
    c. 45 minutes
    d. 60 minutes

Copyright © 2011 by Wolters Kluwer Health I Lippincott Williams & Wilkins. *Study Guide for Focus on Nursing Pharmacology.*

CHAPTER 58

Drugs Affecting Gastrointestinal Motility

■ LEARNING OBJECTIVES

Upon completion of this chapter, you will be able to:

1. Describe the underlying processes in diarrhea and constipation and correlate this with the types of drugs used to treat these conditions.

2. Describe the therapeutic actions, indications, pharmacokinetics, contraindications and cautions, most common adverse reactions, and important drug–drug interactions associated with laxatives and antidiarrheal drugs.

3. Discuss the use of laxatives and antidiarrheal agents across the life span.

4. Compare and contrast the prototype laxatives and antidiarrheals with other agents in their class and with other classes of laxatives and antidiarrheals.

5. Outline the nursing considerations, including important teaching points, for patients receiving laxatives and antidiarrheal agents.

■ ASSESSING YOUR UNDERSTANDING

LABELING

Place the name of the following drugs in the appropriate box under the correct drug class.

Bisacodyl   Glycerin

Cascara   Lactulose

Castor oil   Magnesium citrate

Docusate   Psyllium

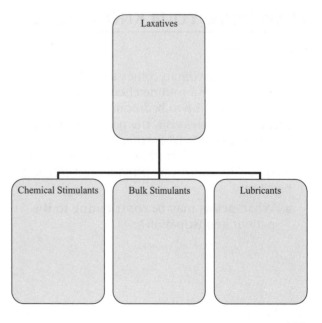

SHORT ANSWER

Supply the information requested.

1. Describe how gastrointestinal (GI) stimulants work.

2. Explain the three methods of action of antidiarrheal agents.

3. Define the term *lubricant* as it refers to GI motility.

4. Compare the action of chemical stimulant laxatives with bulk laxatives.

5. Explain what is meant by cathartic dependence.

6. Describe the action of docusate.

■ APPLYING YOUR KNOWLEDGE

CASE STUDY

A 78-year-old woman comes to the health care agency for a routine checkup. She lives alone in a small two-bedroom senior apartment. During the visit, the patient states that she is "constipated." Further inquiry reveals that she has not had a bowel movement for 2 days. The health care provider recommends psyllium.

a. What factors may be contributing to the patient's constipation?

b. What information would be important to stress with this patient about psyllium?

■ PRACTICING FOR NCLEX

Circle the letter that corresponds to the best answer for each question.

1. A patient is receiving metoclopramide intravenously prior to cancer chemotherapy. The nurse would expect this drug to begin acting within which time frame?
   a. 1 to 5 minutes
   b. 5 to 15 minutes
   c. 15 to 30 minutes
   d. 30 to 45 minutes

2. A group of students are reviewing information about the indications for laxatives. The students demonstrate understanding of the information when they identify which of the following as an indication?
   a. Adjunct to peptic ulcer therapy to eradicate *Helicobacter pylori*
   b. Enhance straining efforts after surgery
   c. Remove ingested poisons from the lower GI tract
   d. Increase secretions and overall activity of the GI tract

3. After teaching a group of students about laxatives, the instructor determines that the teaching has been successful when the students identify which agent as an example of a bulk laxative?
   a. Bisacodyl
   b. Senna
   c. Docusate
   d. Polycarbophil

4. A patient is taking bisacodyl to treat constipation. The nurse suggests that the patient take the drug at which time?
   a. In the morning before breakfast
   b. After eating lunch
   c. At any time during the day
   d. Before going to bed

Copyright © 2011 by Wolters Kluwer Health I Lippincott Williams & Wilkins. *Study Guide for Focus on Nursing Pharmacology.*

5. The nurse is preparing to administer cascara to a patient. The nurse anticipates administering this drug by which route?

   a. Oral

   b. Rectal, via enema

   c. Rectal, via suppository

   d. Intramuscular

6. When reviewing the medical record of a patient who is to receive a chemical stimulant laxative, the nurse would monitor the patient closely if he had which condition?

   a. Appendicitis

   b. Diverticulitis

   c. Coronary artery disease

   d. Ulcerative colitis

7. A patient is prescribed polyethylene glycol–electrolyte solution in preparation for a colonoscopy. The nurse would instruct the patient to do which of the following?

   a. "Take one glassful of the liquid."

   b. "Mix a packet in a glass of cold water."

   c. "Take one to eight spoonfuls in a day."

   d. "Drink 8 ounces every 10 minutes."

8. A patient who is taking magnesium citrate experiences sweating, palpitations, and flushing. The nurse understands that this is most likely related to which of the following?

   a. Direct stimulation of the nerve plexus in the abdominal wall

   b. Sympathetic stress reaction due to intense GI tract neurostimulation

   c. Detergent action on the surface of the intestinal bolus

   d. Formation of a slippery coat on the contents of the intestinal tract

9. The nurse is teaching the patient about possible adverse effects associated with mineral oil. Which of the following would be most important for the nurse to include?

   a. Leakage

   b. Abdominal cramping

   c. Diarrhea

   d. Sweating

10. The nurse is preparing to administer dexpanthenol to a patient based on the understanding that this drug acts in which manner?

   a. Blocking dopamine receptors

   b. Increasing acetylcholine levels

   c. Exerting an osmotic pull on fluids

   d. Acting directly on the muscles of the GI tract

11. Which of the following would the nurse expect to administer to a patient with traveler's diarrhea?

   a. Metoclopramide

   b. Loperamide

   c. Bismuth subsalicylate

   d. Opium derivative

12. After describing the drugs used to treat irritable bowel syndrome, the students demonstrate understanding of the information when they identify alosetron as which of the following?

   a. Anticholinergic

   b. Serotonin antagonist

   c. Chloride channel activator

   d. Selective opioid antagonist

13. A patient is diagnosed with traveler's diarrhea, and the health care provider prescribes rifaximin. The nurse describes this drug as which of the following?

   a. Antidiarrheal

   b. GI stimulant

   c. Antibiotic

   d. Opium derivative

14. A patient who is diagnosed with terminal cancer has been using opioids for pain relief and experiencing constipation despite numerous drug therapies and interventions for relief. The nurse anticipates the use of which agent for this patient?

   a. Lubiprostone

   b. Psyllium

   c. Mineral oil

   d. Methylnaltrexone

15. After teaching a class about irritable bowel syndrome, which statement indicates that the teaching has been successful?

   a. The disorder is relatively rare.

   b. It occurs more often in women than in men.

   c. Diarrhea is the predominant complaint.

   d. The cause is primarily stress related.

Copyright © 2011 by Wolters Kluwer Health I Lippincott Williams & Wilkins. *Study Guide for Focus on Nursing Pharmacology.*

59

Antiemetic Agents

LEARNING OBJECTIVES

Upon completion of this chapter, you will be able to:

1. Outline the vomiting reflex, including factors that stimulate it and mechanisms for measures used to block it.

2. Describe the therapeutic actions, indications, pharmacokinetics, contraindications and cautions, most common adverse reactions, and important drug–drug interactions associated with each of the classes of antiemetic agents.

3. Discuss the use of antiemetics across the life span.

4. Compare and contrast the prototype antiemetics with other agents in their class and with other classes of antiemetics.

5. Outline the nursing considerations, including important teaching points, for patients receiving antiemetics.

■ ASSESSING YOUR UNDERSTANDING

LABELING

Place the name of the following drugs in the appropriate box under the correct drug class.

Buclizine	Ondansetron
Dolasetron	Perphenazine
Meclizine	Prochlorperazine

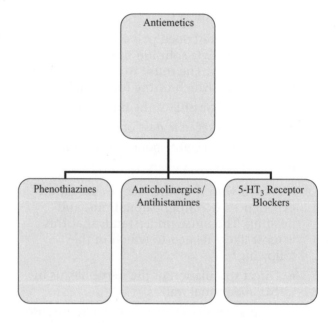

SHORT ANSWER

Supply the information requested.

1. Name the two most common phenothiazines used as antiemetics.

2. Describe the two ways that antiemetics achieve their action.

3. Explain the action of cyclizine.

4. Identify the drug that is used in combination with aprepitant.

5. Name the two drugs that contain the active ingredient of cannabis.

■ APPLYING YOUR KNOWLEDGE

CASE STUDY

A 54-year-old man comes to the emergency department with his wife. His wife states that he started hiccupping earlier that afternoon and has not stopped since that time despite numerous attempts to control the hiccups. "He had this twice before, and they gave him something intravenously and it worked. It always seems to happen when he gets stressed." The patient also has a history of gastroesophageal reflux for which he takes omeprazole. The physician administers chlorpromazine intravenously with relief. The patient is given a prescription for oral chlorpromazine.

a. What would the nurse understand about the patient's condition?

b. What information would be important for the nurse to include when teaching the patient and his wife about chlorpromazine?

■ PRACTICING FOR NCLEX

Circle the letter that corresponds to the best answer for each question.

1. After reviewing the various agents used as antiemetics, a group of students demonstrate understanding of the information when they identify which agent as a 5-HT$_3$ receptor blocker?

a. Chlorpromazine

b. Cyclizine

c. Granisetron

d. Aprepitant

2. When describing the action of prochlorperazine, which of the following would the nurse include as being affected?

a. Local response to stimuli

b. Chemoreceptor trigger zone

c. Cerebrum

d. Medulla

3. When reviewing the medical record of a patient who is to receive promethazine, which of the following would indicate to the nurse that the patient needs to be monitored closely?

a. Active peptic ulcer disease

b. Severe hypotension

c. Brain injury

d. Coma

4. A patient is receiving a phenothiazine antiemetic. The nurse instructs the patient to use the call light if he needs to get out of bed to go to the bathroom based on the understanding that this group of drugs is associated with which of the following?

a. Gastrointestinal overstimulation

b. Central nervous system effects

c. Urinary abnormalities

d. Endocrine effects

5. A patient is receiving an antiemetic. Which of the following would be most appropriate to facilitate the patient's comfort?

a. Offering carbonated drinks

b. Encouraging rapid, shallow breaths

c. Distracting the patient with activities

d. Offering mouth care every 4 to 6 hours

6. A patient receives prochlorperazine rectally at 6:00 PM. The nurse would expect the drug to begin acting at approximately which time?

a. 6:15 PM

b. 6:45 PM

c. 7:15 PM

d. 8:00 PM

Copyright © 2011 by Wolters Kluwer Health I Lippincott Williams & Wilkins. *Study Guide for Focus on Nursing Pharmacology.*

7. A patient is to start receiving chemotherapy at 10:00 AM. The patient has an order for intravenous metoclopramide. The nurse would expect to give the drug at which time?

   a. 9:00 AM

   b. 9:30 AM

   c. 10:15 AM

   d. 11:00 AM

8. The nurse would expect a patient with motion sickness to receive which of the following?

   a. Promethazine

   b. Dolasetron

   c. Perphenazine

   d. Cyclizine

9. A patient is receiving meclizine. The nurse would caution the patient to avoid which of the following?

   a. Caffeine

   b. Chocolate

   c. Alcohol

   d. Aged cheese

10. A patient who received palonosetron prior to a chemotherapy session asks the nurse if she can have a prescription for this drug in case she has nausea and vomiting over the next several days. Which of the following would the nurse need to keep in mind when responding to the patient?

    a. Seven days must pass before a repeat dose can be given.

    b. The drug is a controlled substance.

    c. The drug is limited to the days that chemotherapy is given.

    d. The drug can be given for two or three more doses.

11. The nurse is assessing a patient who is receiving aprepitant for adverse effects. Which of the following would the nurse expect to find? Select all that apply.

    a. Dizziness

    b. Dry mouth

    c. Constipation

    d. Anorexia

    e. Headache

    f. Irritability

12. Which agent would the nurse identify as acting directly in the central nervous system to block receptors associated with nausea and vomiting with little to no effect on serotonin, dopamine, or corticosteroid receptors?

    a. Metoclopramide

    b. Aprepitant

    c. Meclizine

    d. Granisetron

13. A patient is receiving palonosetron. The nurse would expect to administer this drug by which route?

    a. Oral

    b. Intramuscular

    c. Subcutaneous

    d. Intravenous

14. After reviewing information about various antiemetic agents, a group of students demonstrate understanding of the information when they identify which drug as similar to antihistamines but not as sedating?

    a. Hydroxyzine

    b. Nabilone

    c. Trimethobenzamide

    d. Dronabinol

15. When describing dronabinol to a group of students, the instructor emphasizes that this antiemetic is classified as which class of controlled substance?

    a. C-I

    b. C-II

    c. C-III

    d. C-IV

Answers

CHAPTER 1

■ ASSESSING YOUR UNDERSTANDING

MATCHING

1. b   **2.** d   **3.** e   **4.** a   **5.** c

SEQUENCING

$$4 \rightarrow 1 \rightarrow 3 \rightarrow 2 \rightarrow 5$$

FILL IN THE BLANKS

1. Pharmacotherapeutics
2. Plant
3. Genetic engineering
4. Teratogenic
5. A
6. Orphan

■ APPLYING YOUR KNOWLEDGE

CASE STUDY

a. Knowledge of generic and brand names would help the nurse identify if any of the medications were duplicates of the same drug. Some prescribers specify that a drug prescription be "dispensed as written" such that the brand-name product be used. If the patient was taking medications that were the same but one was a generic form while another was the brand-name form, then he would be at high risk for overdose or toxicity.

b. It would be important to obtain a thorough drug history for this patient. Of special emphasis would be his use of any over-the-counter (OTC) medications. Often patients do not consider OTC drugs to be medications. However, OTC drugs can mask signs and symptoms of underlying disease. They also can cause drug interactions and interfere with drug therapy when taken with prescription drugs. Moreover, not taking these drugs as indicated could result in serious overdoses.

■ PRACTICING FOR NCLEX

1. **Answer: a**
   RATIONALE: An adverse effect is considered a negative effect of a drug, one that is undersirable or potentially dangerous. The intended or therapeutic effect is the response that occurs when the drug is given—that is, the helpful effect. A teratogenic effect is a negative effect on a fetus that occurs when a drug is given.

2. **Answer: c**
   RATIONALE: Clinical pharmacology or pharmacokinetics addresses two key concerns: The drug's effects on the body and the body's response to the drug. The biologic effect of chemicals or drugs relates to pharmacology, which also involves the administration of drugs and the processes used by the body to handle the drugs, such as elimination.

3. **Answer: d**
   RATIONALE: Insulin for treating diabetes was obtained exclusively from the pancreas of cows and pigs, but now genetic engineering has allowed scientists to produce human insulin by altering *Escherichia coli* bacteria. Digitalis, opium, and morphine are derived from plant sources.

4. **Answer: b**
   RATIONALE: Ferrous sulfate, or iron, is a drug derived from the iron salt, an inorganic compound. Thyroid hormone, although created synthetically, may be obtained from animal thyroid tissue. Codeine is obtained from the poppy plant; castor oil is derived from *Ricinus communis*, also a plant.

5. **Answer: d**
   RATIONALE: A drug may be removed from further testing during a phase II study if it produces unacceptable adverse effects, is less effective than anticipated, is too toxic when used with patients, and has a low benefit-to-risk ratio.

6. **Answer: a**
   RATIONALE: During preclinical trials, drugs are tested on laboratory animals. A phase I study uses human volunteers for testing. A phase II study allows investigators to try out the drug in patients who have the disease that the drug is designed to treat. A phase III study involves the use of the drug in a vast clinical market.

7. **Answer: b**
   RATIONALE: Levothyroxine sodium is the generic name. L-thyroxine would be the chemical name; Levothroid or Synthroid would be the brand names.

8. **Answer: d**
   RATIONALE: Phase IV study is a phase of continual evaluation in which prescribers are obligated to report to the Food and Drug Administration (FDA) any untoward or unexpected adverse effects associated with the drugs being used. A phase I study uses human volunteers for testing. A phase II study allows investigators to try out the drug in patients who have the disease that the drug is designed to treat. A phase III study involves the use of the drug in a vast clinical market.

9. **Answer: b**
   RATIONALE: A drug identified as category A would be safest because studies of such a drug have not demonstrated a risk to the fetus in the first trimester of pregnancy and no evidence of risk in later trimesters. A category X drug is one in which studies have demonstrated fetal abnormalities or adverse reactions with reported evidence of fetal

risks. A category B drug is one in which animal studies have not demonstrated a risk to the fetus but there are no adequate studies in pregnant women, or animal studies have shown an adverse effect but adequate studies in pregnant women have not demonstrated a risk to the fetus during the first trimester of pregnancy and there is no evidence of risk in later trimesters. A category C drug is one in which animal studies have shown an adverse effect on the fetus, but there are no adequate studies in humans.

10. **Answer: c**
   RATIONALE: Women are not good candidates for phase I studies because the chemicals may exert unknown and harmful effects on a woman's ova, and too much risk is involved in taking a drug that might destroy or alter the ova. Women do not make new ova after birth. Men produce sperm daily, so there is less potential for complete destruction or alteration of the sperm. Women are not more unreliable, and men are not more consistent in body build or less likely to develop toxic effects.

11. **Answer: d**
   RATIONALE: Small amounts of narcotics such as codeine used as antitussives (cough suppressants) or antidiarrheal agents are classified as schedule V (C-V) controlled substances, which indicates that there is little abuse potential. Schedule II (C-II) drugs, such as narcotics, amphetamines, and barbiturates, have a high abuse potential. Schedule III (C-III) drugs, such as nonbarbiturate sedatives or nonamphetamine stimulants, have less abuse potential than C-II. Schedule IV (C-IV) drugs, such as some sedatives, antianxiety agents, and nonnarcotic analgesics, have less abuse potential than C-III drugs.

12. **Answer: d**
   RATIONALE: The Kefauver–Harris Act of 1962 gave the FDA regulatory control over the testing and evaluating of drugs and set standards for efficacy and safety. The Pure Food and Drug Act of 1906 prevented the marketing of adulterated drugs and required labeling to eliminate false or misleading claims. The Federal Food, Drug, and Cosmetic Act of 1938 mandated tests for drug toxicity and provided means for recall of drugs and gave the FDA the power of enforcement. The Durham–Humphrey Amendment of 1951 tightened control over certain drugs and required specification of drugs to be labeled "may not be distributed without a prescription."

13. **Answer: c**
   RATIONALE: The Drug Enforcement Agency, a part of the U.S. Department of Justice, is the agency responsible for enforcing the control of substances with abuse potential. The FDA, an agency in the U.S. Department of Health and Human Services, is responsible for studying drugs and determining their abuse potential.

14. **Answer: d**
   RATIONALE: Genetic engineering is a technologically advanced technique that allows drugs to be created. Plants, animals, and inorganic compounds are examples of natural sources for drugs.

15. **Answer: b**
   RATIONALE: In a phase II study, clinical investigators try out the drug in patients who have the disease that the drug is designed to treat. Preclinical trials involve the use of animal testing of a drug. A phase I study involves the use of human volunteers, usually healthy young men, to test a drug. A phase III study involves the use of the drug in a vast clinical market.

CHAPTER 2

■ ASSESSING YOUR UNDERSTANDING
SEQUENCING

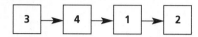

MATCHING
1. c   **2.** d   **3.** b   **4.** a

FILL IN THE BLANKS
1. Pharmacodynamics
2. Pharmacokinetics
3. Agonist
4. Passive diffusion
5. Biotransformation

■ APPLYING YOUR KNOWLEDGE
CASE STUDY

a. Several factors would be most important for the nurse to consider. First, the patient's age may affect all aspects of pharmacokinetics due to the myriad physical changes that occur as part of the aging process. Second, the patient's weight may be a factor necessitating a larger dose to obtain a therapeutic effect. Third, the patient's history of kidney disease may be a factor necessitating a lower dose due to possible interference with the drug's excretion.

b. Other factors that might play a role include the patient's gender (women have more fat cells than men do; thus, drugs depositing in fat may be slowly released and cause prolonged effects); physiologic factors such as hydration status, which could affect the way a drug works on the body; and environmental factors, which could exacerbate or decrease the effectiveness of the drug, in particular antihypertensive agents. In addition, the genetic, immunologic, and psychological factors may play a role in altering the effectiveness of the prescribed therapy.

■ PRACTICING FOR NCLEX

1. **Answer: a**
   RATIONALE: Pharmacodynamics, or how drugs affect the body, involves the action of enzyme systems and receptor sites. Critical concentration, dynamic equilibrium, and protein binding are associated with pharmacokinetics.

2. **Answer: c**
   RATIONALE: Generally, drugs given by the oral route are absorbed more slowly than those given parenterally. Of the parenteral routes, intravenously administered drugs are absorbed the fastest.

3. **Answer: b**
   RATIONALE: Drugs that are tightly bound to protein are released very slowly and have a very long duration of action because they are not free to be broken down or excreted. Drugs that are loosely bound tend to act quickly and to be excreted quickly. Drugs that compete with each other for protein binding sites alter the effectiveness or cause toxicity when the two drugs are given together.

4. **Answer: c**
   RATIONALE: Drugs that are taken orally are usually absorbed from the small intestine directly into the portal venous system (the blood vessels that flow through the liver on their way back to the heart). The portal veins deliver these absorbed molecules into the liver, which immediately transforms most of the chemicals delivered to it by a series of liver enzymes that break the drug into

Copyright © 2011 by Wolters Kluwer Health I Lippincott Williams & Wilkins. *Study Guide for Focus on Nursing Pharmacology.*

metabolites, some of which are active and cause effects in the body and some of which are deactivated and can be readily excreted from the body. As a result, a large percentage of the oral dose is destroyed at this point and never reaches the tissues. This phenomenon is known as the first-pass effect. The portion of the drug that gets through the first-pass effect is delivered to the circulatory system for transport throughout the body. Injected drugs and drugs absorbed from sites other than the gastrointestinal tract undergo a similar biotransformation when they pass through the liver. However, some of the active drug already has had a chance to reach the reactive tissues before reaching the liver.

5. **Answer: d**
   RATIONALE: Phase II biotransformation usually involves a conjugation reaction that makes the drug less polar and more readily excreted by the kidneys. Phase I biotransformation involves oxidation, reduction, or hydrolysis of the drug via the cytochrome P450 system of enzymes.

6. **Answer: c**
   RATIONALE: Ketoconazole is an example of a drug that inhibits the activity of the cytochrome P450 enzyme system. Nicotine, alcohol, and glucocorticoids, such as cortisone, increase the activity of this enzyme system.

7. **Answer: b**
   RATIONALE: Although the skin, saliva, lungs, bile, and feces are some of the routes used to excrete drugs, the kidneys play the most important role in drug excretion.

8. **Answer: c**
   RATIONALE: For each 8 hours, the drug would be reduced by one-half. Thus, after 8 hours, there would be 125 mg remaining; after the next 8 hours (16 hours later), there would be 62.5 mg (125/2) remaining; and after the next 8 hours (or 24 hours later), there would be 31.25 mg (62.5/2) remaining.

9. **Answer: a**
   RATIONALE: A loading dose, which is used to obtain needed effects quickly, uses a higher dose than usual to reach critical concentration. A loading dose does not enhance absorption, prevent drug breakdown by stomach acid, or prolong the half-life.

10. **Answer: c**
    RATIONALE: The liver is the single most important site of drug metabolism. If it is not functioning properly, the drug may not be metabolized correctly and may reach toxic levels in the body. Liver disease does not affect absorption or distribution. Kidney disease would affect drug excretion.

11. **Answer: b**
    RATIONALE: Passive diffusion is the major process through which drugs are absorbed into the body. Active transport, although not very important in the absorption of most drugs, is very important in drug excretion. Filtration also is an important process used in drug excretion, not absorption. Protein binding is an important mechanism involved in distribution of a drug.

12. **Answer: d**
    RATIONALE: A patient with a history of vascular disease or low blood pressure may experience an alteration in the distribution of a drug, preventing it from being delivered to the reactive tissue. A history of gastrointestinal disorders can affect the absorption of many drugs; liver disease may affect the way a drug is biotransformed; and kidney disease may affect the way a drug is excreted.

13. **Answer: a**
    RATIONALE: Pharmacogenomics is a new area of study that explores unique differences in response to drugs that an individual possesses based on genetic makeup. Pharmacodynamics refers to how the drug affects the body; pharmacokinetics refers to how the body acts on drugs. Pharmacology refers to the study of the biologic effects of chemicals.

14. **Answer: c**
    RATIONALE: The receptor site is the area on a cell membrane where many drugs are thought to act. The process is similar to how a key works in a lock, where the chemical (the key) approaches a cell membrane and finds a perfect fit (the lock) at a receptor site. The enzyme system acts as a catalyst for various chemical reactions. An agonist is a drug that interacts directly with receptors sites to cause the same activity that natural chemicals would cause at this site.

15. **Answer: b**
    RATIONALE: Penicillin affecting only bacterial cells is an example of selective toxicity, the property of a drug that affects only systems found in foreign cells without affecting healthy human cells. Critical concentration is the concentration a drug must reach in the tissues that respond to the particular drug to cause the desired effect. First-pass effect is a phenomenon in which drugs given orally are carried directly to the liver after absorption, where they may be largely inactivated by liver enzymes before they can enter the general circulation. Enzyme induction is the process by which the presence of a chemical that is biotransformed by a particular enzyme system in the liver causes increased activity of that enzyme system.

CHAPTER 3

■ ASSESSING YOUR UNDERSTANDING

MATCHING

1. d   **2.** b   **3.** c   **4.** d

SHORT ANSWER

1. Reasons that adverse effects may occur include the following: The drug may have other effects on the body besides the therapeutic effect; the patient is sensitive to the drug being given; the drug's action on the body causes other responses that are undesirable or unpleasant; or the patient is taking too much or too little of the drug, leading to adverse effects.

2. Before administering any drug to a patient, it is important to review the contraindications and cautions associated with that drug as well as the anticipated adverse effects of the drug. This information will direct your assessment of the patient, helping you to focus on particular signs and symptoms that would alert you to contraindications or to proceed cautiously and to establish a baseline for that patient so that you will be able to identify adverse effects that occur.

3. One of the most common occurrences in drug therapy is the development of adverse effects from simple overdosage. In such cases, the patient suffers from effects that are merely an extension of the desired effect.

4. Drug allergies fall into four main classifications: anaphylactic reactions, cytotoxic reactions, serum sickness, and delayed reactions.

5. One of the body's protective mechanisms is the wide variety of bacteria that live within or on the surface of the body. This bacterial growth is called *normal flora*. The normal flora protect the body from invasion by other bacteria, viruses, fungi, and so on. Several kinds of drugs (especially antibiotics) destroy the normal flora, leading to

the development of superinfections or infections caused by the usually controlled organisms.

6. Blood dyscrasia refers to bone marrow depression caused by drug effects on the rapidly multiplying cells of the bone marrow.

7. The electrolyte that can cause the most serious effects when it is altered, even a little, is potassium.

8. Anticholinergic effects may include dry mouth, altered taste perception, dysphagia, heartburn, constipation, bloating, paralytic ileus, urinary hesitancy and retention, impotence, blurred vision, cycloplegia, photophobia, headache, mental confusion, nasal congestion, palpitations, decreased sweating, and dry skin.

■ APPLYING YOUR KNOWLEDGE

CASE STUDY

a. The use of antihistamines is associated with the development of anticholinergic effects. These may include dry mouth, altered taste perception, dysphagia, heartburn, constipation, bloating, paralytic ileus, urinary hesitancy and retention, impotence, blurred vision, cycloplegia, photophobia, headache, mental confusion, nasal congestion, palpitations, decreased sweating, and dry skin. The nurse should focus the assessment on these effects.

b. The nurse would need to question the patient further about what signs and symptoms she experienced specifically related to the use of codeine. For example, the nurse could ask, "What exactly happens when you take codeine?" Many people state that they have a drug allergy because of the effects of the drug. For example, a rash may suggest an allergy, but sleepiness or sedation may reflect the therapeutic effect or, if excessive, a hypersensitivity to the drug's effect. Additional questions may include asking the patient how often she has taken the codeine and whether this (these) reaction(s) occurred only once or with subsequent use. For a true allergy, the patient develops antibodies to a particular drug.

■ PRACTICING FOR NCLEX

1. **Answer: b**
   RATIONALE: Secondary actions are effects that are inevitable and undesired but not related to the desired pharmacologic effects. Nausea and diarrhea are examples of secondary actions due to an antibiotic's effect on the gastrointestinal tract. Primary actions are those associated with the therapeutic effect. Drug allergy involves the formation of antibodies to a particular drug. Hypersensitivity refers to an excessive response to either primary or secondary effects of a drug.

2. **Answer: c**
   RATIONALE: For a patient experiencing a cytotoxic reaction, the prescriber is notified and the drug is discontinued. Subcutaneous epinephrine is used to treat an anaphylactic reaction. The patient is also encouraged to wear some type of Medic-alert identification denoting the allergy. Antipyretics would be used to treat serum sickness reaction.

3. **Answer: d**
   RATIONALE: Serum sickness reaction is manifested by an itchy rash, high fever, swollen lymph nodes, swollen and painful joints, and edema of the face and limbs. Hives and difficulty breathing would be associated with an anaphylactic reaction. Decreased white blood cell count would be associated with a cytotoxic reaction.

4. **Answer: c**
   RATIONALE: For stomatitis, the nurse should recommend frequent mouth care with a nonirritating solution. This may include frequent rinsing with cool liquids. The patient should consume frequent small meals rather than three large meals. An astringent mouthwash or a firm toothbrush would be too irritating.

5. **Answer: a**
   RATIONALE: Superinfection is caused by several kinds of drugs, especially antibiotics (which destroy the normal flora). Antihistamines, antihypertensives, and antineoplastics are not typically associated with superinfection.

6. **Answer: a, b, f**
   RATIONALE: Manifestations of blood dyscrasia include anemia, thrombocytopenia, sore throat, fever, chills, back pain, dark urine, leukopenia, and a reduction of all cellular elements of the complete blood count.

7. **Answer: d**
   RATIONALE: Renal injury is reflected by elevated blood urea nitrogen and creatinine concentration. Liver injury would be reflected by elevated liver enzymes such as aspartate aminotransferase (AST) and alanine aminotransferase (ALT). Hypoglycemia would be indicated by decreased blood glucose levels. Hyperkalemia would be reflected by elevated potassium levels (greater than 5.0 mEq/L).

8. **Answer: b**
   RATIONALE: Drugs with anticholinergic effects often cause dry mouth, constipation, dehydration, and decreased sweating. The patient should be instructed to drink fluids to prevent dehydration and to avoid overly warm or hot environments. In addition, the patient should use sugarless lozenges and perform frequent mouth care to combat dry mouth. A high-fiber diet would be indicated to prevent constipation. Diarrhea is an anticholinergic effect.

9. **Answer: c**
   RATIONALE: Neuroleptic malignant syndrome is manifested by extrapyramidal symptoms, including slowed reflexes, rigidity, and involuntary movements; hyperthermia; and autonomic disturbances, such as hypertension, fast heart rate, and fever.

10. **Answer: a**
    RATIONALE: The manifestations exhibited reflect Parkinson-like syndrome commonly associated with many of the antipsychotic and neuroleptic drugs. These symptoms are not associated with antidiabetic agents, general anesthetics, or anticholinergic agents.

11. **Answer: d**
    RATIONALE: All drugs are potentially dangerous. Even though chemicals are carefully screened and tested in animals and in people before they are released as drugs, drug products often cause unexpected or unacceptable reactions when they are administered. Drugs are chemicals, and the human body operates by a vast series of chemical reactions. Consequently, many effects can be seen when just one chemical factor is altered. Today's potent and amazing drugs can cause a great variety of reactions, many of which are more severe than ever seen before.

12. **Answer: c**
    RATIONALE: A patient taking an antihistamine who experiences drowsiness is an example of a secondary action. The antihistamine is very effective in drying up secretions and helping breathing—the therapeutic effect. Bleeding associated with anticoagulant therapy or a patient taking a recommended dose of antihypertensive who becomes dizzy or weak is an example of a primary action. Urinary

Copyright © 2011 by Wolters Kluwer Health l Lippincott Williams & Wilkins. *Study Guide for Focus on Nursing Pharmacology*.

retention in a patient with an enlarged prostate taking an anticholinergic agent is an example of hypersensitivity.

13. **Answer: a, b, e**
    RATIONALE: Anaphylactic reaction would be manifested by hives, rash, difficulty breathing, increased blood pressure, dilated pupils, diaphoresis, panic feeling, increased heart rate, and respiratory arrest. High fever and swollen joints would be associated with serum sickness reaction.

14. **Answer: d**
    RATIONALE: A delayed allergic reaction is manifested by rash, hives, and swollen joints, similar to the reaction to poison ivy. Skin care, comfort measures, antihistamines, or topical steroids may be used. Epinephrine would be used to treat an anaphylactic reaction. Antipyretics and anti-inflammatory agents may be used to treat serum sickness reaction.

15. **Answer: a**
    RATIONALE: Signs of hypoglycemia, or low blood glucose level, include fatigue; drowsiness; hunger; anxiety; headache; cold, clammy skin; shaking and lack of coordination (tremulousness); increased heart rate; increased blood pressure; numbness and tingling of the mouth, tongue, and/or lips; confusion; and rapid and shallow respirations. In severe cases, seizures and/or coma may occur. Increased urination, fruity breath odor, and increased hunger are signs of hyperglycemia.

CHAPTER 4

■ ASSESSING YOUR UNDERSTANDING
MATCHING
1. b **2.** e **3.** a **4.** c **5.** d
SHORT ANSWER
1. Application of the nursing process with drug therapy ensures that the patient receives the best, safest, most efficient, scientifically based, holistic care.
2. Two major aspects associated with assessment are the patient's history (past illnesses and the current problem) and examination of his or her physical status.
3. The seven rights are as follows: right drug, right storage, right route, right dosage, right preparation, right time, and right recording.
4. Areas to address when obtaining a patient's history include chronic conditions, drug use, allergies, level of education and understanding, social supports, financial supports, and pattern of health care.
5. Patients often neglect to mention over-the-counter drugs or alternative therapies because they do not consider them to be actual drugs or they may be unwilling to admit their use to the health care provider.
6. A patient's weight helps determine whether the recommended drug dosage is appropriate. Because the recommended dosage typically is based on a 150-pound adult male, patients who are much lighter or much heavier often need a dosage adjustment.
7. The specific parameters that need to be assessed depend on the disease process being treated as well as the expected therapeutic and adverse effects of the drug therapy. Assessing these factors before drug therapy begins provides a baseline level to which future assessments can be compared to determine the effects of drug therapy.
8. The placebo effect refers to the anticipation that a drug will be helpful.

LABELING

Assessment	Nursing Diagnosis
b, d, e	a, h
Implementation	**Evaluation**
c, g	f

■ APPLYING YOUR KNOWLEDGE
CASE STUDY
a. The patient's history of heart disease and diabetes are possible factors that could affect the pharmacokinetics and pharmacodynamics of a drug. The nurse would need to research the specific drug to determine if these conditions would be contraindications to use or require cautious use.
b. The patient is somewhat underweight for his height. Thus, the typical recommended dose may be too great for this patient. The nurse would need to obtain the patient's weight and compare it with the standard weight (150 pounds) used for drug therapy. If the patient's weight is much lighter, a dosage reduction might be necessary.
c. Several issues may affect the patient's compliance. The patient's ability to understand explanations and teaching may be hampered by his limited ability to speak English. The nurse would need to include the patient's friend in any teaching and explanation to ensure that the patient understands the information. The patient also has limited social supports, such that he lives alone and the nearest relative is about an hour away. Financial supports also may be limited.

■ PRACTICING FOR NCLEX
1. **Answer: a**
   RATIONALE: Gathering information is the first step—assessment—of the nursing process. Nursing diagnosis is a statement about the patient's status from a nursing perspective. Implementation involves planning patient care and intervening. Evaluation determines the effectiveness of the care and therapy.
2. **Answer: d**
   RATIONALE: Implementation involves planning patient care and intervention. Providing patient teaching would be a part of implementation. Developing a problem statement is done during the nursing diagnosis step. Obtaining baseline information about the patient's health patterns and identifying the patient's social support system would be completed during assessment.
3. **Answer: b**
   RATIONALE: The nursing process is a continual dynamic cyclical process of problem solving that occurs as series of steps to ensure that a patient receives the best, safest, most efficient, scientifically based, holistic care. It is not static or linear. Assessment, one step of the nursing process, allows information to be obtained to determine the patient's current status, priority needs, and problems.
4. **Answer: b**
   RATIONALE: Chronic conditions, such as renal disease, heart disease, diabetes, or chronic lung disease, can affect the pharmacokinetics and pharmacodynamics of a drug and may be contraindications to the use of a drug. Or, these conditions may require cautious use or dosage adjustment when administering a certain drug. Pneumonia, near sightedness, or an episode of gastroenteritis would not be as significant as a history of kidney disease.

Copyright © 2011 by Wolters Kluwer Health | Lippincott Williams & Wilkins. *Study Guide for Focus on Nursing Pharmacology.*

5. Answer: d
RATIONALE: Patients typically are not involved with reporting medication errors. Reporting is the responsibility of national- and institutional-level agencies; thus, this information would not be included in patient teaching about drug therapy. Alternative therapies to avoid, timing of administration, and drug toxicity warning signs would be important points to cover in a patient teaching program.

6. Answer: c
RATIONALE: A drug order should never be written as .5 mg because it could be interpreted as 5 mg, which would be 10 times the ordered dose. The proper dosage would be 0.5 mg. An order for 5.0 mg also requires caution because it could be interpreted as 50 mg.

7. Answer: b
RATIONALE: When administering a topical drug, the nurse needs to determine if the skin needs to be prepared in a specific way because topical agents may require specific handling. Reconstitution would apply to parenteral drugs. Crushing refers to oral drugs. The nurse should always apply the ordered dose or amount.

8. Answer: d
RATIONALE: The patient should know what each of the drugs is being used to treat to ensure a better understanding of what to report, what to watch for, and when to report to the health care provider if the drug is not working. The patient should keep a list of all drugs taken, including prescription, over-the-counter, and herbal medications. Medications should be stored in a dry place, away from children or pets. Storage in the bathroom, which may be hot and humid, may cause drugs to break down faster. The patient should read the labels and follow the directions so that if there are specific times to take the drug, they are followed.

9. Answer: d, b, a, c
RATIONALE: Applying the nursing process steps, the nurse would first question the patient about any chronic conditions, then identify problems related to functioning, then teach the patient about ways to minimize adverse effects, and finally determine that the drug is being effective.

10. Answer: b
RATIONALE: Adult medications should never be used to treat a child. The body organs and systems of children are very different from those of an adult. Parents should read all labels before giving a child a drug, especially over-the-counter products because many of these may contain the same ingredients, thereby accidently overdosing the child. Liquid medications should be measured with appropriate measuring devices such as a measured dosing device or spoon from a measuring set. The parents should never use a flatware teaspoon or tablespoon to measure a child's drugs. Health care providers do not always know what a child is taking, so parents need to keep a list of all medications given to a child, including prescription, over-the-counter, and herbal medicines.

11. Answer: a
RATIONALE: The patient is reporting a problem with ingesting adequate food and nutrients. Therefore, imbalanced nutrition: Less than body requirements would be most appropriate. Risk for imbalanced fluid volume may be a problem if the patient were experiencing vomiting or diarrhea that could lead to excess fluid loss. The patient is not verbalizing a problem with feeding himself. Rather, he is reporting difficulty in eating or consuming adequate food. The patient is taking the medication, so he is not noncompliant.

12. Answer: c
RATIONALE: Developing outcomes is a component of the implementation phase of the nursing process. Obtaining information about the patient's drug use, data about financial constraints, and information about the patient's level of understanding are important aspects of the assessment phase.

13. Answer: b, a, d, c
RATIONALE: The nursing process consists of four major steps in this order: assessment, nursing diagnosis, implementation, and evaluation. The steps overlap and are continuous and dynamic.

14. Answer: a
RATIONALE: The nurse questions the patient about the use of alternative therapies because they can interact with prescribed drugs, causing unwanted or even dangerous drug–drug interactions. Depending on the prescribed drug, the alternative therapy may or may not need to be stopped. There is no evidence to support that alternative therapies increase the risk for addiction. Although the patient's use of alternative therapies may provide some clues as to the patient's health beliefs, this is not the reason for questioning the patient about them as they relate to drug therapy.

15. Answer: b
RATIONALE: If a nurse sees or participates in a medication error, the nurse needs to report it to the institution and then report it to the national reporting program. This report would then be shared with the appropriate agencies, such as the Food and Drug Administration, the drug manufacturer, and the Institute for Safe Medication Practices.

CHAPTER 5

■ ASSESSING YOUR UNDERSTANDING

FILL IN THE BLANKS
1. Cubic centimeter
2. Clark's
3. 1,000
4. Ten
5. Unit

CROSSWORD

■ APPLYING YOUR KNOWLEDGE

CASE STUDY

a. The nurse needs to determine if the mother understands the need for accurate dosage and the prescribed dosage amount to be given to minimize the risk to the child. In addition, the nurse needs to determine if the mother has an appropriate measuring device (a standardized measuring device) in the home for accurate dosage. The nurse should question the mother about what she uses to give liquid medications to her child.

b. The nurse would need to emphasize the need for using a standardized measuring device for the dosage. The nurse should explain that the typical flatware teaspoon or tablespoon or drinking cup varies tremendously in the volume contained. The nurse needs to urge the mother not to use these devices for measuring. Instead, the nurse should instruct the mother to use a standardized measuring device. If the mother does not have one, then the nurse could suggest to the mother where to obtain one or, if appropriate, supply the mother with one. The nurse could also contact the pharmacy where the prescription will be filled to ask if one could be provided with the prescription or assist the mother in finding one. Usually, most pharmacies have these relatively inexpensive devices readily available.

■ PRACTICING FOR NCLEX

1. **Answer: b**
   RATIONALE: The avoirdupois system is an older system that was very popular when pharmacists routinely had to compound medications on their own. The household system of measurement is the system that is commonly found in recipe books. The apothecary system is a very old system of measurement specifically developed for use by apothecaries or pharmacists. The metric system is the most widely used system of measure.

2. **Answer: c**
   RATIONALE: The apothecary system includes units such as grain, dram, ounce, minim, fluidram, and fluid ounce. Liters and kilograms are units in the metric system. Pound is a unit in the household system.

3. **Answer: a**
   RATIONALE: The metric system is the most widely used system of measure. The apothecary system and avoirdupois system are rarely used in the clinical setting. The household system is the measuring system found in most recipe books used at home.

4. **Answer: c**
   RATIONALE: In the metric system, the basic unit of liquid measure is the liter; the basic unit of solid measure is the gram. The kilogram is another unit used for solid measure in the metric system. The minim is the basic unit of liquid measure in the apothecary system.

5. **Answer: b**
   RATIONALE: One grain in the apothecary system of measure is equivalent to 60 mg. Fifteen grains would be equivalent to 1 g or 1,000 mg. One-half grain would be equivalent to 30 mg. Eight fluid ounces would be equivalent to 240 mL in the metric system.

6. **Answer: a**
   RATIONALE: To convert 3 fluid ounces to the metric system, the nurse would set up the following ratio and proportion using the equivalent of 1 fluid ounce = 30 mL:

   $$1/30 = 3/X$$

   Cross multiplying: $1X = 90$; $X = 90$

7. **Answer: b**
   RATIONALE: To determine the amount to give, the nurse would set up the following ratio and proportion using Amount of drug available/One tablet or capsule = Amount of drug prescribed/Number of tablets/Capsules to give:

   $$5 \text{ gr}/1 \text{ tablet} = 10 \text{ gr}/X$$

   Cross multiplying: $5X = 10$; solving for X: $X = 2$

8. **Answer: a**
   RATIONALE: To determine the amount to give, the nurse would set up the following ratio and proportion using Amount of drug available/Volume available = Amount of drug prescribed/Volume to administer:

   $$500 \text{ mg}/5 \text{ mL} = 250 \text{ mL}/X$$

   Cross multiplying: $500X = 1,250$; solving for X: $X = 2.5$ mL

9. **Answer: d**
   RATIONALE: To determine the amount to give, the nurse would set up the following ratio and proportion using Amount of drug available/Volume available = Amount of drug prescribed/Volume to administer:

   $$500 \text{ mL}/1 \text{ mL} = 250 \text{ mL}/X$$

   Cross multiplying: $250X = 500$; solving for X: $X = 2$

10. **Answer: b**
    RATIONALE: To determine the flow rate (gtts/minute), the nurse would set up the following ratio using mL of solution prescribed per hour × Drops delivered per mL/60 minutes/1 hour:

    $$X = \frac{1,000 \text{ mL}/8 \text{ hours} \times 15 \text{ gtts/minute}}{60 \text{ minutes}/1 \text{ hour}}$$

    $$X = \frac{125 \text{ mL/hour} \times 15 \text{ gtts/minute}}{60 \text{ minutes/hour}}$$

    $$X = \frac{1,875 \text{ drops/hour}}{60 \text{ minutes/hour}}$$

    $X = 31.25$ gtts/minute or 32 gtts/minute

11. **Answer: d**
    RATIONALE: Today, the body surface area (nomogram) is considered the most accurate way for determining dosages. The Clark, Fried, and Young rules are rarely used today.

12. **Answer: a, c**
    RATIONALE: To use Clark's rule (Weight of child in pounds/150 pounds X Average adult dose), the nurse needs to know the child's weight in pounds and average adult dose. The child's age in years would be important for using Young's rule. The child's height in centimeters is needed to determine body surface area. Body surface area is not used with the Fried, Clark or Young rules. It is a separate method for calculating pediatric dosages.

13. **Answer: d**
    RATIONALE: Using the mg/kg method, the nurse would set up the problem as follows:

    $$1.1 \text{ mg}/1 \text{ kg} = X \text{ mg}/22 \text{ kg}$$

    Cross multiplying: $1X = 24.2$; solving for X: $X = 24.2$, which would be rounded down to 24 mg.

14. **Answer: b**
    RATIONALE: In 1995, the U.S. Pharmacopeia Convention established standards requiring that all prescriptions, regardless of the system used in drug dosage, include the metric measure for quantity and strength. The Food and Drug Administration and the Institute for Safe Medication Practices are involved with medication errors. The Drug Enforcement Agency enforces control over drugs with abuse potential.

Copyright © 2011 by Wolters Kluwer Health | Lippincott Williams & Wilkins. *Study Guide for Focus on Nursing Pharmacology.*

15. Answer: a, b, d, e
RATIONALE: Units in the household system of measurement include pint, quart, gallon, ounces, cups, tablespoons, teaspoons, drops, and pounds. Dram is a unit of measure in the apothecary system. Milliliter is a unit of measure in the metric system.

CHAPTER 6

■ ASSESSING YOUR UNDERSTANDING

MATCHING

1. d	**2.** e	**3.** g	**4.** c	**5.** b
6. j	**7.** h	**8.** f	**9.** i	**10.** a

SHORT ANSWER

1. One factor involved in the review process is the ability of the patient for self-care, which is the act of self-diagnosing and determining one's own treatment needs.
2. Patients often do not mention the use of alternative therapies to the health care provider. Some patients believe that the health care provider will disapprove of the use of these products and do not want to discuss it; others believe that these are just natural products and do not need to be mentioned.
3. Areas impacting health care including drug therapy in the 21st century include consumers having access to medical and pharmacologic information from many sources and taking steps to demand specific treatments and considerations; offering and advertising of alternative therapies at a record pace, causing people to rethink their approach to medical care and the medical system; financial pressures leading to early discharge of patients from health care facilities and to provision of outpatient care for patients who, in the past, would have been hospitalized and monitored closely; health care providers being pushed to make decisions about patient care and prescriptions based on finances in addition to medical judgment; events of 9/11 and the increased threat of terrorism leading to serious concerns about dealing with exposure to biological or chemical weapons; increasing illicit drug use (at an all-time high), bringing increased health risks and safety concerns; and increasing concerns about the environment and the need to protect it from contamination.
4. Possible health consequences of anabolic steroid abuse include hypertension, hyperlipidemia, acne, cancer, and cardiomyopathy.
5. A biological weapon, or germ warfare, uses bacteria, viruses, and parasites on a large scale to incapacitate or destroy a population.

■ APPLYING YOUR KNOWLEDGE

CASE STUDY

a. The nurse needs to caution the patient about the information he received from his neighbor. Each person responds to medications differently, so what might seem to work for one patient might not work for another. In addition, the nurse needs to talk with the patient about the Internet as a source for information, informing the patient that not all information presented is accurate or reputable.
b. The nurse should help the patient sift through the information to determine if it is appropriate or relevant to this patient. The nurse also could provide the patient with a list of reputable Internet resources that the patient can use to search for information. In addition, the nurse should provide the patient with tips for evaluating Web sites—for example, the way to identify appropriate sources through their Web address, recent updates of information, information that is supported by other sites, and credentials of the author or contributor.
c. The nurse must inform the patient that herbal remedies are not controlled or tested by the Food and Drug Administration (FDA) and as such are considered dietary supplements. Other concerns that need to be addressed include lack of testing of the active ingredients in these products and that if test results are available, they typically were for only a very small number of people with no reproducible results; lack of information about the incidental ingredients in many of these products (some may come directly from plants or from a natural state, the fertilizer used for the plant, the time of the year when the plant was harvested, and the other ingredients that are compounded with the product), which have a direct effect on efficacy; and the increased risk for possible interactions or serious complications when used with prescription medications.

If the patient wishes to use an alternative therapy with the medication regimen prescribed, then the patient and nurse need to talk with the health care prescriber because drug dosages or timing of the various drugs may need to be changed.

■ PRACTICING FOR NCLEX

1. **Answer: c**
RATIONALE: It is not unusual for the media to make current medical research or reports into news. Advertisements of prescription drugs directly to the public became legal in the 1990s. Federal guidelines are present to determine what can be said in an advertisement, but in some cases this further confuses the issue for many consumers. Many standard talk shows include a medical segment that presents just a tiny bit of information frequently out of context—for example, the "disease of the week," which opens a whole new area of interest for the viewer.
2. **Answer: a**
RATIONALE: Due to cost, patients may be tempted to stop taking an antibiotic in order to save the remaining pills for the next time they feel sick and to save the costs of another health care visit and a new prescription. This practice has contributed to the problem of resistant bacteria, which is becoming more dangerous all the time. The creation of a matrix delivery system for many medications can lead to toxicity or ineffectiveness if the patient attempts to split the drug. Generic drug availability in many cases reduces the cost of a drug but is unrelated to the development of resistant bacteria. Drugs obtained via the Internet may be cheaper, but the FDA has found many discrepancies between what was ordered and what is in the product.
3. **Answer: d**
RATIONALE: The Centers for Disease Control and Prevention (CDC) posts regularly updated information on signs and symptoms of infection by various biological agents, guidelines for management, and ongoing research. The FDA Web site would be helpful for information about

Copyright © 2011 by Wolters Kluwer Health | Lippincott Williams & Wilkins. *Study Guide for Focus on Nursing Pharmacology.*

drugs, including those obtained via the Internet and off-label use of drugs. Drug Facts and Comparisons provides a cost comparison of drugs in each class. The National Center for Complementary and Alternative Medicine is a reputable source for information on alternative therapies.

4. **Answer: b**
RATIONALE: Using a drug for off-label use involves using the drug for a situation not on the approved list for which it may be effective. Such use may eventually lead to a new approval of the drug for the new indication. Liability surrounding off-label use is unclear. Drugs often used for off-label indications include the drugs used to treat various psychiatric problems. Off-label use occurs after the drug has received FDA approval for the specific therapeutic indications and then is used for situations that are not part of those stated for approval.

5. **Answer: c**
RATIONALE: Gamma-hydroxybutyrate, or GHB, is a depressant. Cocaine or methamphetamine is considered a stimulant. LSD or MDA is considered a hallucinogen. Fentanyl, morphine, or OxyContin is an opioid.

6. **Answer: d**
RATIONALE: Although ordering drugs on the Internet (often from other countries) may be cheaper, do not require the patient to see a health care provider (many of these sites simply have customers fill out a questionnaire that is reviewed by a doctor), and are delivered right to the patient's door, there are many discrepancies in these drugs when compared with those obtained through usual methods, such as a pharmacy.

7. **Answer: c**
RATIONALE: The patient should take any unused, unneeded, or expired prescription drugs out of their original containers, mix them with an undesirable substance (such as coffee grounds or kitty litter), and put them in an impermeable, nondescript container such as an empty can or sealable bag and then throw the closed container in the trash. Prescription drugs should be flushed only if the patient information specifically instructs that this is safe to do.

8. **Answer: b**
RATIONALE: St. John's wort, a highly advertised and popular alternative therapy, has been found to interact with oral contraceptives, digoxin (a heart medication), the selective serotonin reuptake inhibitors (used for depression), theophylline (a drug used to treat lung disease), various antineoplastic drugs used to treat cancer, and the antivirals used to treat AIDS. It has not been shown to interact with acetaminophen or ibuprofen. Insulin or other antidiabetic agents interact with juniper berries, ginseng, garlic, fenugreek, coriander, dandelion root, and celery to cause hypoglycemia.

9. **Answer: a, b, c**
RATIONALE: If a drug advertisement states what the drug is used for, it must also state adverse effects, contraindications, and precautions. Doses and route of administration are not required to be included.

10. **Answer: d**
RATIONALE: Gone is the era when the health care provider was seen as omniscient and always right. The patient now comes into the health care system burdened with the influence of advertising, the Internet, and a growing alternative therapy industry. Many patients no longer calmly accept whatever medication is selected for them. They often come with requests and demands, and they partake of a complex array of over-the-counter (OTC) and alternative medicines that further complicate the safety and efficacy of standard drug therapy.

11. **Answer: c**
RATIONALE: When using the Internet, sites that are reputable or accurate are ones in which there is a mechanism for feedback or interaction, the preparer is listed with his or her qualifications, the site has been reviewed and recently updated (more than in the last 10 years), and the information is supported by other sites and is in agreement with other sources reviewed.

12. **Answer: a**
RATIONALE: OTC drugs are safe when used as directed, but many times the directions are not followed or even read. However, they can mask the signs and symptoms of an underlying problem, making it difficult to arrive at an accurate diagnosis if the condition persists. OTC drugs do interact with prescription drugs. Many OTC drugs were "grandfathered in" as drugs when stringent testing and evaluating systems became law and have not been tested or evaluated to the extent that new drugs are tested or evaluated today.

13. **Answer: b**
RATIONALE: A patient who abuses ketamine experiences paralysis, loss of sensation, disorientation, and psychic changes. Hallucinations, memory loss, and hypotension would be assessed in a patient abusing MDA (Ecstasy).

14. **Answer: b**
RATIONALE: For cutaneous anthrax, ciprofloxacin or doxycycline would be used. Ribavirin would be used for hemorrhagic fever; streptomycin or gentamicin would be used for tularemia.

15. **Answer: d**
RATIONALE: PCP is a hallucinogen. Amyl nitrate is a stimulant; heroin is an opioid; and rohypnol is an amnesiac.

Copyright © 2011 by Wolters Kluwer Health I Lippincott Williams & Wilkins. *Study Guide for Focus on Nursing Pharmacology.*

CHAPTER 7

■ ASSESSING YOUR UNDERSTANDING
LABELING

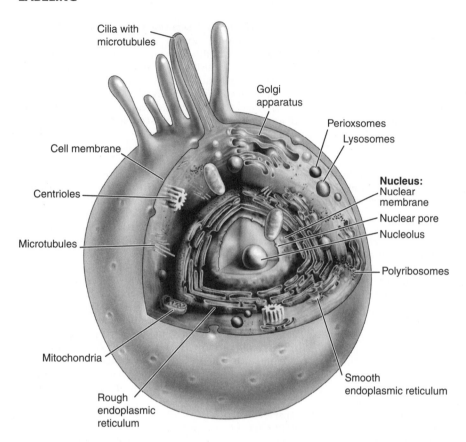

Cilia with microtubules

Golgi apparatus

Perioxsomes

Lysosomes

Cell membrane

Nucleus:
Nuclear membrane

Nuclear pore

Centrioles

Nucleolus

Microtubules

Polyribosomes

Mitochondria

Smooth endoplasmic reticulum

Rough endoplasmic reticulum

FILL IN THE BLANKS
1. Cell
2. Genes
3. Lipids, proteins
4. Organelles
5. Energy
6. Homeostasis
7. Four
8. Nucleus

MATCHING
1. d   2. e   3. c   4. b   5. a

■ APPLYING YOUR KNOWLEDGE
CASE STUDY

a. The students would need to demonstrate the four active phases and the resting phase. For the resting phase, the students would demonstrate typical functioning of the cell or the cell going about its usual actions; for the G_1 phase, the students would show synthesis of substances for DNA formation, collecting materials to make these substances; for the S phase, the students would show DNA synthesis, including doubling of DNA; for the G_2 phase, the students would show production of substances needed for making the mitotic spindles; and for the M phase, the students would show cell division.

b. The students could demonstrate the G_0 phase by walking around and performing usual activities, such as moving

substances, getting nutrition and oxygen, repairing things, and so forth.

c. The students could demonstrate the M phase by having two students side by side and then separating to show the creation of two identical daughter cells or by having a student hold two identical items attached and then splitting the items into two identical ones.

■ PRACTICING FOR NCLEX

1. **Answer: c**
   RATIONALE: The cell membrane contains cholesterol, along with phospholipids and glycolipids as well as proteins. Ribosomes are membranous structures involved in protein production within a cell; free ribosomes are found floating free in the cytoplasm, while others are attached to the surface of the endoplasmic reticulum. Genes are located in the nucleus. The mitochondria are found within the cytoplasm and produce energy as adenosine triphosphate (ATP).

2. **Answer: a**
   RATIONALE: DNA necessary for cell division is found on long strains called *chromatin*. The nucleus is encapsulated in its own membrane. A series of dense fibers and proteins are found within the nucleolus and eventually will become ribosomes. The cell membrane is composed of lipids and proteins.

3. **Answer: b**
   RATIONALE: Histocompatibility antigens or human leukocyte antigens (HLAs) are proteins that the body uses to

Copyright © 2011 by Wolters Kluwer Health I Lippincott Williams & Wilkins. *Study Guide for Focus on Nursing Pharmacology.*

identify a cell as a self-cell or one belonging to that individual. Receptor sites react with a specific chemical outside the cell to stimulate a reaction. Channels allow for the passage of small substances in and out of the cell. Organelles, located in the cytoplasm, are structures with specific functions.

4. **Answer: d**
RATIONALE: The mitochondria is responsible for energy production to allow the cell to function. Proteins are produced by the endoplasmic reticulum and free ribosomes. Cholesterol is produced by the endoplasmic reticulum. Hormone processing occurs in the Golgi apparatus.

5. **Answer: b**
RATIONALE: Lysosomes contain specific digestive enzymes that can break down proteins, nucleic acids, carbohydrates, and lipids and are responsible for digesting worn or damaged sections of a cell when the membrane ruptures and the cell dies. Free ribosomes produce proteins that are important to the cell's structure. The Golgi apparatus prepares hormones or other substances for secretion by processing them and packaging them in vesicles to be moved to the cell membrane for excretion. The endoplasmic reticulum (ER) functions to produce proteins, phospholipids, and cholesterol (rough ER) and to produce lipid and cholesterol and cell products (smooth ER).

6. **Answer: c**
RATIONALE: Active transport requires the expenditure of energy to transport substances. Facilitated diffusion, osmosis, and diffusion are passive transport mechanisms that require no energy for transport.

7. **Answer: d**
RATIONALE: Facilitated diffusion involves the use of a carrier molecule such as an enzyme to move in and out of a cell. Diffusion is the movement of a substance from an area of higher concentration to a lower one due to the concentration gradient. No carrier molecule is needed. Active transport requires the use of energy to move a substance against a concentration gradient. Osmosis is the movement of water from an area of low solute concentration to a higher solute concentration.

8. **Answer: b**
RATIONALE: An isotonic solution has the same solute concentration as human plasma. A hypertonic solution is one that contains a higher concentration of solutes than human plasma. A hypotonic solution contains a lower concentration of solutes than human plasma. Osmotic is not a classification for solutions or fluids.

9. **Answer: a**
RATIONALE: If a red blood cell were placed in a hypotonic solution, the cell would swell and burst because water moves from the solution into the cell. If the cell were placed in a hypertonic solution, the cell would shrink and shrivel because the water inside the cell diffuses out of the cell into the solution. A red blood cell placed in an isotonic solution would remain the same.

10. **Answer: d**
RATIONALE: The life cycle of a cell consists of four active phases and a resting phase. The genetic makeup of a cell determines the rate at which the cells can multiply. Regardless of the rate of reproduction, each cell has approximately the same life cycle. The cells found in breast milk reproduce very slowly, usually over a few months.

11. **Answer: b**
RATIONALE: The G_1 phase starts with stimulation of the cell and ends with the formation of DNA. The formation of two identical daughter cells after cell division occurs in the M phase. Doubling of DNA marks the end of the S phase.

12. **Answer: c**
RATIONALE: Cells in the kidneys use active transport to excrete drugs from the body. Osmosis, facilitated diffusion, and diffusion are not used.

13. **Answer: b**
RATIONALE: Polar regions of the cell membrane (of the phospholipid layer) mix well with water, while the nonpolar regions lying within the cell repel water. The freely moving nature of the cell membrane allows it to adjust to the changing shape of the cell for areas of the membrane to move together to repair itself. Receptor sites are located on the cell membrane, and cholesterol is found in large quantities in the cell membrane, working to keep the phospholipids in place and the cell membrane stable.

14. **Answer: d**
RATIONALE: Exocytosis involves the removal of substances from a cell by pushing them through the cell membrane. Endocytosis involves the incorporation of material into the cell by extending the cell membrane around the substance. Pinocytosis refers to the engulfing of specific substances that have reacted with a receptor site on the cell membrane. Phagocytosis allows the cell to engulf bacterium or a foreign protein and destroy it within the cell by secreting digestive enzymes into the area.

15. **Answer: a**
RATIONALE: The G_0 phase is the resting phase when the cell is stable. The G_1 phase lasts from the time of stimulation from the resting phase until the formation of DNA. The S phase involves the actual synthesis of DNA. In the G_2 phase, the cell produces all substances needed for manufacture of the mitotic spindles.

CHAPTER 8

■ ASSESSING YOUR UNDERSTANDING
MATCHING
1. b **2.** d **3.** c **4.** a **5.** e
SHORT ANSWER
1. The overall goal of anti-infective agents is to interfere with the normal function of the invading organism to prevent it from reproducing and to cause cell death without affecting the host cell.
2. Bactericidal refers to agents that actually cause the death of the cells that they affect. Bacteriostatic refers to agents that interfere with the ability of the cells to reproduce or divide.
3. Spectrum of activity refers to the effectiveness against invading organisms. Some agents, those with a narrow spectrum of activity, are highly selective in their action, making them effective against only a few microorganisms with a very specific metabolic pathway or enzyme. Other agents, those with a broad spectrum of activity, interfere with the biochemical reactions in many different kinds of microorganisms, making them useful in the treatment of a wide variety of infections.
4. The correct identification of the organism causing an infection is an important first step in determining which anti-infective agent should be used.
5. Health care providers can help prevent the emergence of resistant strains by not using antibiotics inappropriately; assuring that the anti-infective is taken at a high enough dose for a long enough period of time; and avoiding the use of newer, powerful anti-infectives if other drugs would be just as effective.

Copyright © 2011 by Wolters Kluwer Health | Lippincott Williams & Wilkins. *Study Guide for Focus on Nursing Pharmacology.*

■ APPLYING YOUR KNOWLEDGE

CASE STUDY

a. The patient's wound, which according to the patient was healing, now does not appear to be healing. There is purulent drainage coming from the wound, suggesting that an infection is still present. The wound should probably be recultured to determine if the infection is the same as on the previous visit or if the patient has developed another infection or possibly an infection involving a resistant organism. If a new or resistant infection has developed, then the anti-infective agent may need to be changed.

b. The patient needs to understand the prescribed medication therapy regimen, especially the need to take the medication exactly as prescribed for the time period prescribed to ensure complete eradication of the infection. In addition, the nurse needs to stress to the patient that he is to continue the medication even if he is feeling better or the wound looks better.

■ PRACTICING FOR NCLEX

1. **Answer: b**
   RATIONALE: Trimethoprim-sulfamethoxazole prevents the cells of the invading organism from using substances essential to their growth and development, leading to an inability to divide and eventually to cell death. Penicillins interfere with the bacterial cell wall. Aminoglycosides, macrolides, and chloramphenicol interfere with protein synthesis. Some antibiotics, antifungals, and antiprotozoal drugs alter the permeability of the cell membrane.

2. **Answer: c**
   RATIONALE: Destruction of the normal flora by anti-infectives commonly leads to superinfection, an infection that occurs when opportunistic pathogens that were kept in check by the normal bacteria have the opportunity to invade the tissues. Neurotoxicity involves damage or interference with the function of nerve tissue, usually in areas where drugs tend to accumulate in high concentrations. Hypersensitivity or allergic reactions result from antibody formation. Resistance refers to the ability over time to adapt to an antibiotic and produce cells that are no longer affected by a particular drug.

3. **Answer: d**
   RATIONALE: Combination therapy may be used when an infection is caused by more than one organism and each pathogen may react to a different anti-infective agent. Combined effects of different drugs sometimes delay the emergence of resistant strains. Typically, combination therapy involves the use of a smaller dosage of each drug, leading to fewer adverse effects while still having a therapeutic impact on the pathogen. Some drugs are synergistic, meaning that they are more powerful when given in combination.

4. **Answer: c**
   RATIONALE: The least commonly encountered adverse effect associated with the use of anti-infective agents is respiratory toxicity. The most commonly encountered adverse effects are direct toxic effects on the kidney, gastrointestinal tract, and nervous system along with hypersensitivity and superinfections.

5. **Answer: a**
   RATIONALE: Aminoglycosides collect in the eighth cranial nerve and can cause hearing loss, dizziness, and vertigo. Lethargy and hallucinations may be associated with other anti-infective agents. Visual changes such as blindness are associated with chloroquine use.

6. **Answer: b**
   RATIONALE: The use of broad-spectrum anti-infectives may result in superinfections—infections occurring when opportunistic pathogens kept in check by normal flora invade the tissues. The patient's complaint of vaginal discharge with itching suggests a superinfection. Bronchodilator therapy, oral contraceptives, and multivitamins would be unrelated to the patient's current complaint.

7. **Answer: d**
   RATIONALE: An anticoagulant interferes with blood clotting and is not an anti-infective agent. Antibiotics, anthelmintics, antiprotozoals, antivirals, and antifungals are all anti-infective agents.

8. **Answer: c**
   RATIONALE: An anti-infective with a narrow spectrum of activity is selective in its action; thus, it is effective against only a few microorganisms with a very specific metabolic pathway or enzyme. Broad-spectrum activity refers to effectiveness against a wide variety of pathogens. Bactericidal refers to a highly aggressive drug that causes cell death. Bacteriostatic refers to a drug's effectiveness in interfering with a cell's ability to reproduce or divide.

9. **Answer: d**
   RATIONALE: Microorganisms develop resistance by producing a chemical that acts as an antagonist to the drug. In addition, the microorganism can produce an enzyme that deactivates the drug, change cellular permeability so that the drug cannot enter the cell, and alter binding sites to no longer accept the drug.

10. **Answer: b**
    RATIONALE: The use of antibiotic prescription for viral illnesses or infections is a contributing factor to the development of resistance. A high enough drug dosage and long enough duration of therapy helps to ensure complete eradication of even slightly resistant organisms. Around-the-clock dosage scheduling eliminates peaks and valleys in drug concentration and helps to maintain a constant therapeutic level to prevent the emergence of resistant microbes.

11. **Answer: a**
    RATIONALE: Penicillins interfere with the biosynthesis of the bacterial cell wall. Sulfonamides, antimycobacterial drugs, and trimethoprim-sulfamethoxazole prevent the cells of the invading organism from using substances essential to their growth and development, leading to cell death. Aminoglycosides and macrolides interfere with the steps involved in protein synthesis. Fluoroquinolones interfere with DNA synthesis in the cell.

12. **Answer: b**
    RATIONALE: Performing sensitivity testing on cultured microbes is important to evaluate the bacteria and determine which drugs are capable of controlling the particular organism. Once the sensitivity testing is completed, then the decision for the drug can be made. Combination therapy is used when appropriate after culture and when sensitivity testing has been completed. Checking patient allergies also would be done after sensitivity testing but before administering the drug. The bactericidal effects of a drug may or may not play a role in the selection of the drug.

13. **Answer: c**
    RATIONALE: Gastrointestinal toxicity would be manifested by diarrhea, nausea, vomiting, or stomach upset. Dizziness and vertigo would reflect neurotoxicity. Rash may suggest a hypersensitivity or allergic reaction.

Copyright © 2011 by Wolters Kluwer Health I Lippincott Williams & Wilkins. *Study Guide for Focus on Nursing Pharmacology.*

14. **Answer: b**
    RATIONALE: Chloroquine can accumulate in the retina and optic nerve and cause blindness. Therefore, a patient complaining of changes in vision would be a cause for concern. Trouble hearing, feeling like the room is spinning, and dizziness are associated with problems involving the eighth cranial nerve.
15. **Answer: c**
    RATIONALE: Anti-infectives that adversely affect the liver and kidneys must be used with caution in older patients, who may have decreased organ function. Older patients often do not present with the same signs and symptoms of infection that are seen in younger people. The older patient is susceptible to severe adverse gastrointestinal, renal, and neurologic effects and must be monitored for nutritional status and hydration during drug therapy. Adults, not older adults, often demand anti-infectives for a "quick cure" of various signs and symptoms.

CHAPTER 9

■ ASSESSING YOUR UNDERSTANDING

FILL IN THE BLANKS

1. Anaerobic
2. Gram-positive
3. Synergistic
4. Bactericidal
5. Cefaclor

LABELING

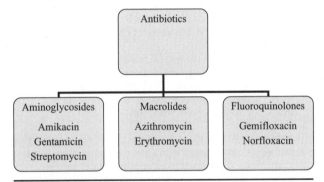

■ APPLYING YOUR KNOWLEDGE

CASE STUDY

a. Ciprofloxacin, a fluoroquinolone, is indicated for treatment of infections caused by susceptible strains of gram-negative bacteria, such as *Escherichia coli*. These infections commonly include the urinary tract, respiratory tract, and skin infections.
b. Ciprofloxacin belongs to the group of antibiotics known as fluoroquinolones. This group acts by entering the bacterial cell by passive diffusion through channels in the cell membrane. Once inside, the drug interferes with the action of DNA enzymes that are necessary for the bacteria's growth and reproduction. This leads to cell death because the bacterial DNA is damaged and the cell cannot be maintained.
c. Although the adverse effects associated with ciprofloxacin are relatively mild, the nurse would still need to address the most common ones, such as headache, dizziness, insomnia, nausea, vomiting, and dry mouth. The nurse would also need to caution the patient about possible bone marrow suppression and photosensitivity, urging the

patient to report any signs and symptoms of an infection, to avoid sun and ultraviolet light exposure, and to wear protective clothing and use sunscreens.
d. Antacids can interfere with the therapeutic effect of the drug, making it less effective. Therefore, the nurse should instruct the patient to make sure that at least 4 hours have passed between the time she takes the ciprofloxacin and the antacid.

■ PRACTICING FOR NCLEX

1. **Answer: c**
   RATIONALE: Gentamicin is classified as an aminoglycoside. Levofloxacin is a fluoroquinolone; clarithromycin is a macrolide; and cefaclor is a cephalosporin.
2. **Answer: b**
   RATIONALE: Telithromycin is a ketolide, which is structurally similar to macrolides. It is not structurally related to penicillins, cephalosporins, or lincosamides.
3. **Answer: d**
   RATIONALE: Streptomycin is an aminoglycoside that is available only for intramuscular use.
4. **Answer: b**
   RATIONALE: Gentamicin, like other aminoglycosides, can cause ototoxicity leading to irreversible hearing loss. Therefore, it would be most important to determine the patient's auditory function to establish a baseline for comparison. Gentamicin can affect the gastrointestinal (GI) tract, leading to nausea, vomiting, diarrhea, and weight loss, which in turn can affect nutrition. However, the patient's GI function and nutritional status would be less of a priority to assess. Gentamicin may cause numbness, tingling, and weakness. However, assessing the patient's muscle strength would be a lower priority.
5. **Answer: a**
   RATIONALE: Rifampin, along with isoniazid, pyrazinamide, ethambutol, streptomycin, and rifapentine, are considered first-line agents for treating tuberculosis. Kanamycin, ciprofloxacin, and capreomycin are second-line agents.
6. **Answer: c**
   RATIONALE: Cefuroxime is a cephalosporin. Doripenem, imipenem-cilastatin, and ertapenem are carbapenems.
7. **Answer: a**
   RATIONALE: Although headache and dizziness, superinfections, and phlebitis (with intravenous administration) can occur, the most common adverse effects of cephalosporins involve the GI tract and include vomiting, diarrhea, nausea, anorexia, abdominal pain, and flatulence.
8. **Answer: a**
   RATIONALE: The patient is exhibiting signs and symptoms of a disulfiramlike reaction that occurs when a cephalosporin such as cefaclor interacts with alcohol. Concurrent use of cefaclor with an oral anticoagulant may increase the patient's risk for bleeding. Concurrent use of cefaclor with another antibiotic such as an aminoglycoside can increase the patient's risk for nephrotoxicity. Adequate fluid intake, although important in maintaining hydration and nutrition, is unrelated to what the patient is experiencing.
9. **Answer: d**
   RATIONALE: Penicillin was the first antibiotic introduced for clinical use. Sir Alexander Fleming produced the original penicillin in the 1920s.
10. **Answer: b**
    RATIONALE: Food in the stomach decreases the absorption of oral macrolides such as erythromycin. Therefore, the drug should be taken on an empty stomach with a full,

8-oz glass of water, 1 hour before or at least 2 to 3 hours after meals. The patient may experience diarrhea with this drug, but it should not be bloody. Bloody diarrhea is associated with pseudomembranous colitis, which needs to be reported to the health care provider immediately. Due to its long half-life, azithromycin is usually ordered as a once-daily dose.

11. **Answer: a**

    RATIONALE: When rifampin and isoniazid are used in combination, the possibility of toxic liver reactions increases, requiring close monitoring. Urine culture would not need to be monitored. Audiometric studies would be monitored for patients receiving ototoxic drugs such as aminoglycosides. Although pulmonary function studies may be indicated to evaluate the patient's respiratory function, these would not be as important as monitoring liver function studies.

12. **Answer: c**

    RATIONALE: Ceftazidime is considered a third-generation cephalosporin. Cefazolin and cephalexin are considered first-generation cephalosporins. Cefaclor is a second-generation cephalosporin.

13. **Answer: b**

    RATIONALE: Clindamycin is considered the prototype lincosamide. Erythromycin and clarithromycin are macrolide antibiotics. Lincomycin is also a lincosamide but not the prototype.

14. **Answer: d**

    RATIONALE: Nafcillin and oxacillin are penicillinase-resistant antibiotics. Amoxicillin, ticarcillin, and carbenicillin are penicillins.

15. **Answer: a**

    RATIONALE: Tetracyclines should be used with caution in children younger than age 8 years because the drugs can potentially damage developing teeth and bones. They do not affect hearing or vision. They are excreted in the urine, so caution is necessary if the patient has underlying renal dysfunction; however, this is not the main reason for avoiding use in children.

CHAPTER 10

■ ASSESSING YOUR UNDERSTANDING

LABELING

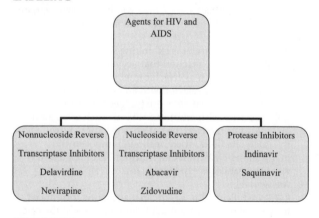

MATCHING

1. e   2. d   3. b   4. c   5. a

■ APPLYING YOUR KNOWLEDGE

CASE STUDY

a. The nurse needs to explain to the patient about her condition in a calm, nonjudgmental, supportive manner. The nurse must emphasize that although the medication can help alleviate the current infection, it does not cure the condition.

b. The nurse needs to instruct the patient that she should take the medication exactly as prescribed for the exact duration of therapy, usually 5 days. In addition, the nurse needs to teach the patient about her infection, including the fact that the drug is not curative. The nurse also should instruct the patient about possible adverse effects, most commonly, nausea, vomiting, headache, depression, paresthesias, neuropathy, rash, and hair loss. Offering suggestions as to how to cope with these effects, such as maintaining adequate food and fluid intake, would be important. The nurse needs to emphasize avoiding sexual activity during a current outbreak and to use safe sex practices to prevent disease transmission.

■ PRACTICING FOR NCLEX

1. **Answer: c**

    RATIONALE: Foscarnet is available only for intravenous use.

2. **Answer: a**

    RATIONALE: Oseltamivir is used as treatment for influenza if the patient has been symptomatic for fewer than 2 days.

3. **Answer: d**

    RATIONALE: Fosamprenavir is a protease inhibitor that may be indicated as part of combination therapy for symptomatic HIV infection. Entecavir, telbivudine, and adefovir are indicated for the treatment of chronic hepatitis B.

4. **Answer: b**

    RATIONALE: Nucleoside reverse transcriptase inhibitors, such as didanosine and zidovudine, were the first class of drugs developed to treat HIV infection. Of the classes listed, fusion inhibitors would be the newest class of drugs developed for HIV infection.

5. **Answer: b**

    RATIONALE: HIV mutates over time, presenting a slightly different configuration with each new generation. Thus, multiple drugs are used to attack the virus at various points in the life cycle to achieve the maximum effectiveness with the least amount of toxicity. Sensitivity is not an issue. The virus needs to enter the cell to cause infection. Adverse effects are numerous with anti-HIV drugs and the use of combination therapy can increase the patient's risk for these adverse effects, including further depression of the immune response.

6. **Answer: c**

    RATIONALE: Of the drugs listed, only zidovudine has been proven safe for use during pregnancy.

7. **Answer: a**

    RATIONALE: Nevirapine is associated with gastrointestinal-related effects, most commonly, dry mouth, dyspepsia, constipation or diarrhea, nausea, and abdominal pain. Rimantadine is more commonly associated with lightheadedness and dizziness. Tenofovir and fosamprenavir are associated with changes in body fat distribution, leading to buffalo hump and thin arms and legs. Maraviroc is associated with paresthesias and fever.

8. **Answer: c**

    RATIONALE: Zanamivir is delivered by a Diskhaler device and is absorbed through the respiratory tract.

Copyright © 2011 by Wolters Kluwer Health | Lippincott Williams & Wilkins. *Study Guide for Focus on Nursing Pharmacology.*

9. Answer: d

RATIONALE: Ibuprofen has not been found to interact with rimantadine. However, anticholinergics such as atropine and drugs such as acetaminophen and aspirin have been associated with an increase in anticholinergic effects and decreased effectiveness, respectively.

10. Answer: a

RATIONALE: Nelfinavir, if used with midazolam, pimozide, rifampin, or triazolam, can lead to severe toxic effects and life-threatening arrhythmias. Delavirdine, if used with warfarin, clarithromycin, or quinidine, can lead to life-threatening effects.

11. Answer: b

RATIONALE: Maraviroc is classified as a CCR5 co-receptor antagonist. Enfuvirtide is categorized as a fusion inhibitor; raltegravir is categorized as an integrase inhibitor; and didanosine is categorized as a nucleoside reverse transcriptase inhibitor.

12. Answer: c

RATIONALE: Although patient teaching about adverse effects, follow-up laboratory testing, and measures to reduce infection transmission are important, it is essential that the patient ensure that he or she has a continuously available and adequate supply of the drug because there is a risk for an acute exacerbation of hepatitis B when the drug is stopped.

13. Answer: a

RATIONALE: If the patient develops a severe local reaction or if open lesions occur near the site of administration, then the drug needs to be stopped to prevent systemic absorption and adverse effects. Localized burning, stinging, and discomfort are associated with the use of docosanol. Since the drug is applied locally, it is not absorbed systemically. The drug does not cure the disease but should help alleviate discomfort.

14. Answer: b

RATIONALE: Oseltamivir is the only antiviral agent found to be effective in the treatment of Avian flu.

15. Answer: d

RATIONALE: Cidofovir is given by intravenous infusion over 1 hour. It is not given orally, topically, or subcutaneously.

CHAPTER 11

■ ASSESSING YOUR UNDERSTANDING

CROSSWORD

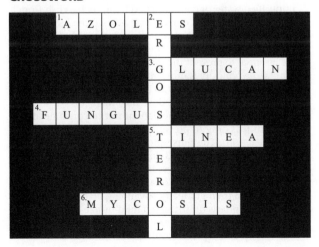

SHORT ANSWER

1. Ketoconazole and fluconazole strongly inhibit the cytochrome P450 (CYP450) enzyme system in the liver.
2. Topical antifungal agents should not be used over open or draining areas, because doing so increases the risk for systemic absorption.
3. The incidence of fungal infections has increased due to the rising number of immunocompromised individuals, such as those with AIDS and AIDS-related complex, those taking immunosuppressant drugs, those who have undergone transplant surgery or cancer treatment, and those with advancing age (the growing number of older adults) who are no longer able to protect themselves from the many fungi found throughout the environment.
4. Three major types of local fungal infections include vaginal infections, oral yeast infections, and a variety of tinea infections.
5. The composition of the protective layer of the fungal cell (the rigid cell wall of chitin and polysaccharides and cell membrane containing ergosterol) makes the organism resistant to antibiotics.

■ APPLYING YOUR KNOWLEDGE

CASE STUDY

a. The nurse should instruct the patient to apply the cream to the affected area in a thin layer twice a day for approximately 2 to 4 weeks. The cream is available over the counter, so it would be essential to ensure that the patient understands how to use the medication properly to avoid possible systemic absorption.
b. The nurse should reinforce the need for the patient to use the cream exactly as recommended and to follow the manufacturer's instructions about use. In addition, the nurse should tell the patient not to apply an occlusive dressing over the area, because this would increase the risk for systemic absorption. The nurse should also tell the patient not to apply the cream to any open or weeping areas and to stop using the drug if he develops blisters or a rash that is severe.
c. Additional instructions would include proper foot-care measures, including cleaning the feet with soap and water and patting them dry before applying the cream; wearing clean, dry cotton socks and keeping the feet dry; avoiding scratching of the area; and using cool compresses to help decrease the itching.

■ PRACTICING FOR NCLEX

1. **Answer: c**

RATIONALE: Ketoconazole blocks the activity of a sterol in the fungal wall. Posaconazole and voriconazole inhibit the synthesis of ergosterol, which in turn leads to an inability of the fungus to form a cell wall, resulting in cell death. Terbinafine inhibits a CYP2D6 enzyme system, which may make it a better choice for patients who need to take drugs metabolized by the CYP450 system; it also inhibits the formation of ergosterol.

2. **Answer: a**

RATIONALE: *Mycosis* is a term used to describe a disease that is caused by a fungus. So both parties are correct, and the nurse's response appropriately addresses the patient's concerns. Mycosis may be related to immunosuppression, but it refers to the disease caused by a fungus. Suggesting that the nurse and patient talk to the doctor indicates that there is some discrepancy between what the doctor said and what the patient thought, which is not the case.

Although the infection may be minor and treatable, telling the client not to worry does not address his concerns.

3. Answer: d

RATIONALE: Ketoconazole can be used systemically and topically to treat fungal infections. Butoconazole and clotrimazole are for topical use only. Voriconazole is for systemic use only.

4. Answer: b

RATIONALE: Amphotericin B is associated with bone marrow suppression, so it would be especially important for the nurse to monitor the patient's complete blood count for changes. The drug does not affect coagulation. Although the drug can cause gastrointestinal (GI) irritation with nausea, vomiting, and potentially severe diarrhea, monitoring bowel sounds would not be as important as monitoring the blood count. Amphotericin B does not affect respiratory function.

5. Answer: b

RATIONALE: Fluconazole, when given intravenously, peaks in 1 hour (60 minutes) and has a duration of action of 2 to 4 hours.

6. Answer: a

RATIONALE: The nurse should arrange for an appropriate culture and sensitivity test before beginning the therapy to ensure that the appropriate drug is being used. This should be done first. Once the specimen has been obtained, the nurse would evaluate renal and hepatic function test to determine baseline function and to determine the risk for possible toxicity during therapy. Not all systemic antifungals are administered intravenously, so inserting an intravenous access device may or may not be necessary.

7. Answer: c

RATIONALE: Topical antifungal agents are agents that are too toxic to be used systemically but are effective in the treatment of local infections. Typically, topical agents should be applied as a thin film. These agents can cause serious local irritation, burning, and pain. Systemic, not topical, antifungal agents are associated with many drug–drug interactions.

8. Answer: d

RATIONALE: Caspofungin is an example of an echinocandin antifungal. Terbinafine is an example of an azole antifungal agent. Nystatin and amphotericin B are examples other antifungals.

9. Answer: a

RATIONALE: Ketoconazole is not the drug of choice for patients with endocrine problems such as diabetes or those with fertility problems. Fluconazole is not associated with the endocrine problems seen with ketoconazole. Itraconazole and terbinafine are associated with liver failure and toxicity.

10. Answer: a, b, d

RATIONALE: Itraconazole has a black box warning regarding the potential for serious cardiovascular effects if it is given with simvastatin, midazolam, pimozide, lovastatin, triazolam, or dofetilide. Increased serum level of warfarin, digoxin, and cyclosporine occur when they are administered with ketoconazole due to the drug's strong inhibition of the cytochrome P450 enzyme system.

11. Answer: b

RATIONALE: Voriconazole should not be used with ergots alkaloids because ergotism can occur. In this situation, the nurse should recommend that the patient not use the ergot until the antifungal therapy is finished.

12. Answer: d

RATIONALE: Serum flucytosine levels greater than 100 mcg/mL are associated with toxicity.

13. Answer: c

RATIONALE: Patients receiving amphotericin B should not take other nephrotoxic drugs such as gentamicin unless absolutely necessary because of the increased risk of severe renal toxicity. Penicillin, amantadine, and aztreonam are not associated with an increased risk for renal dysfunction if given with amphotericin B.

14. Answer: b

RATIONALE: If the patient experiences GI upset, the nurse should suggest that the patient take the drug with food or meals and to try eating small frequent meals instead of three large meals. There is no need to call the prescriber to change the drug unless the patient experiences severe nausea and vomiting, which could interfere with his nutritional status. Advising the patient to sit upright may or may not be helpful.

15. Answer: c

RATIONALE: Sulconazole should not be used longer than 6 weeks due to the risk of adverse effects and possible emergency of resistant strains of fungi. Naftifine, oxiconazole, sertaconazole nitrate, and terbinafine should not be used longer than 4 weeks.

CHAPTER 12

■ ASSESSING YOUR UNDERSTANDING

FILL IN THE BLANKS

1. Trophozoite
2. Malaria
3. Trichomoniasis
4. Trypanosomiasis
5. Protozoan

SEQUENCING

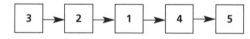

■ APPLYING YOUR KNOWLEDGE

CASE STUDY

a. The nurse needs to ask the patient about what he had to drink and eat during his camping trip. Giardiasis is transmitted through contaminated water or food. It would be important to find out if the patient had consumed unpurified water or contaminated food, such as fish from a contaminated stream or river or if he used the local water for cooking. The nurse also needs to inquire about hygiene facilities when camping because personal hygiene measures are essential to prevent the transmission of disease.

b. Tinidazole typically is ordered as a one-time single dose of 2 g. The nurse would need to instruct the patient to take this medication as a single dose with food.

c. The nurse should warn the patient not to consume alcohol with this drug to prevent severe adverse effects (disulfiram reaction). The nurse should advise the patient to avoid alcohol for at least 3 days after taking the single dose. Other areas to address include measures to ensure adequate fluid and nutritional intake, such as clear fluids initially and then gradually advancing diet as tolerated, with an emphasis on increased fluid intake and small frequent meals; possible adverse effects such as central nervous system effects; and warning signs that need to be

Copyright © 2011 by Wolters Kluwer Health | Lippincott Williams & Wilkins. *Study Guide for Focus on Nursing Pharmacology.*

reported, such as an increase in his gastrointestinal (GI) symptoms or development of signs and symptoms of another infection, like fever and chills.

■ PRACTICING FOR NCLEX

1. Answer: c
RATIONALE: Antimalarial drugs are usually given in combination form to attack the parasite at various stages of its life cycle, thereby preventing the acute malarial reaction in individuals who have been infected with the parasite. Currently, chloroquine is the mainstay of antimalarial treatment. Quinine was the first drug found to be effective against malaria, but it is no longer available. Combination therapy is recommended because many strains of the parasite are developing resistance to chloroquine.

2. Answer: a
RATIONALE: Chloroquine enters the human red blood cells and changes the metabolic pathways necessary for reproduction. It is also directly toxic to the parasites that absorb it and, due to its acidity, decreases the ability of the parasite to create DNA. Mefloquine increases the acidity of the plasmodial food vacuoles, causing cell rupture and death. Pyrimethamine blocks the use of folic acid in protein synthesis. Primaquine disrupts the mitochondria.

3. Answer: b
RATIONALE: Pregnancy should be avoided during treatment with any of the antimalarial agents. For mefloquine, the patient should avoid pregnancy during therapy and for 2 months after the completion of therapy. Antimalarial agents are contraindicated for use with lactating women, so another method of feeding should be chosen if treatment is absolutely necessary.

4. Answer: a, b, f
RATIONALE: Cinchonism may occur with high levels of primaquine and is manifested by tinnitus, vomiting, vertigo, and nausea. Fever, dyspepsia, and rash are adverse effects associated with antimalarial agents not suggestive of cinchonism.

5. Answer: b
RATIONALE: Ophthalmologic evaluation would be most important, because these drugs are associated with visual changes including possible blindness due to retinal damage from the drug. Assessment of the patient's respiratory status and pupillary response would not be crucial. Assessing the patient's nutritional status would be helpful to establish a baseline if the patient experiences adverse GI effects. However, this assessment would be a lower priority than an ophthalmologic evaluation.

6. Answer: c
RATIONALE: Trichomoniasis is usually spread during sexual intercourse by men who have no signs and symptoms of the infection. A mosquito bite can transmit malaria. The common housefly is responsible for transmitting Chagas' disease. Drinking contaminated water is associated with giardiasis.

7. Answer: d
RATIONALE: Metronidazole combined with oral anticoagulants can lead to increased bleeding, necessitating dosage adjustments with the anticoagulant. Abdominal cramps, ataxia, and peripheral neuropathy (as manifested by paresthesias) are adverse effects that are associated with antiprotozoal agents and are unrelated to the use of the warfarin.

8. Answer: b
RATIONALE: Pentamidine is given as an inhalation or intramuscular or intravenous injection. It is not given orally, transdermally, or subcutaneously.

9. Answer: c
RATIONALE: A patient should not consume alcohol if he or she is taking metronidazole or tinidazole. Interaction with alcohol is not associated with pentamidine, atovaquone, or nitazoxanide use.

10. Answer: a
RATIONALE: Atovaquone is indicated for the prevention and treatment of *Pneumocystis carinii* pneumonia (PCP). Metronidazole or tinidazole is used to treat giardiasis, amebiasis, and trichomoniasis. Pentamidine can be used to treat trypanosomiasis.

11. Answer: d
RATIONALE: Leishmaniasis is treated with systemic pentamidine. Amebiasis is treated with metronidazole or tinidazole. Giardiasis may be treated with nitazoxanide. PCP is treated with oral atovaquone.

12. Answer: a
RATIONALE: Malaria results from the bite of an infected mosquito, most specifically the *Anopheles* mosquito. Consuming food grown in contaminated soil can lead to amebiasis. Consumption of unpurified spring water is associated with giardiasis. The bite of an infected tsetse fly leads to trypanosomiasis (African sleeping sickness).

13. Answer: b
RATIONALE: Protozoal infections are most common in tropical areas, where many people experience multiple infestations at the same time. Protozoa also survive and reproduce in any area where people live in very crowded and unsanitary conditions. Insect control has helped to control the various insects associated with these infections; however, the rise of insecticide-resistant insects such as mosquitoes has allowed the infections to continue to flourish.

14. Answer: a
RATIONALE: The person who is bitten by an infected mosquito is injected with thousands of sporozoites that then undergo asexual cell division and reproduction. Trophozoites form, which lead to the formation of schizonts and then merozoites, which enter the circulation and invade red blood cells.

15. Answer: a
RATIONALE: Chloroquine is considered a potent schizonticidal agent. Hydroxychloroquine has limited action at this phase. Primaquine is considered a potent gametocytocidal agent. Primaquine and pyrimethamine are considered important prophylactic agents.

CHAPTER 13

■ ASSESSING YOUR UNDERSTANDING

SHORT ANSWER

1. Infections by nematodes include pinworms, whipworms, threadworms, Ascaris, and hookworms.
2. Pinworms are the most common helminthic infection in school-age children in the United States.
3. Nematodes are roundworms; platyhelminths are flatworms. Both cause intestine-invading worm infections.
4. A helminth is a worm that can cause disease by invading the body.
5. Trichinosis is the disease that is caused by the ingestion of the encysted larvae of the roundworm in undercooked pork.

MATCHING

1. c   2. d   3. a   4. e   5. b

Copyright © 2011 by Wolters Kluwer Health l Lippincott Williams & Wilkins. *Study Guide for Focus on Nursing Pharmacology.*

■ APPLYING YOUR KNOWLEDGE
CASE STUDY

a. Pinworms spread rapidly among children in schools, summer camps, and other institutions. Inadequate hygiene measures at the summer camp and the close proximity of children in the camp, possibly sharing clothing or other items, may have contributed to the transmission of the infection. The worm eggs are ingested either from transfer by touching the eggs when they are shed to clothing, toys, or bedding or by inhaling the eggs that become airborne and then are swallowed.

b. The nurse needs to respond to the mother in a supportive and nonjudgmental manner, emphasizing that the infection is not a reflection of hygiene measures or lifestyle. The nurse needs to clarify any misconceptions that the mother may have, reminding the mother that pinworms is the most common helminthic infection among school-age children.

c. The child is to receive mebendazole (available in chewable form), which is given orally in the morning and evening for three consecutive days. If necessary, the nurse should assist the mother in making up a schedule to ensure compliance with the therapy, informing the mother that the regimen may need to be repeated in 3 weeks if the infection does not clear. In addition, the nurse should review the common adverse effects of the drug, such as abdominal discomfort, diarrhea, or pain and suggest to the mother to give the drug with meals or food to minimize any gastrointestinal upset that may occur. Other instructions should address hygiene measures such as frequent hand washing, especially after using the toilet; keeping the child's nails short; showering in the morning to remove any eggs deposited in the anal area; changing and washing undergarments, bed linens, and other clothing every day; and disinfecting the toilet facilities.

■ PRACTICING FOR NCLEX

1. Answer: d
RATIONALE: Tapeworms are cestodes—segmented flatworms that cause infection. Pinworms, whipworms, and Ascaris are roundworm infections.

2. Answer: b
RATIONALE: Trichinosis is caused by the ingestion of encrusted larvae of the roundworm in undercooked pork. Consumption of unwashed vegetables would lead to Ascaris. A recent insect bite would be associated with causing filariasis. Swimming in a contaminated lake could lead to schistosomiasis.

3. Answer: c
RATIONALE: Mebendazole is considered the prototype anthelmintic agent.

4. Answer: a
RATIONALE: Ascaris is an intestinal-invading worm infection. Trichinosis, filariasis, and schistosomiasis are examples of tissue-invading worm infections.

5. Answer: c
RATIONALE: Pyrantel may be preferred especially for patients who have trouble remembering to take medications or following drug regimens because it is administered as a single one-time dose. It is not administered monthly. All anthelmintic agents are effective in eradicating the infection. Mebendazole is available in chewable form.

6. Answer: c
RATIONALE: Mebendazole is not metabolized in the body. Very little of the drug is absorbed systemically, so adverse effects are few. Most of the drug is excreted unchanged in the feces.

7. Answer: c
RATIONALE: Praziquantel is administered orally in three doses every 4 to 6 hours over a period of 1 day. Mebendazole, a chewable tablet, is administered every morning and evening for a period of 3 days. Ivermectin and pyrantel are administered as a single one-time dose.

8. Answer: b
RATIONALE: Albendazole is associated with bone marrow depression and renal failure. Stevens–Johnson syndrome is associated with thiabendazole use. Diarrhea and fever are adverse effects associated with mebendazole and pyrantel.

9. Answer: d
RATIONALE: Filariasis occurs when worm embryos enter the body via insect bites. Swimming in contaminated water with snail-deposited larvae causes schistosomiasis. Consuming undercooked fish containing the larvae of cestodes leads to a tapeworm infection. Eating unwashed vegetables grown in contaminated soil can cause Ascaris.

10. Answer: c
RATIONALE: The drug of choice for treating a threadworm infection is thiabendazole. Ivermectin is a second choice for treatment. Pyrantel is used to treat pinworms and roundworms. Praziquantel is used to treat a wide number of schistosomes or flukes.

11. Answer: a
RATIONALE: With a whipworm infection, bloody diarrhea and colic may be noted. Pneumonia is associated with a threadworm infection. Fatigue suggests a hookworm infection. Weight loss is associated with a tapeworm infection.

12. Answer: d
RATIONALE: For proper diagnosis of a helminthic infection, a stool examination for ova and parasites is essential. A complete blood count may help to identify anemia associated with a hookworm infection. A urinalysis may be done to establish a baseline but would provide no information about the infection. Liver function tests would be appropriate before administering therapy to ensure adequate liver function and evaluate for possible toxicity related to drug therapy but would not provide information about the helminthic infection.

13. Answer: a
RATIONALE: Toilets should be cleaned daily. Other measures including thorough and frequent hand washing, especially after using the bathroom; consistently washing any fresh fruits and vegetables, and using hot, chlorine-treated water for laundering clothes and bed linens.

14. Answer: b
RATIONALE: Threadworm infections can cause more damage to the human than most other helminths, possibly leading to death from pneumonia or from lung or liver abscesses that result from larval invasion. Ascaris is the most prevalent helminthic infection worldwide. Schistosomiasis is a common problem in parts of Africa, Asia, and certain South American and Caribbean countries. Pinworm infection is the most common helminthic infection among school-age children.

15. Answer: c
RATIONALE: Trichinosis is caused by the ingestion of undercooked pork, so the nurse should emphasize the need to thoroughly cook any pork products. Washing hands after working with soil would help to minimize the risk for threadworm or whipworm infections. Avoiding swimming in waters that may be contaminated would be helpful in preventing schistosomiasis. Protection from insect bites would be helpful in preventing filariasis.

Copyright © 2011 by Wolters Kluwer Health | Lippincott Williams & Wilkins. *Study Guide for Focus on Nursing Pharmacology.*

CHAPTER 14

■ ASSESSING YOUR UNDERSTANDING

CROSSWORD

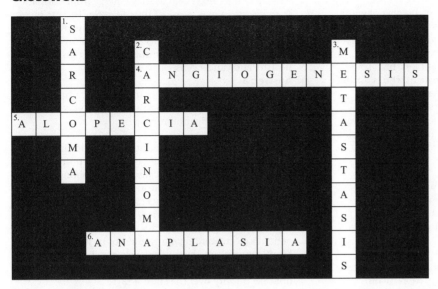

SHORT ANSWER

1. The two major groups of cancer are solid tumors and hematologic malignancies.
2. All cancers start with a single cell that is genetically different from other cells in the surrounding tissue. The cell divides, passing it abnormalities to daughter cells and eventually producing a tumor or neoplasm that has characteristics quite different from the original tissue.
3. Antineoplastic drugs work by affecting cell survival or by boosting the immune system in its efforts to combat abnormal cells.
4. Most cancer patients are not considered cured until they have been cancer free for a period of 5 years due to the possibility that cancer cells will emerge from dormancy to cause new tumors or problems. No cells yet have been identified that can remain dormant for longer than 5 years, so the chances of the emergence of one after that time are very slim.
5. Alkylating agents can affect cells even in the resting phase of the cell cycle, thus they are said to be non–cell cycle specific.
6. Mitotic inhibitors kill cells as the process of mitosis begins in the M phase of the cell cycle.

■ APPLYING YOUR KNOWLEDGE

CASE STUDY

a. The nurse needs to respond to the patient's concerns honestly and with empathy. The nurse should acknowledge the patient's concern and then provide the patient with information about the possible adverse effects of the two drugs. Cisplatin is an alkylating agent; paclitaxel is a mitotic inhibitor. Both are associated with neurologic adverse effects and hypersensitivity reactions. Alopecia and bone marrow suppression may occur with both drugs. In addition, cisplatin can be nephrotoxic, and paclitaxel can be cardiotoxic.

The patient is visibly anxious, so it would be appropriate to provide the patient with written handouts and pamphlets about her therapy so that the patient can review them and then ask questions on the next visit. The patient also needs information about the usual protocol, including how the drugs will be given and any special devices, such as a central venous access device (port) that may need to be inserted for administration. The nurse also needs to provide the patient with information about measures to address the typical adverse effects such as frequent rest periods, small frequent meals, increased fluid intake, and scarves/wigs for hair loss. In addition, the nurse should explain any medications that may be ordered to manage the adverse effects, such as using antiemetics before chemotherapy sessions to reduce the risk of nausea and vomiting and the use of amifostine to protect the healthy cells from the toxic effects of cisplatin. Some protocols also include the use of intravenous fluids to ensure adequate hydration and antihistamines to reduce the risk of hypersensitivity reactions. The nurse should review the protocols with the patient.

b. Cisplatin is given intravenously every 3 weeks; paclitaxel is administered intravenously over 3 hours every 3 weeks. Therefore, the nurse needs to explain the schedule to the patient and assist her in estimating the amount of time that will be required for the chemotherapy sessions, possibly suggesting some activity such as reading or listening to music to help pass the time. Since the patient may experience some fatigue related to the therapy, it might be helpful for the nurse to suggest that someone be available to transport the patient to and from the facility where the therapy will be administered.

■ PRACTICING FOR NCLEX

1. **Answer: d**
   RATIONALE: Vincristine is classified as a mitotic inhibitor. Fluorouracil and methotrexate are classified as antimetabolites. Chlorambucil is classified as an alkylating agent.
2. **Answer: a**
   RATIONALE: Odansetron blocks serotonin receptors in the chemoreceptor trigger zone (CTZ) and is one of the most

Copyright © 2011 by Wolters Kluwer Health I Lippincott Williams & Wilkins. *Study Guide for Focus on Nursing Pharmacology.*

effective antiemetics. Antihistamines help to reduce the risk of hypersensitivity reactions and decrease secretions; corticosteroids help to relieve inflammation and may aid in reducing possible hypersensitivity.

3. Answer: c

RATIONALE: Leukopenia indicates that the number of white blood cells is low. Subsequently, the patient is at risk for infection because adequate white blood cells are not present to mount a response. Disturbed body image might result from alopecia or significant weight loss. Imbalanced nutrition may be appropriate for the patient who is unable to consume adequate calories or nutrients secondary to nausea and vomiting. Deficient fluid volume would be appropriate for a patient who is experiencing an increase in fluid loss through vomiting or diarrhea or who is unable to consume adequate amounts of fluid by mouth due to nausea or vomiting.

4. Answer: d

RATIONALE: Methotrexate is absorbed well from the gastrointestinal (GI) tract and can be administered orally. Cytarabine, fluorouracil, and gemcitabine must be administered parenterally because they are not absorbed well from the GI tract.

5. Answer: b

RATIONALE: Leucovorin is administered to counteract the effects of treatment with methotrexate. Alprazolam, metoclopramide, and aprepitant are used to help alleviate the nausea and vomiting associated with chemotherapy.

6. Answer: c

RATIONALE: Antimetabolites inhibit DNA production in cells that depend on certain natural metabolites to produce DNA, replacing the needed metabolites, which prevents normal cellular function. Alkylating agents react chemically with portions of the RNA, DNA, or other cellular proteins. Antineoplastic antibiotics interfere with cellular DNA synthesis by inserting themselves between base pairs in the DNA chain. Mitotic inhibitors interfere with the ability of a cell to divide, blocking or altering DNA synthesis.

7. Answer: b

RATIONALE: Imatinib belongs to the group of drugs called *protein tyrosine kinase inhibitors*, which do not affect healthy human cells. Etoposide and vincristine, both mitotic inhibitors, and doxorubicin, an antineoplastic antibiotic, damage both healthy and cancer cells.

8. Answer: d

RATIONALE: Tamoxifen belongs to the group of drugs that are hormones or hormone modulators. These agents are hormone specific. This drug competes with estrogen at the receptor sites, ultimately blocking estrogen. The adverse effects specific to this action would involve menopause-associated effects. Bone marrow suppression, GI toxicity, and hepatic dysfunction occur with this drug, but these are not specific to the drug's action.

9. Answer: a

RATIONALE: The adverse effects associated with imatinib include GI upset, muscle cramps, heart failure, fluid retention, and skin rash. Thus a nursing diagnosis of excess fluid volume would be most likely. The severe bone marrow suppression, alopecia, and severe GI effects associated with the more traditional antineoplastic therapy do not occur.

10. Answer: b

RATIONALE: Cancer cells tend to move through the cell cycle at about the same rate as their cells of origin. Malignant cells that remain in a dormant phase for long periods are difficult to destroy. These cells can emerge long

after cancer treatment has finished—after weeks, months, or years—to begin their division and growth cycle all over again. Therefore, antineoplastic agents are often given in sequence over periods of time, in the hope that the drugs will affect the cancer cells as they emerge from dormancy or move into a new phase of the cell cycle. The use of cycles is unrelated to allowing the body to recover. A person is said to be cured of cancer only after a 5-year period of being cancer free. Most antineoplastic agents destroy healthy and cancer cells.

11. Answer: a

RATIONALE: Mitomycin is an example of an antineoplastic antibiotic. Teniposide, vinblastine, and docetaxel are examples of mitotic inhibitors.

12. Answer: c

RATIONALE: Bleomycin is associated with pulmonary fibrosis. Therefore, the nurse would need to monitor the patient's chest x-ray periodically. Although bone marrow suppression can occur, monitoring the patient's platelet count would be less of a concern when compared to the risks associated with pulmonary fibrosis. The drug is not associated with cardiac toxicity, so monitoring the patient's electrocardiogram would not be warranted. Monitoring serum electrolyte levels may be indicated if the patient is experience severe GI effects, but this would not take priority over the chest x-rays.

13. Answer: d

RATIONALE: The majority of agents used to control nausea and vomiting secondary to chemotherapy directly block the CTZ. They do not affect neurotransmitters, gastric acidity, or the gag reflex.

14. Answer: a

RATIONALE: Imatinib is administered orally.

15. Answer: b

RATIONALE: Angiogenesis refers to the process in which abnormal cells release enzymes that generate blood vessels in the area to supply both oxygen and nutrients to the cells. Metastasis refers to process of traveling from the place of origin to develop new tumors in other areas of the body. Autonomy refers to the process of growing without the usual homeostatic restrictions that regulate cell growth and control. Anaplasia refers to the process in which the cells lose their ability to differentiate and organize, which leads to a loss in their ability to function normally.

CHAPTER 15

■ ASSESSING YOUR UNDERSTANDING

MATCHING

1. b	**2.** e	**3.** c	**4.** g	**5.** h
6. a	**7.** d	**8.** f		

FILL IN THE BLANKS

1. Kinin
2. Mast
3. Antibodies or immunoglobulins
4. Chemotaxis
5. Phagocytosis

■ APPLYING YOUR KNOWLEDGE

CASE STUDY

a. The patient is exhibiting three of the four cardinal signs of an inflammatory reaction. The patient's throat is red (rubor), swollen (tumor), and he has pain (dolor). The

Copyright © 2011 by Wolters Kluwer Health | Lippincott Williams & Wilkins. *Study Guide for Focus on Nursing Pharmacology*.

throat is not touched to determine if it is warm (calor). In addition, the patient also has a fever, which is most likely due to the release of a natural pyrogen by the neutrophils engulfing and digesting the invader. In addition, leukotrienes are being released to induce slow-wave sleep as an energy conservation measure, which is reflected by the patient's malaise and complaints of feeling tired.

b. Pathogens introduced in the body via the respiratory tract will meet up with B cells in the tonsils and begin an immune response. Other mediators also may be involved. For example, interleukins, which stimulate the T and B cells, also cause fever and slow-wave sleep induction.

■ PRACTICING FOR NCLEX

1. **Answer: d**
RATIONALE: The major histocompatibility complex is the body's last barrier of defense, which involves the ability to distinguish between self-cells and foreign cells. The skin is considered the body's first line of defense. The mucous membranes and gastric acid are also two other body defenses.

2. **Answer: c**
RATIONALE: Lymphocytes include T cells, B cells, and natural killer cells. Neutrophils and monocytes or macrophages are types of myelocytes.

3. **Answer: a**
RATIONALE: Neutrophils are capable of engulfing and digesting foreign material, or phagocytosis. Basophils contain chemical mediators important for initiating and maintaining an immune or inflammatory response. The exact function of eosinophils is unknown. Macrophages release chemicals necessary to elicit a strong inflammatory reaction.

4. **Answer: d**
RATIONALE: Histamine is a substance released when a cell membrane is injured and is not considered lymphoid tissue. Bone marrow, the thymus gland, and the spleen are lymphoid tissues.

5. **Answer: b**
RATIONALE: Bradykinin causes local vasodilation and also stimulates nerve endings to cause pain. Vasoconstriction and platelet aggregation result from the action of thromboxanes. Swelling results from the change in capillary permeability resulting from leukotrienes and histamine.

6. **Answer: a**
RATIONALE: Cell injury causes activation of the Hageman factor, which in turn activates kallikrein, leading to the conversion of kininogen to bradykinin. Bradykinin causes the release of arachidonic acid, which also causes the release of autocoids, such as prostaglandins, leukotrienes, and thromboxanes.

7. **Answer: b**
RATIONALE: Warmth or heat and redness are due to vasodilation. Activation of the nerve fibers would be noted as pain. Fluid leakage into tissues would be assessed as swelling. Pyrogen release would result in a fever.

8. **Answer: a**
RATIONALE: T cells provide cell-mediated immunity. B cells provide humoral immunity, which involves antibody or immunoglobulin production. Neutrophils are not associated with either cell-mediated or humoral immunity.

9. **Answer: a**
RATIONALE: Immunoglobulin M is the first immunoglobulin released and contains antibodies produced at the first exposure to the antigen. Immunoglobulin G contains antibodies made by the memory cells. Immunoglobulin A is secreted by plasma cells in the gastrointestinal and respiratory tracts and in epithelial cells. Immunoglobulin E appears to be involved with allergic responses and activation of mast cells.

10. **Answer: c**
RATIONALE: Interleukin-1 stimulates T and B cells to initiate an immune response. Thymosin is a thymus hormone that is important in the maturation of T cells and cell-mediated immunity. Tumor necrosis factor is a chemical released by macrophages that inhibits tumor growth. Interferons are chemicals secreted by cells that have been invaded by viruses to prevent viral replication and also suppress malignant cell replication and tumor growth.

11. **Answer: b**
RATIONALE: Autoimmune disease occurs when the body responds to specific self-antigens to produce antibodies or cell-mediated immune responses against its own cells. Rejection occurs in response to foreign cells introduced into the body. Viral invasion results in an alteration of the cell membrane and antigenic presentation of the cell. Neoplastic growth occurs when mutant cells escape the normal surveillance of the immune system and begin to grow and multiply.

12. **Answer: d**
RATIONALE: Mucus is sticky and traps invaders and inactivates them for later destruction and removal by the body. It does not promote their removal. Cilia sweep away captured pathogens and also move them to an area, causing irritation and leading to removal by coughing or sneezing.

13. **Answer: c**
RATIONALE: Mast cells are basophils that are fixed and do not circulate. Mature leukocytes are monocytes or macrophages. Eosinophils are circulating myelocytic leukocytes. Neutrophils are phagocytes.

14. **Answer: a**
RATIONALE: The lymph nodes store concentrated populations of neutrophils, basophils, eosinophils, and lymphocytes in areas of the body that facilitate their surveillance for and destruction of foreign proteins. The thymus gland is responsible for the final differentiation of T cells and for regulating the actions of the immune system. The bone marrow plays a role in differentiating the cellular components.

15. **Answer: c**
RATIONALE: All transplants, except autotransplantation, produce an immune response. Therefore, matching a donor's HLA markers as closely as possible to those of the recipient for histocompatibility is essential. The more closely the foreign cells can be matched, the less aggressive the immune reaction will be to the donated tissue.

CHAPTER 16

■ ASSESSING YOUR UNDERSTANDING
MATCHING
1. c **2.** b **3.** a **4.** d **5.** e
SHORT ANSWER
1. The prototype salicylate drug is aspirin.
2. Because many anti-inflammatory drugs are available over the counter (OTC), there is a potential for abuse and overdosing. They also block the signs and symptoms of a

Copyright © 2011 by Wolters Kluwer Health l Lippincott Williams & Wilkins. *Study Guide for Focus on Nursing Pharmacology.*

present illness, thus potentially causing the misdiagnosis of a problem. Patients also may combine these drugs and unknowingly induce toxicity.

3. Signs of salicylate toxicity include hyperpnea; tachypnea; hemorrhage; excitement; confusion; pulmonary edema; convulsions; tetany; metabolic acidosis; fever; coma; and cardiovascular, renal, and respiratory collapse.

4. Cyclooxygenase-1 (COX-1) is present in all tissues and seems to be involved in many body functions, including blood clotting, protecting the stomach lining, and maintaining sodium and water balance in the kidneys. COX-1 turns arachidonic acid into prostaglandins as needed in a variety of tissues. Cyclooxygenase-2 (COX-2) is active at sites of trauma or injury when more prostaglandins are needed, but it does not seem to be involved in the other tissue functions.

5. Salicylism is a syndrome that is associated with high levels of salicylates.

■ APPLYING YOUR KNOWLEDGE
CASE STUDY

a. The nurse needs to find out if the patient is experiencing any other signs and symptoms of bleeding, including any prolonged bleeding from cuts, nosebleeds, or upper gastrointestinal (GI) bleeding. The nurse should also test the patient's stool for blood to determine if there is blood in the stool. Changes in stool color may be related to other factors such as food. Additionally, the nurse should inquire about the duration of use for the ibuprofen and the actual frequency as well as how the patient takes the drug. For example, does the patient routinely take the drug every day, three times a day? How long has he been taking it? Does the patient take the drug on an empty stomach, or does he take it with food? The nurse also needs to inquire about any other drugs that the patient may be using that could interact with the ibuprofen. Moreover, the nurse would need to assess the patient's vital signs for changes and monitor laboratory test results, such as complete blood count, and coagulation studies to determine if the patient is experiencing blood loss leading to anemia or to evaluate his clotting abilities.

b. Teaching should address administration measures such as taking the drug with food or meals to prevent gastric irritation, safety measures to prevent injury and bruising, oral care measures such as using a soft toothbrush and gentle brushing, and danger signs and symptoms such as increased bleeding as well as any follow-up laboratory testing that may be necessary. Depending on the evaluation, the ibuprofen may need to be stopped, and another analgesic may need to be prescribed. If this is the case, then patient teaching would focus on the new drug and the reasons for stopping the ibuprofen.

■ PRACTICING FOR NCLEX

1. **Answer: c**
   RATIONALE: Acetaminophen has analgesic and antipyretic properties but does not exert an anti-inflammatory effect. Therefore, it would not be indicated for joint inflammation. Ibuprofen, naproxen, and diclofenac have anti-inflammatory properties and would be appropriate for use.

2. **Answer: d**
   RATIONALE: Mesalamine or olsalazine would be appropriate for a patient with inflammatory bowel disease. Diflunisal is indicated for the treatment of moderate pain and arthritis in adults; aspirin is used for the treatment of fever, pain, and inflammatory conditions. Choline magnesium

trisalicylate is indicated for the relief of mild pain, fever, and arthritis.

3. **Answer: a**
   RATIONALE: All anti-inflammatory drugs available OTC have adverse effects that can be dangerous if toxic levels of the drug circulate in the body. Since these drugs are available OTC, there is a potential for abuse and overdosing. In addition, these drugs block the signs and symptoms of a present illness. OTC agents, if combined with other drugs, can induce toxicity.

4. **Answer: b**
   RATIONALE: Salicylism can occur with high levels of aspirin and be manifested by ringing in the ears, dizziness, difficulty hearing, nausea, vomiting, diarrhea, mental confusion, and lassitude. Excitement, tachypnea, and convulsions suggest acute salicylate toxicity.

5. **Answer: a**
   RATIONALE: Care must be taken to make sure that the child receives the correct dose of any anti-inflammatory agent. This can be a problem because many of these drugs are available in OTC pain, cold, flu, and combination products. Parents need to be taught to read the label to find out the ingredients and the dosage they are giving the child. Aspirin for flulike symptoms in children is to be avoided due to the increased risk for Reye's syndrome. Children are more susceptible to the GI and central nervous system effects of these drugs, so the drugs should be given with food or meals. Acetaminophen is the most used anti-inflammatory drug for children. However, parents need to be cautioned to avoid overdosage, which can lead to severe hepatotoxicity.

6. **Answer: c**
   RATIONALE: Salicylates are contraindicated for patients who have had surgery within the past week because of the increased risk for bleeding. Their use in patients with an allergy to salicylates or tartrazine would increase the risk for an allergic reaction. Their use in patients with impaired renal function may increase the risk for toxicity because the drug is excreted in the urine. There is no associated risk for fluid imbalance and salicylate therapy.

7. **Answer: d**
   RATIONALE: Nonsteroidal anti-inflammatory drugs (NSAIDs) inhibit prostaglandin synthesis. Salicylates block prostaglandin activity. Acetaminophen acts directly on thermoregulatory cells in the hypothalamus. Gold salts inhibit phagocytosis.

8. **Answer: c**
   RATIONALE: Aurothioglucose is administered by intramuscular injection. Auranofin is given orally. Anakinra and etanercept are administered subcutaneously. None of the antiarthritic drugs are given intravenously.

9. **Answer: b**
   RATIONALE: Gold salts do not repair damage but rather help to prevent further damage. They are indicated for patients whose disease has been unresponsive to standard therapy. They are most effective if used early in the disease. Gold salts are highly toxic.

10. **Answer: d**
    RATIONALE: Gold salts should not be combined with penicillamine, cytotoxic drugs, immunosuppressive agents, or antimalarials other than low-dose corticosteroids because of the potential for severe toxicity.

11. **Answer: a**
    RATIONALE: Sulindac is an NSAID. Etanercept, adalimumab, and methotrexate are classified as disease-modifying antirheumatic drugs.

Copyright © 2011 by Wolters Kluwer Health | Lippincott Williams & Wilkins. *Study Guide for Focus on Nursing Pharmacology.*

12. **Answer: c**

RATIONALE: Anakinra blocks the increased interleukin-1 responsible for the degradation of cartilage in rheumatoid arthritis. Etanercept reacts with free-floating tumor necrosis factor released by active leukocytes in autoimmune inflammatory disease to prevent damage caused by tumor necrosis factor. Leflunomide directly inhibits an enzyme, dihydroorotate dehydrogenase (DHODH), that is active in the autoimmune process. Penicillamine lowers immunoglobulin M rheumatoid factor levels.

13. **Answer: d**

RATIONALE: Hyaluronidase derivatives, such as sodium hyaluronate and hylan G-F 20, have elastic and viscous properties. These drugs are injected directly into the joints of patients with severe rheumatoid arthritis of the knee. Aurothioglucose is a gold salt that is administered subcutaneously. Penicillamine is administered orally, and etanercept is administered subcutaneously.

14. **Answer: b**

RATIONALE: COX-2 receptors block platelet clumping. COX-1 receptors maintain renal function, provide for gastric mucosal integrity, and promote vascular hemostasis.

15. **Answer: b**

RATIONALE: Although adequate hydration is important to promote renal function and drug excretion, it would be more important to instruct the patient in the signs and symptoms of GI bleeding. Blacks have a documented decreased sensitivity to the pain-relieving effects of many anti-inflammatory agents and have an increased risk of developing GI adverse effects to these drugs. Increased dosages may be needed to achieve pain relief, but the increased dosage increases the patient's risk for developing adverse GI effects. The drug should not be combined with an OTC salicylate, as this would further increase the patient's risk for adverse GI effects. The patient should be instructed to use nonpharmacologic measures to relieve pain, such as warm soaks and positioning.

CHAPTER 17

■ ASSESSING YOUR UNDERSTANDING

LABELING

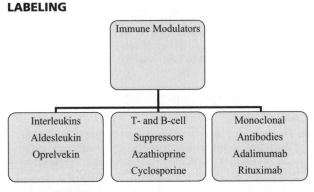

SHORT ANSWER

1. Immune stimulants include the interferons and interleukins.
2. The interleukin receptor antagonist is anakinra.
3. With the exception of erlotinib, which is given orally, all of the monoclonal antibodies are injected either intramuscularly, intravenously, or subcutaneously.
4. The exact mechanism of action of the T- and B-cell suppressors is not clearly understood. It has been shown

that they do block antibody production by B cells, inhibit suppressor and helper T cells, and modify the release of interleukins and T-cell growth factor.
5. Patients receiving immune suppressants have an increased susceptibility to infection and an increased risk of neoplasm.

■ APPLYING YOUR KNOWLEDGE

CASE STUDY

a. The nurse would need to explain to the patient that interferons are considered immune stimulants, and they act like the substances naturally produced and released by the cells in response to a virus or other stimuli. The nurse needs to correlate the drug's action with the underlying pathophysiologic events associated with multiple sclerosis as an autoimmune disorder. In addition, the nurse would explain that these drugs may help to reduce the frequency and duration of the episodes.

b. One of two interferons may be prescribed: interferon beta-1a or interferon beta-1b. Interferon beta-1a is administered intramuscularly once a week; interferon beta-1b is administered subcutaneously every other day.

c. Patient teaching should include information about the drug, its actions, and the method for administration. The patient may need to learn how to self-administer the injection, if indicated. In addition, the nurse needs to teach the patient about possible adverse effects, such as flulike symptoms (due to stimulation of the immune and inflammatory response), and other effects, such as headache, dizziness, bone marrow depression, depression, suicidal ideation, photosensitivity, and liver impairment. If the patient is of childbearing age, the nurse needs to recommend the use of barrier contraception to avoid pregnancy.

■ PRACTICING FOR NCLEX

1. **Answer: a**

RATIONALE: Interferon alfa-2b would be classified as an immune stimulant. Abatacept, mycophenolate, and sirolimus are T- and B-cell suppressors that are immune suppressants.

2. **Answer: c**

RATIONALE: Oprelvekin has been associated with severe hypersensitivity reactions, as manifested by chest tightness, difficulty breathing or swallowing, or swelling. Cardiac arrhythmias and mental status changes are adverse effects associated with interleukin therapy and do not suggest hypersensitivity. Fever is associated with the flulike adverse effects of interleukin therapy, not hypersensitivity.

3. **Answer: b**

RATIONALE: Cyclosporine is administered orally. Alefacept is administered as an intravenous bolus or intramuscularly; glatiramer acetate is administered subcutaneously; and abatacept is given intravenously.

4. **Answer: d**

RATIONALE: Supportive care and comfort measures are appropriate, including drinking plenty of fluids, using acetaminophen for fever or aches and pains, maintaining a comfortable environment such as one that is neither too warm nor too cool, and getting plenty of rest.

5. **Answer: c**

RATIONALE: Cetuximab is antibody specific to epidermal growth factor receptor sites. Muromonab-CD3 is a T-cell–specific antibody. Infliximab and adalimumab are antibodies specific for human tumor necrosis factors.

Copyright © 2011 by Wolters Kluwer Health I Lippincott Williams & Wilkins. *Study Guide for Focus on Nursing Pharmacology.*

6. Answer: a

RATIONALE: Erlotinib, a monoclonal antibody, is administered orally. All other monoclonal antibodies are administered parenterally.

7. Answer: d

RATIONALE: Pulmonary edema would be manifested by dyspnea, chest pain, and wheezing. Fever, chills, and myalgia suggest the development of a flulike adverse effect.

8. Answer: b

RATIONALE: Although safety measures and nutrition are important, it is essential to ensure that the patient is well hydrated because gemtuzumab is associated with fever after the infusion of the drug. A bedside commode would be appropriate if the patient experienced diarrhea and had difficulty getting to the bathroom.

9. Answer: c

RATIONALE: Mycophenolate is a T- and B-cell suppressor that is used in patients having transplants to reduce the risk of rejection. Subsequently, the patient is at high risk for infection. Acute pain, imbalanced nutrition, and deficient knowledge may be appropriate, but the risk for infection would be the priority.

10. Answer: d

RATIONALE: Interferons and interleukins are immune stimulants; monoclonal antibodies, interleukin receptor antagonists, and T- and B-cell suppressors are immune suppressants.

11. Answer: b

RATIONALE: A number of interferons are produced by recombinant DNA technology, including interferon alfacon-1 (Infergen), interferon alfa-2b (Intron A), peginterferon alfa-2a (Pegasys), peginterferon alfa-2b (PEG-INTRON), and interferon beta-1b (Betaseron). Interferon alfa-n3 (Alferon N) is produced by harvesting human leukocytes. Interferon gamma-1b (Actimmune) is produced by *Escherichia coli* bacteria. Interferon beta-1a (Avonex) is produced from Chinese hamster ovary cells.

12. Answer: a

RATIONALE: Photosensitivity is a possible adverse effect, so the patient should avoid exposure to the sun and ultraviolet light, if possible, and wear protective clothing when outside. Fluid intake, use of acetaminophen, and follow-up laboratory testing are appropriate for a patient receiving interferons.

13. Answer: d

RATIONALE: Abatacept is indicated for a reduction in the signs and symptoms and the slowing of structural damage in adults with rheumatoid arthritis who have had inadequate response to other drugs. Alefacept is appropriate for patients with moderate to severe chronic plaque psoriasis who are candidates for systemic therapy. Azathioprine is indicated for the prevention of transplant rejection. Glatiramer is used to reduce the number of relapses in multiple sclerosis patients.

14. Answer: b

RATIONALE: Patients receiving anakinra and etanercept must be monitored closely for severe and even life-threatening infections. The combination is not associated with anemia, bleeding, or hypersensitivity.

15. Answer: a

RATIONALE: Muromonab-CD3 is a T-cell–specific antibody. Adalimumab, certolizumab, and infliximab are antibodies specific for human tumor necrosis factor. Alemtuzumab is an antibody specific for lymphocyte receptor sites. Basiliximab and daclizumab are specific to interleukin-2 receptor sites on activated T cells.

CHAPTER 18

■ ASSESSING YOUR UNDERSTANDING

FILL IN THE BLANKS

1. Antitoxins
2. Vaccines
3. Serum sickness
4. Passive
5. Immunization
6. Smallpox
7. Immunoglobulin G
8. Antivenin

SHORT ANSWER

1. Active immunity occurs when the body recognizes a foreign protein and begins producing antibodies to react with that specific protein or antigen. After plasma cells are formed to produce antibodies, specific memory cells that produce the same antibodies are created. If the specific foreign protein is introduced into the body again, these memory cells react immediately to release antibodies. This type of immunity is thought to be lifelong. Passive immunity occurs when preformed antibodies are injected into the system and react with a specific antigen. These antibodies come from animals that have been infected with the disease or from humans who have had the disease and have developed antibodies. The circulating antibodies act in the same manner as those produced from plasma cells, recognizing the foreign protein and attaching to it, rendering it harmless. Unlike active immunity, passive immunity is limited. It lasts only as long as the circulating antibodies last because the body does not produce its own antibodies.

2. Serum sickness is manifested by fever, arthritis, flank pain, myalgia, and arthralgia.

3. The human papilloma virus (HPV) vaccine, Gardasil, is recommended for girls ages 9 to 26 years, being most effective when given before HPV infection occurs. It is best given before a girl becomes sexually active.

4. Older adults should receive yearly flu and pneumococcal vaccines as well as a tetanus booster every 10 years.

5. The bacillus Calmette-Guérin (BCG) vaccine for tuberculosis is widely used throughout the world, in countries with a high incidence of tuberculosis to limit the spread of the disease. However, the vaccine is not routinely used in the United States because the incidence of tuberculosis is relatively low, and it can induce false-positive tuberculin skin test results.

■ APPLYING YOUR KNOWLEDGE

CASE STUDY

a. There is some controversy surrounding the HPV vaccine. The nurse needs to listen to the mother's concerns and address each of them, specifically providing the mother with accurate information about the vaccine.

b. The nurse should inform the mother that the vaccine is effective against certain but not all types of HPV (types 16 and 18, which account for 70% of cervical cancers, and types 6 and 11, which are responsible for 90% of genital warts). In addition, it is only effective if it is given before HPV infection occurs. The nurse would need to stress that HPV infection is highly prevalent and does not always cause symptoms. Other information that the nurse needs to address is that the vaccine, which requires a series of

Copyright © 2011 by Wolters Kluwer Health | Lippincott Williams & Wilkins. *Study Guide for Focus on Nursing Pharmacology.*

three injections, can be expensive. Additionally, the nurse needs to address the questions posed by others such as the long-term effects and effectiveness of the vaccine, the belief that the vaccine will cause women to stop getting annual pelvic exams and Pap smears, and the misconception that the vaccine will lead to earlier or more frequent sexual activity among women who have had the vaccination.

c. The girl is within the recommended age for the vaccine. The vaccine is administered in a series of three injections. The nurse practitioner could administer the first dose with this visit, then administer the second dose in approximately 2 months, followed by the third dose in about 6 months.

■ PRACTICING FOR NCLEX

1. **Answer: a**
   RATIONALE: Vaccines provide active immunity. They promote the formation of antibodies against a specific disease. The person experiences an immune response without having to suffer the full course of the disease. Severe reactions are rare.

2. **Answer: d**
   RATIONALE: The protein of an immunization could be an actual weakened bacterial cell membrane, the protein coat of a virus, or an actual virus (protein coat with the genetic fragment that makes up a virus) that has been chemically weakened and thus cannot cause disease. Immune sera refers to sera that contains antibodies to specific bacteria or viruses.

3. **Answer: b**
   RATIONALE: The patient would receive an immune sera, most specifically rabies immune globulin. A vaccine would be used to stimulate active immunity due to exposure to a specific disease. An antitoxin would be used to protect the person from toxins released by invading pathogens. Antivenin is used to protect against spider or snake bites.

4. **Answer: b**
   RATIONALE: There is no vaccine available for plague. There is a vaccine for anthrax, but it is available only for military use. There is a vaccine for smallpox and a botulinum toxoid for botulism.

5. **Answer: c**
   RATIONALE: The vaccine for tetanus is a toxoid. The vaccines for haemophilus influenza B and pneumococcal polyvalent are bacterial vaccines. Hepatitis A is a viral vaccine.

6. **Answer: d, e, f**
   RATIONALE: Caution should be used any time a vaccine is given to a child with a history of febrile convulsions or brain injury or in any condition in which a potential fever would be dangerous. Caution also should be used in the presence of any acute infection. An immune deficiency, allergy to a vaccine component, and a blood transfusion within the past 3 months are contraindications to the use of vaccines.

7. **Answer: c**
   RATIONALE: Difficulty breathing may be a sign of a hypersensitivity reaction and should be reported immediately.

Pain or nodule formation at the injection site and moderate fever are common and expected adverse effects that do not require notification of the health care provider.

8. **Answer: a**
   RATIONALE: The nurse should instruct the mother to ensure that the child has ample rest time during the day. Acetaminophen, not aspirin, should be used for fever. Aspirin masks the signs of Reye's syndrome. Warm compresses, not cold, would be better for any pain at the injection site. The child should also rest his arm and avoid overuse.

9. **Answer: c**
   RATIONALE: Antivenin is used to treat snake bites. An antitoxin would be used to treat poisonous substances released by invading pathogens. Toxoids are vaccines. Immune sera typically refers to sera that contain antibodies to specific bacteria or viruses.

10. **Answer: a**
    RATIONALE: Meningococcal infections would be prevented by a vaccine. A toxoid is a type of vaccine made from the toxins produced by the organism. Immune globulins and antivenin are examples of immune sera.

11. **Answer: b**
    RATIONALE: Antithymocyte immune globulin is used to treat acute renal transplant rejection. The varicella virus vaccine would be used to prevent varicella (chicken pox). Hepatitis B immune globulin would be used for postexposure prophylaxis for hepatitis B. Respiratory syncytial virus (RSV) immune globulin would be used to prevent RSV in children younger than 2 years of age with bronchopulmonary dysplasia or premature birth.

12. **Answer: d**
    RATIONALE: Tetanus toxoid is used to provide passive immunization against tetanus as the result of an injury that could potentially precipitate a tetanus infection, such as a puncture wound by a nail. Zoster vaccine would be indicated to prevent herpes zoster (shingles) in a person over age 60 years. Hepatitis A vaccine is indicated for prevention of hepatitis A infection. Lymphocyte immune globulin is indicated for the management of allograft rejection in a patient with renal transplantation.

13. **Answer: c**
    RATIONALE: To prevent Rh factor sensitization, the woman would receive RHO immune globulin (RhoGAM). Crotalidae polyvalent immune fab would be used to treat rattlesnake bites. Cytomegalovirus immune globulin would be used to lessen primary cytomegalovirus disease after renal transplantation. The HPV vaccine would be used to prevent human papilloma virus infection.

14. **Answer: a**
    RATIONALE: The rotavirus vaccine is only administered orally.

15. **Answer: d**
    RATIONALE: The meningococcal polysaccharide vaccine is administered subcutaneously, often into the fatty (adipose) tissue layer of the upper arm. Deep into the muscle of the lateral thigh or upper outer quadrant of the buttocks reflects intramuscular administration. Directly into the dermis layer of the skin reflects intradermal administration.

Copyright © 2011 by Wolters Kluwer Health | Lippincott Williams & Wilkins. *Study Guide for Focus on Nursing Pharmacology.*

CHAPTER 19

■ ASSESSING YOUR UNDERSTANDING
LABELING

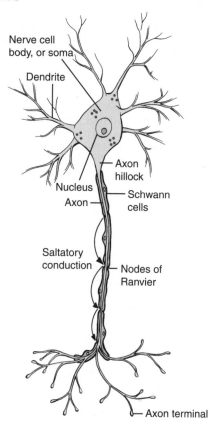

Nerve cell body, or soma

Dendrite

Axon hillock

Nucleus

Axon

Schwann cells

Saltatory conduction

Nodes of Ranvier

Axon terminal

MATCHING

1. e	2. g	3. b	4. i	5. c
6. f	7. h	8. j	9. a	10. d

■ APPLYING YOUR KNOWLEDGE
CASE STUDY

a. The nurse would need to explain to the patient that motor fibers from the brain cross to the other side of the spinal cord before emerging to interact with effector cells in the periphery such as the muscles. As a result, injury to the left side of the brain would lead to motor problems on the opposite side. Thus, the patient's right side is affected.

b. Blood flow to the brain is supplied by the carotid and vertebral arteries, which deliver blood to a common vessel at the bottom of the brain (the circle of Willis). This vessel then distributes blood to the brain as needed. With the mini-strokes, one of the carotid arteries was narrowed, thus supplying less blood to the circle of Willis. Although the blood flow was decreased, the areas of the brain on that side still have an adequate blood supply because the circle of Willis is able to provide blood to the area. The signs and symptoms most likely reflect a slight reduction in blood flow initially, but their quick resolution suggests that the circle of Willis was able to compensate and reestablish adequate blood flow.

■ PRACTICING FOR NCLEX

1. **Answer: c**
   RATIONALE: The neuron is the basic structural unit of the nervous system. The synapse refers to the junction between a nerve and an effector, such as a gland, muscle, or another nerve. Neurotransmitter is a chemical produced by a nerve and released when the nerve is stimulated. Soma refers to the cell body of a neuron.

2. **Answer: b**
   RATIONALE: The axon carries information from a nerve to be transmitted to effector cells. The dendrite brings information into the neuron from other neurons. The soma is the cell body of the neuron. Ganglia are groups of nerve bodies located in specific areas.

3. **Answer: d**
   RATIONALE: The nervous system does not prevent stimulus exposure. Rather, the nervous system is responsible for analyzing incoming stimuli, controlling the functions of the human body, and integrating internal and external responses.

4. **Answer: c**
   RATIONALE: Efferent fibers are nerve axons that carry nerve impulses from the central nervous system to the periphery to stimulate muscles or glands. The presynaptic nerve is the nerve that releases a chemical, a neurotransmitter, into the synaptic cleft. Schwann cells are cells located at specific intervals along nerve axons to allow nerve conduction.

5. **Answer: c**
   RATIONALE: For an action potential to occur, a stimulus of sufficient strength must be present and the nerve membrane must be able to respond—that is, when it has repolarized. Sodium ions rush into the cell when the neuron is stimulated, termed *depolarization*. The nerve cell membrane is permeable to potassium ions when the cell is at rest.

6. **Answer: d**
   RATIONALE: Epinephrine and norepinephrine are catecholamines released by nerves in the sympathetic branch of the autonomic nervous system and are classified as hormones when released by the adrenal medulla. Dopamine is a neurotransmitter involved with the coordination of motor and intellectual impulses and responses. Gamma-aminobutyric acid (GABA) inhibits nerve activity. Acetylcholine aids in communication between nerves and muscles.

7. **Answer: b**
   RATIONALE: Serotonin is an important neurotransmitter involved in arousal and sleep. GABA is important in preventing overexcitability or stimulation of nerve activity. Norepinephrine is a catecholamine involved in the fight-or-flight response. Dopamine is involved in the coordination of impulses and responses, both motor and intellectual.

8. **Answer: b**
   RATIONALE: The blood–brain barrier is a functioning boundary that keeps toxins, proteins, and other large structures out of the brain and prevents their contact with the sensitive and fragile neurons. It is not the mechanism for blood delivery to the brain or the center responsible for controlling vital functions.

9. **Answer: c**
   RATIONALE: The hindbrain contains the brain stem, where the pons and medulla oblongata are located. The thalamus and limbic system are part of the midbrain. The cerebrum is part of the forebrain.

Copyright © 2011 by Wolters Kluwer Health | Lippincott Williams & Wilkins. *Study Guide for Focus on Nursing Pharmacology.*

10. **Answer: a**
    RATIONALE: The spinal cord is made up of 31 pairs of spinal nerves.
11. **Answer: d**
    RATIONALE: The extrapyramidal system coordinates unconscious motor activity that regulates control of posture and position. Motor function control is regulated by sensory nerves and motor nerves along with the pyramidal system, which coordinates voluntary movement, and the extrapyramidal system. The cerebral cortex is involved in processing intellectual and emotional information, but the exact mechanism is not known.
12. **Answer: c**
    RATIONALE: Stimulation of a neuron causes depolarization, which allows sodium to rush into the cell, changing the resting membrane potential (cell is relatively negative [containing more potassium ions] compared to the outside of the cell [containing more sodium ions]). This sudden reversal creates an action potential, leading to repolarization, which returns the cell to its resting membrane potential.
13. **Answer: a, d**
    RATIONALE: The cerebrum contains motor and sensory neurons and the speech/communication areas. Cranial nerves and the chemoreceptor trigger zone are part of the hindbrain. Spinal nerve roots are found in the spinal cord.
14. **Answer: b**
    RATIONALE: The nodes of Ranvier are areas of uncovered nerve membrane that allow electrical impulses to "leap" or be conducted along the fiber. Schwann cells are myelinated areas along nerve axons that are resistant to electrical stimulation. Myelin is a substance that speeds electrical conduction and protects the nerves from fatigue due to frequent formation of action potentials. Synapse is the area where nerves communicate with each other.
15. **Answer: c**
    RATIONALE: The midbrain contains the hypothalamus, thalamus, and midbrain. The hindbrain contains the reticular activating system, respiratory control center, and swallowing center.

CHAPTER 20

■ ASSESSING YOUR UNDERSTANDING

FILL IN THE BLANKS

1. Anxiety
2. Hyponosis
3. Awareness
4. Sympathetic
5. Benzodiazepines
6. Gamma-aminobutyric acid (GABA)
7. Increased
8. Melatonin

SHORT ANSWER

1. Barbiturates, once the mainstay for the treatment of anxiety as well as for sedation and sleep induction, are not used frequently today because they are associated with potentially severe adverse effects and many drug–drug interactions. In addition, the risk for addiction and dependence is high.
2. Parenteral forms of benzodiazepines place the patient at increased risk for adverse effects, especially central nervous system (CNS) depression. The patient should be switched to oral forms as soon as possible.

3. The response of a child to anxiolytic may be unpredictable. Commonly, inappropriate aggressiveness, crying, irritability, and tearfulness can occur.
4. Drugs used as hypnotics act on the reticular activating system and block the brain's response to incoming stimuli.
5. Some blacks are genetically predisposed to delayed metabolism of benzodiazepines, leading to increased serum drug levels and increased sedation and incidence of adverse effect.

■ APPLYING YOUR KNOWLEDGE

CASE STUDY

a. The nurse would need to gather information related to the patient's usual routine and sleep hygiene activities. For example, the nurse should question the patient about naps during the day, level of activity and exercise, use of stimulants such as caffeine (including when and how much), and usual routine before going to bed.
b. The patient is an older adult who will probably need a dosage reduction for several reasons. He may have age-related changes in liver and/or renal function that may increase his risk for toxicity related to the drug. Older adult patients also have been found to be especially sensitive to this drug, thus necessitating a lower dosage.
c. Education should include the following: information about the drug, such as the drug name, dosage, and time for administration (taking the drug before bed); need to ensure at least 4 to 8 hours for sleep; signs and symptoms of adverse drug effects; safety measures to reduce the risk for injury; need for daily exercise and avoidance of daytime naps; and sleep hygiene measures such as a consistent routine, use of warm milk before bed, avoidance of caffeine-containing products after dinner, and avoidance of stimulating activities.

■ PRACTICING FOR NCLEX

1. **Answer: c**
   RATIONALE: Ramelteon should be taken ½ hour before going to bed.
2. **Answer: b**
   RATIONALE: Flurazepam would be used as a hypnotic. Lorazepam, diazepam, and alprazolam would be use as anxiolytics.
3. **Answer: a**
   RATIONALE: Benzodiazepines make GABA more effective, which leads to the anxiolytic effect. The drug does not affect action potentials. Depression of the cerebral cortex and motor output are associated with the use of barbiturates.
4. **Answer: c**
   RATIONALE: Patients who receive parenteral benzodiazepines should be monitored in bed for a period of at least 3 hours. Thus, the patient would be allowed out of bed at approximately 2 PM.
5. **Answer: d**
   RATIONALE: Intra-arterial administration of benzodiazepines would result in arteriospasm and gangrene. CNS depression, blurred vision, and urinary retention are adverse effects associated with benzodiazepines in general.
6. **Answer: a**
   RATIONALE: When giving diazepam intravenously, it should not be mixed in solution with any other drugs. Therefore, it would be best to start an intravenous line in another

Copyright © 2011 by Wolters Kluwer Health I Lippincott Williams & Wilkins. *Study Guide for Focus on Nursing Pharmacology.*

area, such as the opposite arm, so that the patient can receive the full benefits of both drugs. Notifying the prescriber that the diazepam cannot be given or waiting until the other drug is completed before giving the diazepam is inappropriate. Adding it to the current infusion is inappropriate because potentially serious drug–drug interactions can occur.

7. **Answer: b**
RATIONALE: Signs and symptoms of benzodiazepine withdrawal include nightmares, nausea, headache, and malaise. Dry mouth, hypotension, and urinary retention are adverse effects associated with benzodiazepine use.

8. **Answer: c**
RATIONALE: The effects of benzodiazepines are increased when taken with oral contraceptives, necessitating a change in dosage of the benzodiazepine. The effects of benzodiazepines are decreased when taken with theophylline and ranitidine, which might result in the need for an increased dosage of the benzodiazepine. Alcohol should not be used with benzodiazepines because the combination increases the risk of CNS depression.

9. **Answer: b**
RATIONALE: Diazepam peaks in approximately 1 to 2 hours, so the maximum effect of the drug would be seen between 5 and 6 PM.

10. **Answer: d**
RATIONALE: It would be appropriate to have the patient void before administering the medication to reduce the patient's risk for injury if the patient attempts to get out of bed after the drug is given. Raising the side rails, instituting a bowel program, and dimming the lights would be appropriate after giving the drug.

11. **Answer: c**
RATIONALE: Flumazenil is the antidote for benzodiazepines and is used to reverse the sedation of benzodiazepines used for diagnostic procedures. Temazepam and triazolam are benzodiazepines used as hypnotics. Promethazine is an antihistamine with sedative effects.

12. **Answer: d**
RATIONALE: Phenobarbital is considered the prototype barbiturate.

13. **Answer: b**
RATIONALE: When given intravenously, barbiturates can result in bradycardia, hypotension, hypoventilation, respiratory depression, and laryngospasm. Bleeding is not associated with barbiturate therapy.

14. **Answer: a**
RATIONALE: Although taking the drug with meals, increasing fiber intake (to prevent constipation), and using additional measures to promote relaxation would be helpful instructions, it would be most important for the nurse to warn the patient not to stop the drug abruptly. There is a risk for withdrawal if anxiolytics, both benzodiazepines and barbiturates, are stopped abruptly.

15. **Answer: c**
RATIONALE: Buspirone has no sedative, anticonvulsant, or muscle relaxant properties, but it does reduce the signs and symptoms of anxiety. Diphenhydramine is an antihistamine that can be sedating. Zaleplon causes sedation and is used for short-term treatment of insomnia. Meprobamate has some anticonvulsant properties and CNS-relaxing effects.

CHAPTER 21

■ ASSESSING YOUR UNDERSTANDING
LABELING

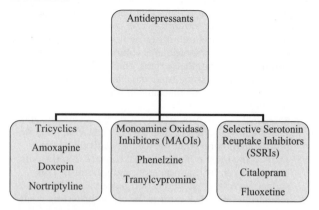

SHORT ANSWER

1. The three biogenic amines are norepinephrine, dopamine, and serotonin.
2. Tricyclic antidepressants all reduce the uptake of serotonin and norepinephrine.
3. Affect refers to the feelings that people experience when they respond emotionally.
4. When ingested while taking MAOIs, tyramine may be absorbed in high concentrations, resulting in increased blood pressure. In addition, tyramine causes the release of stored norepinephrine from nerve terminals, which contributes to high blood pressure and hypertensive crisis.
5. Amitriptyline is associated with a marked sedative and anticholinergic effect.
6. SSRIs do not have the many adverse effects associated with tricyclic antidepressants and MAOIs.

■ APPLYING YOUR KNOWLEDGE
CASE STUDY

a. The nurse would most likely suspect that the patient is experiencing a hypertensive crisis due to ingestion of foods containing tyramine while receiving MAOIs or a possible drug–drug interaction with the patient's current MAOI and a tricyclic antidepressant (imipramine).
b. The nurse would need to assess for additional manifestations of hypertensive crisis, including palpitations, neck stiffness, sweating, dilated pupils, photophobia, tachycardia, and chest pain. In addition, the nurse needs to gather information about the patient's recent food intake to determine if the patient ingested foods containing tyramine, which can precipitate a hypertensive crisis with MAOIs. Another area that the nurse needs to investigate is if the patient is still taking the imipramine, a tricyclic antidepressant with phenelzine. These drugs can interact, leading to hypertensive crisis. In addition, the nurse should obtain information about any other medications that the patient may be taking—for example, sympathomimetics, which could lead to an increase in sympathomimetic effects such as vasoconstriction, pupillary dilation, and increased heart rate as well as increased blood pressure.

Copyright © 2011 by Wolters Kluwer Health I Lippincott Williams & Wilkins. *Study Guide for Focus on Nursing Pharmacology.*

c. The nurse would need to teach the patient to check with his health care provider before taking any other over-the-counter drugs or prescription medications because MAOIs interact with many of them. If the patient was still taking the imipramine, then the nurse would need to tell the patient to stop the drug to prevent further interaction. In addition, the nurse needs to teach the patient about foods that contain tyramine and the importance of avoiding them. The nurse could give the patient a written list of the foods so that he can refer to it in the future.

■ PRACTICING FOR NCLEX

1. Answer: b
RATIONALE: Bupropion is an antidepressant that is also used for smoking cessation in lower dosages. Venlafaxine is used to treat and prevent depression in generalized anxiety disorder, as treatment for social anxiety disorder, and to help decrease addictive behaviors. Mirtazapine and selegiline are used to treat depression.

2. Answer: c
RATIONALE: Although studies have been done, the Food and Drug Administration has concluded that there is not enough evidence to link suicidal ideation to antidepressant use. However, all of the drugs should be used with caution, and prescriptions should be written in the smallest quantity feasible. Only a few tricyclic antidepressants have established pediatric dosages for children over age 6 years; the use of MAOIs should be avoided; and SSRIs are associated with serious adverse effects in children. Antidepressant use with children is challenging because the child's response is unpredictable.

3. Answer: a
RATIONALE: The adverse effects of nortriptyline, such as sedation, anticholinergic effects, hypotension, and cardiovascular effects, are negligible. Amitriptyline exhibits marked sedation, anticholinergic effects, and hypotension. Clomipramine is associated with moderate sedation, anticholinergic effects, hypotension, and cardiovascular effects. Doxepin is associated with moderate sedative and anticholinergic effects as well as mild hypotension and cardiovascular effects.

4. Answer: a
RATIONALE: Tricyclic antidepressants are administered in oral form.

5. Answer: c
RATIONALE: Only clomipramine is indicated for the treatment of obsessive-compulsive disorder.

6. Answer: d
RATIONALE: A recent myocardial infarction would be a contraindication for use because of the potential occurrence of reinfarction or extension of the infarction due to the drug's cardiac effects. Cautious use and close monitoring would be appropriate for the patient with glaucoma and prostatic hypertrophy due to the anticholinergic effects. Cautious use in renal dysfunction also is warranted because the drugs are excreted in the urine.

7. Answer: c
RATIONALE: Transdermal selegiline should be applied to dry intact skin on the upper arm, upper thigh, or upper torso. The patient should always remove the old patch before applying a new one to prevent inadvertent overdose. Transdermal selegiline is associated with central nervous system (CNS) and gastrointestinal (GI) effects.

8. Answer: d
RATIONALE: Trazodone is associated with a risk for low blood pressure and priapism (a sustained, painful

erection). CNS effects, such as dizziness and sedation, occur with this drug but are not a cause for notifying the health care provider.

9. Answer: a, b, c, f
RATIONALE: Isocarboxazid is an MAOI, which necessitates avoiding foods containing tyramine such as aged cheeses, red wines, smoked meats (i.e., pepperoni), and sour cream.

10. Answer: b
RATIONALE: Fluoxetine is associated with respiratory changes such as cough, GI effects such as dry mouth, CNS effects such as drowsiness, and genitourinary effects such as impotence.

11. Answer: d
RATIONALE: It may take up to 4 weeks before the full effect of an SSRI is noted.

12. Answer: c
RATIONALE: Sertraline is an SSRI. Doxepin is a tricyclic antidepressant. Nefazodone and bupropion are other antidepressants that are not classified as tricyclic antidepressants, SSRIs, or MAOIs.

13. Answer: b
RATIONALE: Paroxetine, a SSRI, and phenelzine, an MAOI, should not be given together because of the risk for serotonin syndrome. At least 4 to 6 weeks should be allowed between the use of the two drugs when switching from one to the other.

14. Answer: a, b
RATIONALE: The nurse should inform the patient to take the tricyclic antidepressant once daily in the morning as prescribed to ensure the maximum benefit. The dosage could be divided if the patient experiences severe GI effects. Sugar-free hard candies and gums would help to alleviate the dry mouth that may occur. A high-fiber diet would be appropriate if the patient develops constipation. The nurse should instruct the patient to control the lighting, temperature, and stimuli of the environment to address possible CNS effects.

15. Answer: c
RATIONALE: MAOIs interact with oral antidiabetic agents, increasing the patient's risk for hypoglycemia. Diabetic ketoacidosis would be associated with hyperglycemia. Orthostatic hypotension, urinary retention, dysuria, and incontinence may occur with MAOI therapy, but these are not associated with the interaction of an oral antidiabetic agent and an MAOI.

CHAPTER 22

■ ASSESSING YOUR UNDERSTANDING

SHORT ANSWER

1. The most common type of psychosis is schizophrenia.
2. Psychotherapeutic agents are used to treat perceptual and behavioral disorders, targeting action at thought processes rather than affective states. They do not cure the disorder but help patients function in a more acceptable manner and carry out activities of daily living.
3. Antipsychotic agents are called neuroleptic agents because of the associated neurologic adverse effects.
4. Antipsychotic agents are no longer called major tranquilizers because the primary action of these drugs is not sedation but a change in neuron stimulation and response.
5. Antipsychotic drugs are classified as typical or atypical antipsychotics.

Copyright © 2011 by Wolters Kluwer Health | Lippincott Williams & Wilkins. *Study Guide for Focus on Nursing Pharmacology.*

LABELING

Dopamine	Serotonin	Norepinephrine
Aripiprazole Chlorpromazine Clozapine Lithium Molindone Pimozide Quetiapine Ziprasidone	Aripiprazole Clozapine Quetiapine Ziprasidone	Lithium

■ APPLYING YOUR KNOWLEDGE

CASE STUDY

a. Since the patient is experiencing mania, obtaining the information from the patient at this time would probably be quite difficult. The nurse could question the patient but would need to keep in mind that the patient may not be a reliable source of information. Since the patient is known to the staff, the nurse could review the patient's medical record to gather information about the patient's medications (including herbal therapies such as psyllium, which could interact with lithium and lead to nontherapeutic drug levels) and previous episodes. In addition, the medical record could provide the nurse with the name of a family member or contact person who could help provide information. If the nurse determines that the patient has been taking lithium in the past, the nurse could obtain a serum drug level to determine if the drug level was therapeutic. If the level was not therapeutic, then the nurse might conclude that the patient had stopped taking the medication.

b. In most cases, the drug of choice would be lithium. However, other agents can be used for acute manic episodes such as olanzapine or ziprasidone.

c. The nurse would need to provide clear, simple explanations to the patient at the present time, emphasizing what is being done and why. Any other teaching would need to be postponed until the patient's mania is controlled. Once this occurs, the nurse would need to implement a teaching plan that addresses the medication prescribed, including the importance of compliance and follow-up to monitor drug levels. The nurse may need to involve a family member or support person in this teaching to ensure that the patient understands the information. It may be necessary to initiate a social service referral to assist the patient in complying with the therapy.

■ PRACTICING FOR NCLEX

1. Answer: a
RATIONALE: Pseudoparkinsonism is manifested by cogwheel rigidity, muscle tremors, drooling, a shuffling gait, and slow movements. Abnormal eye movements, neck spasms, and excessive salivation would suggest dystonia.

2. Answer: b
RATIONALE: Therapeutic serum lithium levels range from 0.6 mEq/L to 1.2 mEq/L, so a level of 0.8 mEq/L would be considered therapeutic. A level of 0.2 mEq/L would be nontherapeutic. Levels above 1.2 mEq/L would be considered toxic.

3. Answer: c
RATIONALE: Clozapine is classified as an atypical antipsychotic. Haloperidol, loxapine, and pimozide are considered typical antipsychotics.

4. Answer: d
RATIONALE: Fluphenazine is considered a highly potent antipsychotic. Chlorpromazine, thioridazine, and prochlorperazine are considered low-potent antipsychotics.

5. Answer: a
RATIONALE: After administering parenteral forms of antipsychotic agents, the nurse should keep the patient recumbent for approximately ½ hour to reduce the risk of orthostatic hypotension.

6. Answer: b
RATIONALE: Phenothiazines such as fluphenazine often turn the urine pink to reddish-brown as a result of excretion. Fatal arrhythmias are associated with thioridazine, mesoridazine, and ziprasidone. Nasal congestion, not rhinorrhea, is a possible adverse effect. The risk for developing diabetes is associated with atypical antipsychotics. Fluphenazine is a typical antipsychotic.

7. Answer: c
RATIONALE: Clozapine is associated with significant leukopenia. Subsequently, is it available only through the Clozaril Patient Management System, which involves monitoring white blood cell count and compliance issues with only a 1-week supply being given at a time. Aripiprazole, olanzapine, and quetiapine are not associated with leukopenia.

8. Answer: b
RATIONALE: A thiazide diuretic–lithium combination increases the risk of lithium toxicity because sodium is lost and lithium is retained. Lithium effectiveness is decreased with tromethamine and antacids. Psyllium interferes with the absorption of lithium, leading to nontherapeutic levels.

9. Answer: a, c, e
RATIONALE: A patient with a serum lithium level between 1.5 to 2.0 mEq/L would exhibit central nervous system (CNS) problems such as electrocardiogram changes, slurred speech, and polyuria. Hypotension, hyperreflexia, and seizures would be assessed with levels between 2.0 to 2.5 mEq/L.

10. Answer: c
RATIONALE: The last dose of methylphenidate should be administered before 6 PM to reduce the incidence of insomnia.

11. Answer: d
RATIONALE: Modafinil would be indicated for the treatment of narcolepsy. Atomoxetine, dexmethylphenidate, and lisdexamfetamine are indicated for the treatment of attention deficit disorders.

12. Answer: a
RATIONALE: Tardive dyskinesia involves abnormal muscle movements such as lip smacking, tongue darting, slow and aimless arm and leg movements, and chewing movements. Akathisia is manifested by continued restlessness and an inability to sit still. Pseudoparkinsonism is manifested by muscle tremors, cogwheel rigidity, drooling, shuffling gait, and slow movements. Dystonia is manifested by spasms of the tongues, neck, back, and legs.

13. Answer: a
RATIONALE: Nasal congestion is a manifestation of anticholinergic effects. Neuroleptic malignant syndrome reflects the drug's effect on the CNS. Laryngospasm is a respiratory effect; arrhythmia is a cardiovascular effect.

14. Answer: b
RATIONALE: Periodically, the drug therapy needs to be interrupted to determine if the child experiences a recurrence of symptoms, which would indicate the need for continued treatment.

Copyright © 2011 by Wolters Kluwer Health | Lippincott Williams & Wilkins. *Study Guide for Focus on Nursing Pharmacology.*

15. Answer: c
RATIONALE: Haloperidol is associated with the greatest increased risk of extrapyramidal adverse effects. Sedation, anticholinergic effects, and hypotension can occur, but the risk for these is much less when compared with the risk for extrapyramidal effects.

16. Answer: d
RATIONALE: Aripiprazole is indicated for the treatment of mania and schizophrenia. Lithium and lamotrigine are indicated only for the treatment of mania. Risperidone is indicated only for the treatment of schizophrenia.

CHAPTER 23

■ ASSESSING YOUR UNDERSTANDING

MATCHING

1. g	**2.** f	**3.** b	**4.** d	**5.** a
6. e	**7.** c			

SHORT ANSWER

1. The five types of generalized seizures are tonic-clonic, absence, myoclonic, febrile, jacksonian, and psychomotor.
2. Simple partial seizures occur in a single area of the brain and may involve a single muscle movement or sensory alteration. Complex partial seizures involve a series of reactions or emotional changes, complex sensory changes such as hallucinations, mental distortion, changes in personality, loss of consciousness, and loss of social inhibitions. Motor changes may include involuntary urination, chewing motions, diarrhea, and so on. The onset of complex partial seizures usually occurs by the late teens.
3. Drugs used to treat generalized seizures most often lead to sedation and other central nervous system (CNS) effects.
4. The succinimides and drugs that modulate gamma-aminobutyric acid (GABA) are most frequently used to treat absence seizures.
5. Phenobarbital has very low lipid solubility, giving it a slow onset and very long duration of action.
6. The drugs used to control partial seizures stabilize nerve membranes in two ways—either directly, by altering sodium and calcium channels, or indirectly, by increasing the activity of GABA, an inhibitory neurotransmitter, and thereby decreasing excessive activity.

■ APPLYING YOUR KNOWLEDGE

CASE STUDY

a. The nurse needs to allow the mother and father to verbalize their concerns and fears and then correct any misconceptions that they may have about their son's condition. The nurse also would then begin to teach the parents about the disorder and his treatment, including the drug therapy regimen, emphasizing that consistency and compliance with the therapy is essential in controlling the disorder. In addition, the nurse would begin teaching the parents how to manage a seizure if it does occur to avoid injury to the child while at the same time remaining calm. Written instructions in this case would probably be very helpful so that the parents can review the information and then ask questions that they may have. Information about the drug's adverse effects and the need for follow-up testing of serum drug levels would be important. Knowing that the child's drug level is therapeutic is helpful in alleviating some of the anxiety related to the child having another seizure.

b. The nurse would recommend that the child wear Medic-alert identification that lists his condition and the therapy he is taking. Additional recommendations and suggestions may include having the parents talk with parents of other children with seizures as well as having the parents join a support group. In addition, the nurse would encourage the parents to talk with child's teacher and school nurse about dealing with the seizures as well as talk with the child's classmates and friends about his condition and what to do if a seizure occurs. Talking with the school nurse would be very important because the child may need to take medication while at school.

■ PRACTICING FOR NCLEX

1. Answer: c
RATIONALE: Levetiracetam is available for oral or intravenous use. Carbamazepine, gabapentin, and felbamate are administered orally.

2. Answer: b
RATIONALE: The therapeutic serum phenytoin levels range from 10 to 20 mcg/mL. Thus, a level of 12 mcg/mL would fall within this range.

3. Answer: d
RATIONALE: Hydantoins may cause gingival hyperplasia, severe liver toxicity, and bone marrow suppression. Physical dependence and withdrawal syndrome are associated with benzodiazepines.

4. Answer: c
RATIONALE: The barbiturates and barbituratelike drugs depress motor nerve output, inhibit impulse conduction in the ascending reticular activating system (RAS), depress the cerebral cortex, and alter cerebellar function. They stabilize nerve membranes throughout the CNS directly by influencing ionic channels in the cell membrane, thereby decreasing excitability and hyperexcitability to stimulation.

5. Answer: d
RATIONALE: Although phenobarbital is available in oral and parenteral forms, status epilepticus is an emergency situation that requires the drug to be given intravenously to achieve a rapid onset of action.

6. Answer: a
RATIONALE: Lamotrigine has been associated with very serious to life-threatening rashes, and the drug should be discontinued at the first sign of any rash. Somnolence and confusion are typical CNS effects; anorexia is a common gastrointestinal effect.

7. Answer: b
RATIONALE: Pregabalin has a controlled substance rating of category V because it causes feelings of well-being and euphoria. Subsequently, its use should be limited in patients who have a history of abuse of medications and alcohol. Increased CNS depression would occur if the patient ingested alcohol with either topiramate, felbamate, or tiagabine.

8. Answer: a
RATIONALE: Therapeutic serum carbamazepine levels range from 4 to 12 mcg/mL. Therefore, a level under 4 mcg/mL would suggest that the drug has not reached therapeutic levels, so the dosage may need to be increased.

9. Answer: b
RATIONALE: The patient is experiencing CNS effects that could lead to injury. Therefore, the nurse would need to implement safety precautions as the priority. Hydration may be needed if the patient were experiencing vomiting

or diarrhea. Skin-care measures would be appropriate for the development of a rash. Emotional support would be appropriate if the patient had verbalized difficulty coping with the condition or drug therapy.

10. **Answer: b**
    RATIONALE: When phenobarbital is given to a child intravenously for treatment of a febrile seizure, a second dose may be repeated in 6 hours, which in this situation would be 4 PM.

11. **Answer: c**
    RATIONALE: Valproic acid is considered the drug of choice for myoclonic seizures and a second choice drug for absence seizures. Clonazepam may be used for myoclonic seizures, but it is not considered the drug of choice. Diazepam and zonisamide are not used for treating myoclonic seizures.

12. **Answer: c**
    RATIONALE: Ethosuximide is most frequently used to treat absence seizures. Mephobarbital, ethotoin, and primidone are typically used for tonic-clonic seizures.

13. **Answer: a**
    RATIONALE: Zonisamide inhibits voltage-sensitive sodium and calcium channels, thus stabilizing the nerve cell membranes and modulating calcium-dependent presynaptic release of excitatory neurotransmitters. Hydantoins decrease the conduction through nerve pathways. Barbiturates and barbituratelike agents depress the cerebral cortex and motor nerve output.

14. **Answer: a**
    RATIONALE: Ethotoin is administered orally.

15. **Answer: d**
    RATIONALE: Although weight loss and anorexia may occur, ethosuximide is associated with bone marrow suppression, including potentially fatal pancytopenia, so it would be most important for the nurse to monitor the patient's complete blood count. The drug is not associated with any cardiovascular effects that would necessitate an electrocardiogram.

CHAPTER 24

■ ASSESSING YOUR UNDERSTANDING

FILL IN THE BLANKS

1. Bradykinesia
2. Substantia nigra
3. Dopamine, cholinergic
4. Dopaminergic, anticholinergic
5. Tyramine

LABELING

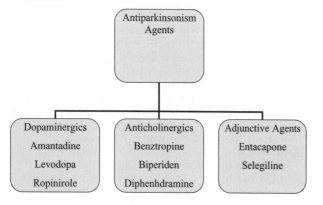

■ APPLYING YOUR KNOWLEDGE

CASE STUDY

a. The nurse might interpret these signs and symptoms as being related to a possible hypertensive crisis that can occur with rasagiline and the ingestion of foods containing tyramine, some drugs, and some herbal preparations.

b. The nurse would need to investigate if the patient has taken any herbal preparations such as St. John's wort or medications such as meperidine or other analgesics. In addition, the nurse would need to ask the patient and his daughter about ingestion of tyramine foods such as aged cheeses; red wine; smoked or pickled meats or fish; certain dairy products, such as sour cream or yogurt; chocolate; or certain fruits, such as figs, raisins, grapes, pineapples, or oranges.

■ PRACTICING FOR NCLEX

1. **Answer: a**
   RATIONALE: Levodopa is a precursor of dopamine that crosses the blood–brain barrier, where it is converted to dopamine, acting like a replacement therapy. Amantadine increases the release of dopamine. Apomorphine directly binds with postsynaptic dopamine receptors. Ropinirole directly stimulates dopamine receptors.

2. **Answer: b**
   RATIONALE: When levodopa is used in combination with carbodopa, the enzyme dopa is inhibited in the periphery, diminishing the metabolism of levodopa in the gastrointestinal tract and in peripheral tissues, thereby leading to higher levels crossing the blood–brain barrier. Because the carbidopa decreases the amount of levodopa needed to reach a therapeutic level in the brain, the dosage of levodopa can be decreased, which reduces the incidence of adverse side effects.

3. **Answer: c**
   RATIONALE: Apomorphine is administered subcutaneously. The other dopaminergic agents are administered orally.

4. **Answer: d**
   RATIONALE: Levodopa is contraindicated in patients with suspicious skin lesions because the drug is associated with the development of melanoma. Cautious use is recommended for patients with myocardial infarction, bronchial asthma, and peptic ulcer disease, as these conditions could be exacerbated by dopamine receptor stimulation.

5. **Answer: c**
   RATIONALE: Adverse effects associated with dopaminergics usually result from stimulation of dopamine receptors and may include nervousness, anxiety, confusion, mental changes, muscle twitching, ataxia, and hypotension.

6. **Answer: d**
   RATIONALE: St. John's wort can lead to hypertensive crisis if taken with rasagiline, not levodopa. Decreased effectiveness of levodopa is seen with the use of pyridoxine (vitamin B_6), phenytoin, and multivitamin supplements.

7. **Answer: a**
   RATIONALE: Trihexyphenidyl is available only in an oral form.

Copyright © 2011 by Wolters Kluwer Health | Lippincott Williams & Wilkins. *Study Guide for Focus on Nursing Pharmacology.*

8. **Answer: b**
   RATIONALE: Anticholinergics are contraindicated for patients with myasthenia gravis, which could be exacerbated by the blocking of acetylcholine receptor sites at the neuromuscular synapses. Hypertension, hepatic dysfunction, and cardiac arrhythmia would require cautious use.

9. **Answer: d**
   RATIONALE: Agitation would be noted due to the blocking of central acetylcholine receptors. Constipation, reduced sweating, and dry mouth may be noted as well.

10. **Answer: c**
    RATIONALE: Bromocriptine is classified as a dopaminergic agent. Diphenhydramine and biperiden are classified as anticholinergics. Tolcapone is considered an adjunctive agent.

11. **Answer: d**
    RATIONALE: The patient is experiencing central nervous system (CNS) effects related to drug therapy, which could predispose the patient to falls. Thus, a risk for injury would be appropriate. Risk for impaired thermoregulation would be related to blockage of reflex sweating mechanism. Disturbed thought processes would be reflected by disorientation, confusion, and memory loss. Deficient knowledge would be appropriate if the patient were asking questions about the drug therapy.

12. **Answer: b**
    RATIONALE: Entacapone inhibits catecholamine-O-methyl transferase, which eliminates catecholamines including dopamine. Lactic dehydrogenase is a liver enzyme. Rasagiline inhibits monoamine oxidase type B. Acetylcholinesterase breaks down acetylcholine.

13. **Answer: b**
    RATIONALE: Apomorphine is associated with a risk for hypotension and a prolonged QT interval. Therefore, the priority would be to monitor the patient's cardiac status closely. The drug is given by subcutaneous injection, not oral administration. Checking for skin lesions would be appropriate for a patient receiving levodopa due to its association with melanoma. Palpating the bladder would be appropriate for any dopaminergic agent because of the risk for urinary retention. However, this would not be the priority.

14. **Answer: c**
    RATIONALE: Biperiden is indicated for the treatment of drug-induced parkinsonism resulting from the drug effects of phenothiazines. Bromocriptine and pramipexole are indicated for the treatment of idiopathic Parkinson's disease. Selegiline is indicated for the treatment of idiopathic Parkinson's disease with levodopa-carbidopa in patients whose response to therapy has decreased.

15. **Answer: b**
    RATIONALE: Blurred vision is considered a peripheral anticholinergic effect. Delirium, agitation, and memory loss are considered central effects affecting the CNS.

CHAPTER 25

■ ASSESSING YOUR UNDERSTANDING
CROSSWORD

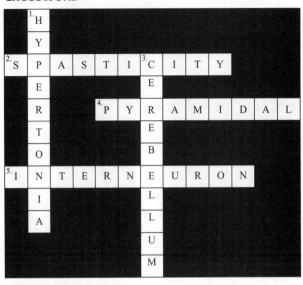

SHORT ANSWER

1. The pyramidal tract controls precise intentional movement; the extrapyramidal tract coordinates unconsciously controlled muscle activity and allows the body to make automatic adjustments in posture or position and balance.
2. Muscle spasticity is caused by nerve damage in the central nervous system (CNS).
3. Muscle spasm often results from injury to the musculoskeletal system.
4. Movement and muscle control are regulated by spinal reflexes and the upper CNS, including the basal ganglia, cerebellum, and cerebral cortex.
5. Centrally acting skeletal muscle relaxants are often referred to as spasmolytics because they lyse or destroy spasm by interfering with the reflexes that are causing the spasm.
6. Baclofen is the prototype centrally acting skeletal muscle relaxant.
7. Direct-acting skeletal muscle relaxants enter the muscle to prevent muscle contraction directly.
8. Botulinum toxin type A is used to improve the appearance of moderate to severe glabellar lines.

■ APPLYING YOUR KNOWLEDGE
CASE STUDY

a. Cyclobenzaprine is a centrally acting skeletal muscle relaxant that is used to relieve the discomfort of acute musculoskeletal conditions. The nurse would need to determine if the patient is to receive the regular or the controlled-release form so that the appropriate schedule can be determined. Typically, the controlled-release form is taken at the same time each day to ensure consistent drug levels. In addition, the nurse would need to teach the patient about the commonly occurring adverse effects such as CNS depression; gastrointestinal (GI) upset, including dry mouth, nausea,

Copyright © 2011 by Wolters Kluwer Health | Lippincott Williams & Wilkins. *Study Guide for Focus on Nursing Pharmacology.*

and constipation; and urinary frequency and urgency. The nurse would also need to instruct the patient to avoid alcohol and other CNS depressants.

b. The nurse would also need to include instructions for care of the injured area such as rest, support for the injured area, heat application, and the use of anti-inflammatory agents. As the area heals, physical therapy may be indicated to help the muscle return to its normal tone. In addition, the nurse should teach the patient about ways to minimize injury in the future, including adequate warm-ups and not overdoing it.

■ PRACTICING FOR NCLEX

1. Answer: b
RATIONALE: Carisoprodol is the centrally acting skeletal muscle relaxant of choice for older patients because it is considered safer than the other agents.

2. Answer: c
RATIONALE: Simple reflex arcs involve sensory receptors in the periphery and spinal motor nerves. Such reflex arcs make up what is known as the spindle gamma loop system. The pyramidal tract is part of the CNS that controls precise intentional movement. The extrapyramidal tract, also a part of the CNS, controls unconscious muscle activity. The basal ganglia is the portion of the brain that is associated with unconscious muscle movements.

3. Answer: a
RATIONALE: Botulinum toxin type A is classified as a direct-acting skeletal muscle relaxant. Diazepam, methocarbamol, and orphenadrine are centrally acting skeletal muscle relaxants.

4. Answer: d
RATIONALE: Centrally acting skeletal muscle relaxants would be contraindicated for treatment of muscle spasms related to a rheumatic disorder. Epilepsy, cardiac disease, or hepatic function would necessitate cautious use.

5. Answer: b
RATIONALE: Baclofen peaks in 2 hours after administration, so maximum effectiveness would be noted at this time, which in this case would be 10 AM.

6. Answer: c
RATIONALE: Dantrolene is indicated for the control of spasticity resulting from upper motor neuron disorders such as amyotrophic lateral sclerosis. Chlorzoxazone, metaxalone, and methocarbamol are used to treat acute musculoskeletal conditions.

7. Answer: a
RATIONALE: Dantrolene interferes with the release of calcium from the muscle tubules, preventing the fibers from contracting. Botulinum toxins A and B bind directly to the receptor sites of motor nerve terminals and inhibit the release of acetylcholine. Centrally acting muscle relaxants interfere with the reflexes that are causing the muscle spasm. Tizanidine is thought to increase inhibition of presynaptic motor neurons in the CNS.

8. Answer: c
RATIONALE: Chlorzoxazone may discolor the urine, becoming orange to purple-red in color. Baclofen, carisoprodol, and tizanidine do not discolor urine.

9. Answer: b
RATIONALE: Botulinum toxin is administered as an injection and should not be given if there is active infection at the site of the intended injection.

10. Answer: d
RATIONALE: Dantrolene therapy must be discontinued at any sign of liver dysfunction. Intermittent GI upset,

visual disturbances, and urinary retention are associated adverse effects of the drug and, although problematic, do not necessitate discontinuing the drug.

11. Answer: b
RATIONALE: Dantrolene is the drug that would be used as prevention and treatment of malignant hyperthermia.

12. Answer: c
RATIONALE: Although deficient knowledge, risk for injury, and disturbed thought processes may apply, the patient with an acute knee strain most likely would be experiencing pain as well as muscle spasms further contributing to the pain, subsequently leading to the use of a centrally acting skeletal muscle relaxant. Thus, a nursing diagnosis of acute pain would be the priority.

13. Answer: b
RATIONALE: The risk for hepatocellular disease is increased in women and all patients over the age of 35 years. Respiratory disease could be exacerbated with the use of dantrolene. Acute infection would be a contraindication to the use of botulinum toxins.

14. Answer: d
RATIONALE: The use of botulinum toxin type A is associated with droopy eyelids (in severe cases), headache, respiratory infections, flulike syndrome, pain, redness, and muscle weakness, which are usually temporary. Abnormal hair growth, acne, and photosensitivity may be associated with dantrolene.

15. Answer: a, c, f
RATIONALE: Adverse effects associated with baclofen therapy include drowsiness, urinary frequency, constipation, hypotension, fatigue, weakness, and dry mouth.

CHAPTER 26

■ ASSESSING YOUR UNDERSTANDING

LABELING

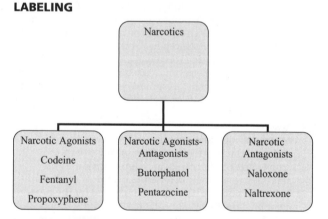

SHORT ANSWER

1. Two small-diameter sensory nerves, called the A-delta and C fibers, respond to stimulation by generating nerve impulses that produce pain sensations.
2. A fibers transmit sensations associated with touch and temperature.
3. Opioid receptors respond to naturally occurring peptins, endorphins, and enkephalins.
4. The three factors may include past experience with pain, learned response, and environmental setting.
5. The three functions of narcotic agonists-antagonists include relief of moderate to severe pain, adjunct to general anesthesia, and pain relief during labor and delivery.

Copyright © 2011 by Wolters Kluwer Health I Lippincott Williams & Wilkins. *Study Guide for Focus on Nursing Pharmacology.*

6. Triptans cause cranial vascular constriction and relief of migraine headaches.

7. The four types of opioid receptors are mu, kappa, beta, and sigma.

■ APPLYING YOUR KNOWLEDGE

CASE STUDY

a. The patient's increase in pain may be due to several factors. The patient's cancer may be progressing, which most likely would increase the amount of pain that he is experiencing. The patient also may be developing a tolerance for the medication, necessitating a larger dose or a more frequent dosing schedule. Additionally, psychological factors may be involved since the patient will not be receiving any further treatment, thus dispelling any hopes for a remission or cure.

b. Possible options include increasing the dosage of the morphine or administering it by another route that may be more effective. Another drug such as fentanyl may be added to the regimen to address the breakthrough pain that the patient is experiencing.

c. The nurse would suggest comfort measures to promote the effectiveness of the medication. For example, the nurse might suggest back rubs or massages, heat or cold therapy, relaxation techniques, and complementary therapies such as music therapy or aromatherapy to aid in relaxation. In addition, it would be important for the nurse to encourage the patient to verbalize his feelings and concerns related to his prognosis so that the patient's pain is not exacerbated by anxiety, fear, or depression. Support groups and hospice care may be appropriate suggestions.

■ PRACTICING FOR NCLEX

1. Answer: b
RATIONALE: Fentanyl is available as a transdermal patch.

2. Answer: b
RATIONALE: The most appropriate method for assessing pain is to have the patient rate his pain by using some type of scale. This provides objective evidence of the severity of the pain and provides a basis for comparison later on.

3. Answer: a
RATIONALE: Typically, codeine or hydrocodone are used to relieve coughing.

4. Answer: a
RATIONALE: Extended-release preparations should be taken as a whole tablet—not cut, crushed, or chewed. Doing so with oxycodone would allow release of the entire drug dose at one time instead of the gradual release over time, as would be appropriate with an extended-release form.

5. Answer: c
RATIONALE: Many sources recommend waiting 4 to 6 hours to breast-feed a baby after receiving a narcotic.

6. Answer: b
RATIONALE: Oral morphine peaks in approximately 1 hour; in this situation, it would be 4:00 PM.

7. Answer: d
RATIONALE: Pentazocine is available in parenteral and oral forms, making it the preferred choice for patients who will be switched from parenteral to oral forms after surgery.

8. Answer: c
RATIONALE: Narcotics are associated with orthostatic hypotension, pupil constriction, constipation, and respiratory depression with apnea.

9. Answer: c
RATIONALE: Naloxone is a narcotic antagonist that is used to reverse the effects of narcotics such as morphine. Butorphanol and buprenorphine are narcotic agonists-antagonists that are used for moderate to severe pain relief. Ergotamine would be used to prevent and treat migraine attacks.

10. Answer: a
RATIONALE: Naltrexone is administered orally.

11. Answer: a
RATIONALE: Migraine headaches are associated with severe unilateral pulsating pain on one side of the head. Sharp steady eye pain with an onset usually during sleep is associated with cluster headaches. A dull band of pain around the head suggests a tension headache.

12. Answer: a
RATIONALE: Ergot derivatives block alpha-adrenergic and serotonin receptor sites in the brain to cause constriction of cranial vessels, a decrease in cranial artery pulsation, and a decrease in the hyperperfusion of the basilar artery bed.

13. Answer: b
RATIONALE: Ergotamine, an ergot derivative, would be most appropriate for the prevention and treatment of an acute migraine attack. Triptans such as sumatriptan and eletriptan are used for treatment of an acute migraine but not prevention. Naloxone is used to reverse the effects of opioids.

14. Answer: c
RATIONALE: Dihydroergotamine is administered intranasally or intramuscularly at the first sign of a headache. Ergotamine could be administered sublingually or via inhalation. All triptans are administered orally except for sumatriptan, which could be administered orally, subcutaneously, or by nasal spray.

15. Answer: c
RATIONALE: With sumatriptan, the patient should take the first dose at the first sign of a headache and then repeat the dose, if needed, in approximately 2 hours.

CHAPTER 27

■ ASSESSING YOUR UNDERSTANDING

CROSSWORD

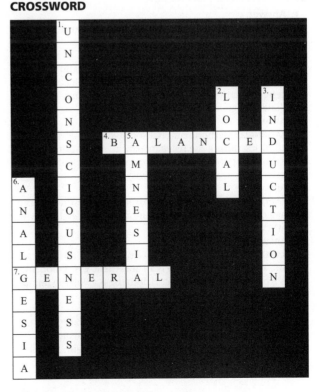

SEQUENCING

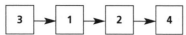

$$3 \rightarrow 1 \rightarrow 2 \rightarrow 4$$

■ APPLYING YOUR KNOWLEDGE

CASE STUDY

a. The nurse needs to approach the patient in a supportive, nonjudgmental manner and slowly explain the events of the day. The nurse needs to determine what the patient knows about the surgical experience and then reinforce this information, correcting any misconceptions or misinformation that she may have. If necessary, the nurse may need to go step-by-step as to what to expect so that the patient does not experience any additional upset or stress. In addition, the patient is visibly anxious, so the nurse need to provide the patient with support to help alleviate her anxiety. Explanations geared to the patient's level of understanding would be the most effective.

b. The nurse needs to underscore the importance of the history and physical examination as well as the tests being done to ensure that the most appropriate choices for anesthesia are used—that is, ones that would be the most effective without causing her undue harm. Information about underlying medical conditions and the use of other drugs is important to prevent additional adverse effects and drug–drug interactions. The anesthesiologist or certified nurse anesthetist is the individual who will decide which anesthetics the patient will receive. It might be helpful to have the anesthesiologist return to talk with the patient about what to expect. This may have already been done, but it does not seem that the patient has understood or heard what was told to her. The nurse would also explain the use of any preoperative sedation that may be given and how that might make her feel as well as what will happen when she is transported to the surgical suite.

■ PRACTICING FOR NCLEX

1. Answer: c
   RATIONALE: Pupillary dilation occurs during stage 3 of surgical anesthesia.

2. Answer: a
   RATIONALE: Although ketamine, midazolam, and propofol exert only mild analgesic effects, thiopental has no analgesic properties, indicating that the patient may need additional analgesics after surgery.

3. Answer: d
   RATIONALE: Methohexital is associated with nausea and vomiting during the recovery period. Adverse effects include hypotension, suppressed respirations, and decreased gastrointestinal activity.

4. Answer: b
   RATIONALE: Combinations of barbiturate anesthestics and narcotics may produce apnea more commonly than with other analgesics.

5. Answer: a
   RATIONALE: Midazolam is an example of a nonbarbiturate anesthetic. Nitrous oxide is an anesthetic gas. Thiopental is a barbiturate anesthetic. Halothane is a volatile liquid anesthetic.

6. Answer: c
   RATIONALE: Ketamine is associated with a bizarre state of unconsciousness in which the patient appears to be awake but is unconscious and cannot feel pain. Propofol produces much less of a hangover effect. Droperidol

produces a state of mental detachment. Etomidate is sometimes used to sedate patients receiving mechanical ventilation.

7. Answer: b
   RATIONALE: Ketamine has an onset of action within 30 seconds; droperidol's onset is within 3 minutes; etomidate's onset occurs within 1 minute; and propofol's onset occurs within 30 to 60 seconds.

8. Answer: d
   RATIONALE: During recovery from etomidate, myoclonic and tonic movements, nausea, and vomiting may occur. Chills, hypertension, hallucinations, and cardiac arrhythmias can occur during recovery from droperidol. Respiratory depression and central nervous system suppression may occur during recovery from midazolam.

9. Answer: b
   RATIONALE: Nitrous oxide can block the reuptake of oxygen after surgery and cause hypoxia. Subsequently, it is always given in combination with oxygen.

10. Answer: a
   RATIONALE: Volatile liquids are liquids that are unstable at room temperature and release gases that are inhaled by the patient, as are gas anesthetics.

11. Answer: c
   RATIONALE: Although monitoring temperature and reflexes, providing comfort measures, and providing pain relief are important, the priority is to ensure that emergency equipment is readily available to allow for prompt intervention should problems arise.

12. Answer: b
   RATIONALE: In increasing concentrations, local anesthetics also cause the loss of the following sensations in this order: temperature, touch, proprioception, and skeletal muscle tone.

13. Answer: b
   RATIONALE: The dermal patch is applied 20 to 30 minutes before the procedure.

14. Answer: a
   RATIONALE: When a local anesthetic is to be applied, it is important to ensure that the area is intact and free of breakdown to prevent inadvertent systemic absorption of the drug.

15. Answer: c
   RATIONALE: Benzocaine is an example of an ester. Mepivacaine, lidocaine, and dibucaine are examples of amide local anesthetic agents.

CHAPTER 28

■ ASSESSING YOUR UNDERSTANDING

FILL IN THE BLANKS

1. Neuromuscular junction (NMJ)
2. Sarcomere
3. Actin, myosin
4. Acetylcholine
5. Nondepolarizing
6. Depolarizing

SEQUENCING

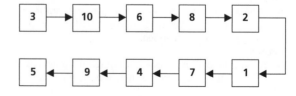

$$3 \rightarrow 10 \rightarrow 6 \rightarrow 8 \rightarrow 2$$
$$5 \leftarrow 9 \leftarrow 4 \leftarrow 7 \leftarrow 1$$

Copyright © 2011 by Wolters Kluwer Health I Lippincott Williams & Wilkins. *Study Guide for Focus on Nursing Pharmacology.*

■ APPLYING YOUR KNOWLEDGE

CASE STUDY

a. The patient is to be intubated; the pancuronium would be used to facilitate passage of the endotracheal tube during the intubation procedure and to minimize the patient's attempt to fight or resist mechanical ventilation.

b. The patient has a history of asthma, which could be exacerbated by the use of pancuronium due to the paralysis of the respiratory muscles altering perfusion and respiratory function. In addition, the drug can cause respiratory obstruction with wheezing and bronchospasm. Therefore, his respiratory status and oxygenation would need to be monitored very closely as he is mechanically ventilated. Also, measures to prevent aspiration would be important to prevent drug-related gastrointestinal effects from further compromising the patient's respiratory status. As a victim of multiple trauma, it is likely that his fluid and electrolyte balanced would be altered. This could affect membrane stability and subsequent muscular function. In addition, hyperkalemia can occur due to changes in the muscle membrane. Close monitoring of fluid and electrolyte status would be essential. Monitoring for hypotension and cardiac arrhythmias would be necessary to determine the patient's ability to adapt to the drugs. Moreover, the drug does not alter the pain perception, so the nurse would need to assess the patient's level of pain frequently.

c. The drug does not allow muscle contraction, so the nurse needs to inform the patient and family that the patient's muscles will be paralyzed. However, the patient may still feel pain and be conscious because the drug does not affect pain perception or consciousness. The nurse needs to work with the patient and family in setting up a means to communicate his needs or changes in his condition because the patient is unable to speak since he is intubated and receiving mechanical ventilation. Additionally, the nurse would inform the patient and family about the need for frequent turning and repositioning to prevent skin breakdown and the use of periodically evaluating muscle response and recovery, including the use of a peripheral nerve stimulator to assess the degree of neuromuscular blockade.

■ PRACTICING FOR NCLEX

1. Answer: d
RATIONALE: Of the NMJ blockers, cisatracurium has the longest duration of action.

2. Answer: a
RATIONALE: Atracurium should not be used before induction of anesthesia.

3. Answer: b
RATIONALE: Calcium channel blockers may greatly increase the paralysis caused by nondepolarizing NMJ blockers. If used together, the dose of the nondepolarizing NMJ agent would be decreased. Cholinesterase inhibitors would decrease the effectiveness of the nondepolarizing NMJ agent. Depolarizing NMJ blockers also interact with calcium channel blockers.

4. Answer: a
RATIONALE: The body's initial reaction to succinylcholine is muscle pain that occurs with the initial muscle contraction reaction. Hyperthemia would suggest malignant hyperthermia but does not occur as a first response. Hypotension and respiratory depression also occur, but these would not be an initial assessment finding.

5. Answer: b
RATIONALE: Conditions associated with a decreased production of cholinesterase, the enzyme necessary to break

down succinylcholine, include cirrhosis, metabolic disorders, cancer, burns, dehydration, malnutrition, hyperpyrexia, thyrotoxicosis, collagen diseases, and exposure to neurotoxic insecticides.

6. Answer: a
RATIONALE: According to the sliding filament theory, acetylcholine interacts with nicotinic receptors, not muscarinic receptors. Acetylcholine is broken down by acetylcholinesterase, freeing the receptor for further stimulation which when stimulated causes depolarization that leads to the release of calcium. Calcium combines with troponin, which then causes the release of actin and myosin binding sites, allowing them to react together. This repeated reaction leads to fiber shortening and muscle contraction.

7. Answer: c
RATIONALE: NMJ blockers, in most cases, do not affect pain perception and consciousness. They cause muscle paralysis without total central nervous system depression and are associated with serious adverse effects. They do not readily cross the blood–brain barrier.

8. Answer: d
RATIONALE: Succinylcholine is associated with the development of malignant hyperthermia in susceptible patients. Pancuronium, vecuronium, and atracurium are not associated with the development of this condition.

9. Answer: b
RATIONALE: Aspirin is useful in relieving the muscle pain that occurs with administration of a NMJ blocker, specifically succinylcholine. Dantrolene would be used to treat malignant hyperthermia that may occur with succinylcholine. Morphine would not be used to alleviate this muscle pain. Naloxone is used to reverse the depression associated with narcotic overdoses.

10. Answer: d
RATIONALE: Depolarizing NMJ blockers cause stimulation of the muscle cell, stay on the receptor site, and prevent repolarization, resulting in muscle paralysis with a muscle that is in a constant contracted state. Nondepolarizing NMJ blockers prevent depolarization of the muscle cells.

11. Answer: a
RATIONALE: Succinylcholine is the only NMJ blocker that may cause increased intraocular pressure.

12. Answer: c
RATIONALE: Pancuronium has an onset of action of approximately 4 to 6 minutes.

13. Answer: b
RATIONALE: Succinylcholine has a short duration of action, lasting approximately 4 to 6 minutes after administration.

14. Answer: a
RATIONALE: Myasthenia gravis would be a contraindication for the use of a nondepolarizing NMJ blocker because blockage of the acetylcholine cholinergic receptors would aggravate the neuromuscular disease. Cirrhosis and malnutrition would require extremely cautious use of succinylcholine, which is a depolarizing NMJ blocker. Glaucoma would be a contraindication to the use of succinylcholine due to the increased intraocular pressure that occurs.

15. Answer: c
RATIONALE: A cholinesterase inhibitor is used to overcome the excessive neuromuscular blockade of a nondepolarizing NMJ blocker. A direct-acting skeletal muscle relaxant, such as dantrolene, would be used to treat malignant hyperthermia associated with a depolarizing NMJ blocker. A peripheral nerve stimulator is used to assess the degree of neuromuscular blockade. A narcotic antagonist would be used to reverse a narcotic's effect.

CHAPTER 29

■ ASSESSING YOUR UNDERSTANDING

CROSSWORD

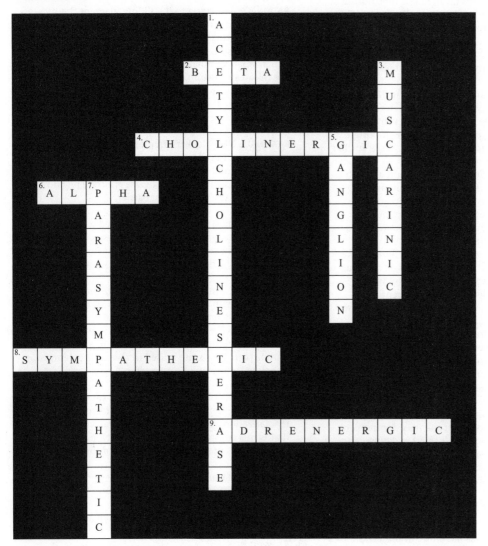

SHORT ANSWER

1. The main nerve centers are located in the hypothalamus, medulla, and spinal cord.

2. Throughout the autonomic nervous system (ANS), nerve impulses are carried from the central nervous system (CNS) to the outlying organs by way of a two-neuron system. In most peripheral nervous system activities, the CNS nerve body sends an impulse directly to an effector organ or muscle. The ANS does not send impulses directly to the periphery. Instead, axons from CNS neurons end in ganglia, or groups of nerve bodies that are packed together, located outside the CNS. These ganglia receive information from the preganglionic neuron that started in the CNS and relay that information along postganglionic neurons. The postganglionic neurons transmit impulses to the neuroeffector cells—muscles, glands, and organs.

3. The sympathetic nervous system (SNS) is also called the thoracolumbar system.

4. Acetylcholine is the neurotransmitter released by the pre-ganglionic nerves of the SNS.

5. The catecholamines include norepinephrine, dopamine, serotonin, and epinephrine.

6. Sympathetic adrenergic receptors are classified as alpha-1, alpha-2, beta-1, and beta-2.

7. Parasympathetic nervous system (PNS) receptors are classified as muscarinic or nicotinic.

8. The two enzymes involved are monoamine oxidase (MAO), and catechol-O-methyl transferase.

■ APPLYING YOUR KNOWLEDGE

CASE STUDY

a. The patient is experiencing an anxiety attack, which in most instances would be similar to a fight-or-flight response. Thus, the patient's SNS is predominating at this point. The patient's heart rate and respiratory rate are increased, and she is experiencing sweating due to the

Copyright © 2011 by Wolters Kluwer Health | Lippincott Williams & Wilkins. *Study Guide for Focus on Nursing Pharmacology.*

increase in metabolic activity that is occurring. The patient's cool and clammy hands are most likely related to the vasoconstriction and diversion of blood away from the area to more vital centers.

b. Additional signs and symptoms would include increased blood pressure, increased depth of respirations, bronchial dilation, pupillary dilation, piloerection, decreased bowel sounds, and decreased urination.

c. The nurse would explain the fight-or-flight response as the basis for what she is experiencing, correlating her anxiety level as a stimulus for the response. The nurse could liken the response to an accelerator that speeds things up for action. The nurse needs to emphasize that this response is a normal body response but that if the body becomes overstimulated, it can lead to system overload and disorders.

■ PRACTICING FOR NCLEX

1. **Answer: a, b, f**
   RATIONALE: The ANS functions to control heart rate, water balance, and respiration. Level of consciousness, sensory perception, and muscle movement are functions of the CNS.

2. **Answer: c**
   RATIONALE: The SNS has short preganglionic nerve fibers and long postganglionic nerve fibers that synapse with neuroeffectors. The cells are located primarily in the thoracic and lumbar sections of the spinal cord. The ganglia are located in chains running alongside the spinal cord.

3. **Answer: d**
   RATIONALE: In the stress or fight-or-flight response, the nurse would assess diminished bowel sounds, tachycardia, hypertension, and pupil dilation.

4. **Answer: a**
   RATIONALE: The release of adrenal hormones, including cortisol, suppress the immune and inflammatory reactions to preserve energy during the fight-or-flight response. Thyroid hormone increases metabolism and efficient use of energy. Aldosterone causes sodium and water retention and potassium excretion. Glucose is formed by glycogenolysis to increase the blood glucose level and provide energy.

5. **Answer: a**
   RATIONALE: Alpha-1 stimulation leads to vasoconstriction and increased peripheral vascular resistance resulting in a rise in blood pressure. Alpha-2 stimulation prevents overstimulation of effector sites and moderate insulin release by the beta cells of the pancreas. Beta-1 stimulation increases myocardial activity. Beta-2 stimulation causes vasodilation and bronchodilation.

6. **Answer: d**
   RATIONALE: Relaxation of the urinary detrusor muscle occurs with stimulation of beta-2 receptors. Alpha-1 receptor stimulation would promote closure of the urinary sphincter. Alpha-2 stimulation prevents overstimulation of effector sites and moderate insulin release by the beta cells of the pancreas. Beta-1 stimulation increases myocardial activity.

7. **Answer: b**
   RATIONALE: With parasympathetic nervous stimulation, gastric motility increases, secretions increase, pupils constrict, and the rectal and urinary sphincters relax to allow elimination.

8. **Answer: c**
   RATIONALE: In the PNS, the neurotransmitter involved in pre- and postganglion activity is acetylcholine. Norepinephrine is involved in postganglionic activity of the SNS. Epinephrine is involved in the adrenergic response, being secreted directly into the bloodstream by the

adrenal medulla. Dopamine is converted to norepinephrine in the adrenergic cells.

9. **Answer: a**
   RATIONALE: The vagus nerve, originating in the cranium, is one of the most important parts of the PNS. Adrenergic receptors, norepinephrine, and MAO are aspects that would be included in the discussion of the SNS.

10. **Answer: b**
    RATIONALE: The SNS preganglionic fibers are short; the PNS preganglionic fibers are long. The SNS ganglia are located in chains along the spinal cord; those of the PNS are located close to or within the effector tissue. The SNS is the system involved in the stress response, while the PNS is the rest and digest system. The PNS contains nicotinic and muscarinic receptors.

11. **Answer: d**
    RATIONALE: Vasodilation, as well as bronchodilation and uterine relaxation, occur as a result of beta-2 stimulation. Piloerection results from stimulation of alpha-1 receptors.

12. **Answer: b**
    RATIONALE: Alpha-2 receptors are found in the beta cells of the pancreas. Alpha-1 receptors are found in blood vessels, the iris, and urinary bladder. Beta-1 receptors are found in cardiac tissue. Beta-2 receptors are found in the smooth muscle of the blood vessels, bronchi, periphery, and uterine muscle.

13. **Answer: c**
    RATIONALE: Cholinergic nerves are located on all preganglionic nerves in the ANS, postganglionic nerves of the PNS and a few SNS nerves, motor nerves on skeletal muscles, and cholinergic nerves within the CNS.

14. **Answer: b**
    RATIONALE: Muscarinic receptors are located in visceral effector organs such as the gastrointestinal tract, bladder, and heart; in sweat glands; and in some vascular smooth muscle. Nicotinic receptors would be found in the adrenal medulla, neuromuscular junction, and CNS.

15. **Answer: b**
    RATIONALE: Norepinephrine is made by the nerve cells using tyrosine, which is obtained in the diet. Dihydroxyphenylalanine (dopa) is produced by a nerve, using tyrosine from the diet and other chemicals. With the help of the enzyme dopa decarboxylase, the dopa is converted to dopamine, which in turn is converted to norepinephrine in adrenergic cells.

CHAPTER 30

■ ASSESSING YOUR UNDERSTANDING

LABELING

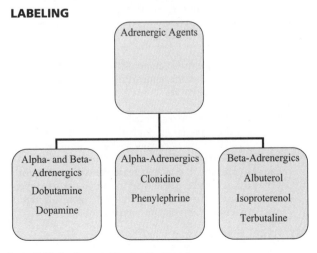

SHORT ANSWER

1. Adrenergic agonists stimulate the adrenergic receptors of the sympathetic nervous system directly by reacting with receptor sites or indirectly by increasing norepinephrine levels.
2. Adrenergic agonists are also referred to as sympathomimetic agents because they mimic or produce the same effects of the sympathetic nervous system.
3. Dopamine is the sympathomimetic drug of choice for treating shock.
4. Clonidine specifically stimulates alpha-2 receptors and is used to treat hypertension because its action blocks release of norepinephrine from nerve axons.
5. A sympathomimetic agent (adrenergic agonist) will lose effectiveness if it is combined with any adrenergic antagonist.
6. Adrenergic agonists cause vasoconstriction. In patients with vascular problems, their use could exacerbate the underlying vascular problem due to the systemic vasoconstriction that occurs.

■ APPLYING YOUR KNOWLEDGE

CASE STUDY

a. The nurse should respond to the patient in a nonjudgmental and supportive manner. The nurse should investigate further about the underlying reasons for the patient's statements. For example, is the patient concerned that there is not a sufficient dosage contained in the patch? Or is the patient more comfortable with taking pills? Possibly, the patient may be anxious about how to apply the patch or apply the patch correctly. He might believe that it is easier to just take a pill.

b. The nurse needs to instruct the patient how the patch works, providing a gradual release of the drug that lasts 7 days, and about how to apply the patch, once every 7 days to a hairless area of the body, such as the upper arm or chest. The nurse also needs to reinforce the need to apply the patch to intact, clean, dry skin and to remove the patch before applying a new one. Additional instructions also should address not stopping the patch abruptly because of possible rebound hypertension. The nurse also needs to warn the patient about possible adverse effects, including central nervous system effects such as bad dreams, sedation, drowsiness, fatigue, and headache. Safety measures including changing positions slowly, lifestyle modifications to control blood pressure, the importance of avoiding over-the-counter (OCT) cold preparations, and compliance with regular follow-ups to evaluate blood pressure would be essential.

■ PRACTICING FOR NCLEX

1. **Answer: b**
   RATIONALE: Dopamine is a naturally occurring catecholamine. Dobutamine, ephedrine, and metaraminol are synthetic catecholamines.

2. **Answer: a**
   RATIONALE: Dobutamine, although it acts at both receptor sites, has a slight preference for beta-1 receptor sites. It is used in the treatment of congestive heart failure because it can increase myocardial contractility without much change in rate and does not increase the oxygen demand of the cardiac muscle. There is an increased risk for hypertension if any alpha- and beta-adrenergic agonist is used with herbal therapies and OTC preparations.

3. **Answer: b**
   RATIONALE: Adverse effects of alpha- and beta-adrenergic agonists include dyspnea, hypertension, and constipation. Personality changes are associated with alpha-specific adrenergic agonists.

4. **Answer: c**
   RATIONALE: The drug of choice for treating shock is dopamine because it stimulates the heart and blood pressure and also causes a renal and splanchnic arteriole dilation that increases blood flow to the kidney, preventing diminished renal blood supply and possible renal shutdown that can occur with epinephrine or norepinephrine. Ephedrine is used to treat hypotensive episodes, but its use is declining because of the availability of less-toxic drugs with more predictable onset and action. Dobutamine is used to treat congestive heart failure.

5. **Answer: a**
   RATIONALE: Alpha- and beta-adrenergic agonists interact with caffeine, ma huang, and OTC cold preparations, increasing the risk for hypertension. St. John's wort has not been shown to interact with these agents.

6. **Answer: d**
   RATIONALE: If extravasation occurs, the nurse should infiltrate the site with 10 mL of saline containing 5 to 10 mg of phentolamine. Hyaluronidase and sodium bicarbonate may be used for extravasation of certain antineoplastic agents. Lactated Ringer's solution would be inappropriate.

7. **Answer: a, d, e**
   RATIONALE: Clonidine is an alpha-specific adrenergic agonist that may cause sensitivity to light (photophobia), personality changes, difficulty urinating, and pupil dilation. Hyperglycemia may occur if the patient has diabetes and takes clonidine.

8. **Answer: c**
   RATIONALE: Intramuscular phenylephrine has an onset of action within 10 to 15 minutes.

9. **Answer: c**
   RATIONALE: The desired effects of isoproterenol include improved contractility and conductivity, increased heart rate, bronchodilation, relaxation of the uterus, and increased blood flow to skeletal muscles and splanchnic beds.

10. **Answer: a**
    RATIONALE: To counteract the effects of isoproterenol, a beta-specific adrenergic agonist, the nurse would administer a beta-adrenergic blocker.

11. **Answer: d**
    RATIONALE: Most of the beta-specific adrenergic agonists are beta-2–specific adrenergic agonists, which are used to treat and manage bronchial spasm, asthma, and other obstructive pulmonary conditions.

12. **Answer: a**
    RATIONALE: Pulmonary hypertension would be a contraindication for isoproterenol because the drug could exacerbate the condition. Glaucoma would be a contraindication for the use of an alpha-specific adrenergic agonist. Pheochromocytoma and hypovolemia would be contraindications for the use of alpha- and beta-adrenergic agonists.

13. **Answer: c**
    RATIONALE: If dopamine or norepinephrine could not be used to prevent hypotension, then metaraminol would be the drug of choice. It increases myocardial contractility and causes peripheral vasoconstriction.

Copyright © 2011 by Wolters Kluwer Health I Lippincott Williams & Wilkins. *Study Guide for Focus on Nursing Pharmacology.*

14. Answer: b
RATIONALE: Midodrine is associated with a serious supine hypertension. Therefore, monitoring blood pressure changes in different positions (standing, sitting, and supine) would be most important. The drug is not associated with respiratory adverse effects. Decreased urinary output and anorexia may occur, but these would not be as important as monitoring the changes in the patient's blood pressure.

15. Answer: b
RATIONALE: Phenylephrine is a common agent found in many OTC cold and allergy products. Ephedra has been banned by the Food and Drug Administration as a drug. Neither metaraminol nor albuterol are found in OTC products.

CHAPTER 31

■ ASSESSING YOUR UNDERSTANDING

LABELING

Nonselective Alpha	Alpha-1 Selective	Nonselective Beta	Beta-1 Selective
Phentolamine	Doxazosin Terazosin	Carteolol Pindolol Propranolol	Atenolol Esmolol

FILL IN THE BLANKS

1. Sympatholytics
2. Norepinephrine
3. Hypoglycemia
4. Hypertension
5. Lowering
6. Postsynaptic
7. Cardiovascular
8. Decreased
9. Two
10. Atenolol

■ APPLYING YOUR KNOWLEDGE

CASE STUDY

a. The patient is receiving carvedilol, a nonselective adrenergic blocker, as well as sotalol, a nonselective beta blocker. Both agents lower blood pressure. The diuretic promotes fluid loss, which also aids in lowering blood pressure. The fluid loss associated with diuretic therapy also may be contributed to possible dehydration, which could lower the blood pressure further. The patient may be experiencing orthostatic hypotension, which is a drop in blood pressure that occurs with position changes.

b. It would be important to obtain additional information by obtaining the following: vital signs; blood pressure evaluation in the lying, sitting, and standing positions (to evaluate any changes in readings with position changes); electrocardiogram (to rule out any underlying cardiac changes that might be contributing to the patient's complaints); evaluation of hydration status (skin turgor, review of fluid intake, and electrolyte levels). In addition, it would be important to ask the patient about any alcohol ingestion, which can contribute to hypotension.

c. The patient needs instructions related to safety measures, such as rising slowly from a sitting position or sitting at the edge of the bed for a few minutes before arising. In addition, the patient needs to ensure that he is taking in adequate amounts of fluid to prevent any dehydration that would further compound the hypotension. Additionally, the patient should be instructed not to stop taking the drugs abruptly because of the possible serious adverse effects that might occur. Additionally, emphasis on compliance with the therapy and follow-up is essential to ensure that the patient's needs and concerns are addressed and to ensure maximum drug therapy effectiveness with the least amount of adverse effects.

■ PRACTICING FOR NCLEX

1. Answer: a
RATIONALE: Monitoring liver function studies would be most important because carvedilol has been associated with hepatic failure. Renal function studies may be appropriate to evaluate for possible renal dysfunction that might necessitate a change in drug dosage, but this would not be the priority. Monitoring complete blood count and coagulation studies would not be necessary.

2. Answer: b
RATIONALE: Sotalol absorption is decreased by the presence of food; to ensure maximum effectiveness of the drug, the patient should take it on an empty stomach, not with an antacid or after a large meal. The dose is typically divided during the day and should not be taken all at once.

3. Answer: b
RATIONALE: Nonselective adrenergic blockers block the effects of norepinephrine at the alpha and beta receptors in the sympathetic nervous system, leading to a slower pulse rate, lowering of blood pressure, increased renal perfusion, and decreased renin levels.

4. Answer: c
RATIONALE: Labetalol, a nonselective adrenergic blocker, increases the effectiveness of antidiabetic agents leading to an increased risk for hypoglycemia. Hypotension would occur if the drug were combined with other drugs that are known to lower blood pressure. Arrhythmias and bronchospasm are adverse effects of nonselective adrenergic blockers and are unrelated to the combination of labetalol and insulin.

5. Answer: b
RATIONALE: Alpha-1 selective adrenergic blockers cause a decrease in vascular tone and vasodilation, which leads to a fall in blood pressure. Because these drugs do not block the presynaptic alpha-2 receptor sites, the reflex tachycardia that accompanies a fall in blood pressure does not occur. They also block smooth muscle receptors in the prostate, prostatic capsule, prostatic urethra, and urinary bladder neck, which lead to a relaxation of the bladder and prostate and improved flow of urine in males.

6. Answer: a
RATIONALE: Tamsulosin, an alpha-1 selective adrenergic blocker, is used for the treatment of benign prostatic hypertrophy. Prazosin, also an alpha-1 selective blocker, is used to treat hypertension. Carteolol, a nonselective beta blocker, is used for the treatment of hypertension. Amiodarone, a nonselective adrenergic blocker, is reserved for use in treating arrhythmias.

7. Answer: b

RATIONALE: Adverse gastrointestinal (GI) effects are associated with the loss of the balancing sympathetic effect on the GI tract and the increased parasympathetic dominance. The drug's effect on liver function would be associated with the development of liver dysfunction and failure. Blockage of norepinephrine in the central nervous system (CNS) would lead to adverse effects such as dizziness, paresthesias, insomnia, fatigue, and vertigo. Loss of vascular tone would be associated with hypotension, heart failure, pulmonary edema, and cerebrovascular accident.

8. Answer: a

RATIONALE: Oral labetalol peaks in 1 to 2 hours.

9. Answer: d

RATIONALE: Although safety measures are important part of the teaching plan for any nonselective beta blocker, they would be a priority for a patient receiving propranolol. The drug crosses the blood–brain barrier, leading to the development of CNS effects. Carteolol, nadolol, and sotalol do not cross the blood–brain barrier; thus, the risk for CNS effects would be less.

10. Answer: b

RATIONALE: A patient receiving propranolol should understand that the drug should not be stopped abruptly but rather should be tapered over a period of 2 weeks. Getting up slowly, spacing activities, and reporting any chest pain or difficulty breathing demonstrate an understanding of the possible adverse effects of the drug and measures to address them.

11. Answer: d

RATIONALE: Atenolol is a beta-1 selective adrenergic blocker. This agent would be preferred for the patient who smokes because the drug does not usually block beta-1 receptor sites. Subsequently, it does not block the sympathetic bronchodilation that would be important for this patient. Timolol, pindolol, and nadolol are nonselective beta-adrenergic blockers that would block this sympathetic bronchodilation.

12. Answer: c

RATIONALE: Beta-1 selective blockers are contraindicated in patients with sinus bradycardia. Diabetes, thyroid disease, and chronic obstructive pulmonary disease are conditions that require cautious use of beta-1 selective blockers.

13. Answer: d

RATIONALE: For acute myocardial infarction, metoprolol is given via intravenous bolus. Three doses, each given at 2-minute intervals, are used and then the patient is started on oral therapy, which is started 15 minutes after the last intravenous dose.

14. Answer: a

RATIONALE: Bisoprolol is often the drug of choice for older patients who require an adrenergic blocker for hypertension because it is not associated with as many problems in this age group and regular dosing profiles may be used.

15. Answer: c

RATIONALE: A beta-1 selective blocker is helpful after a myocardial infarction because it decreases the cardiac workload and myocardial oxygen demand. The drug decreases contractility, excitability, and the heart rate. Although it also decreases blood pressure, it is not this effect that makes it a useful in preventing reinfarction.

CHAPTER 32

■ ASSESSING YOUR UNDERSTANDING

LABELING

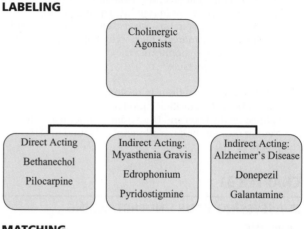

MATCHING

1. d   **2.** a   **3.** e   **4.** c   **5.** b

■ APPLYING YOUR KNOWLEDGE

CASE STUDY

a. The patient is most likely experiencing either a myasthenic crisis in which she needs additional medication or a cholinergic crisis or cholinergic overdose, necessitating withdrawal of the medication. Myasthenia gravis is a condition that is characterized by periods of exacerbations and remissions that are highly unpredictable. Too much pyridostigmine can lead to a cholinergic crisis, whereas as not enough pyridostigmine can lead to a myasthenic crisis. Both conditions are manifested by increasing muscle weakness.

b. To determine whether the patient is experiencing a myasthenic or cholinergic crisis, an edrophonium challenge test would be used. *If* the patient improves after injection of the edrophonium, then she most likely is experiencing a myasthenic crisis. In this case, additional cholinergic medication would be given. If the patient's signs and symptoms do not improve or actually become worse with edrophonium, then the patient most likely is experiencing a cholinergic crisis. In this situation, the pyridostigmine would be stopped.

c. If the patient is experiencing a myasthenic crisis, additional pyridostigmine may be ordered or possibly another indirect-acting cholinergic agonist might be used. The patient would require close monitoring to evaluate for resolution of the signs and symptoms, such as improved swallowing, speech, and breathing. For example, if an increased dosage of pyridostigmine were ordered, improved signs and symptoms would be seen within 5 minutes of intravenous administration and within 35 to 45 minutes of oral administration.

If the patient were experiencing a cholinergic crisis, then the pyridostigmine would be stopped immediately and supportive intensive care, including possible intubation and mechanical ventilation, is necessary to ensure adequate respiratory function.

■ PRACTICING FOR NCLEX

1. Answer: b

RATIONALE: Cholinergic agents cause increased salivation, pupil constriction, decreased heart rate, and increased bladder muscle tone.

Copyright © 2011 by Wolters Kluwer Health l Lippincott Williams & Wilkins. *Study Guide for Focus on Nursing Pharmacology*.

2. **Answer: a**
   RATIONALE: When administered ophthalmically, pilocarpine results in miosis. It does not cause ptosis (drooping) or paralysis of the eye muscles.

3. **Answer: d**
   RATIONALE: Adverse effects associated with direct-acting cholinergic agents include urinary urgency, bradycardia, hypotension, and diarrhea.

4. **Answer: c**
   RATIONALE: For nonobstructive postoperative urinary retention, bethanechol may be ordered. Cevimeline is used to treat dry mouth associated with Sjorgren's syndrome. Pilocarpine is used to relieve intraocular pressure of glaucoma (ophthalmic form) or to treat dry mouth associated with Sjorgren's syndrome. Carbachol is used to relieve increased intraocular pressure.

5. **Answer: b**
   RATIONALE: Indirect-acting cholinergic agonists react chemically with acetylcholinesterase to prevent it from breaking down acetylcholine. This leads to an accumulation of acetylcholine. Direct-acting cholinergic agonists occupy receptor sites for acetylcholine on the membranes of the effectors cells. Cholinergic agonists in general act at the same site as the neurotransmitter acetylcholine and are often called *parasympathomimetic* because their action mimics that of the parasympathetic nervous system.

6. **Answer: d**
   RATIONALE: Donepezil is an indirect-acting cholinergic agent used to treat Alzheimer's disease. Pyridostigmine, neostigmine, and ambenonium would be used to treat myasthenia gravis.

7. **Answer: c**
   RATIONALE: Exposure to nerve gas would be manifested by the following: bronchial and pupil constriction, slow heart rate, muscle contraction, and increased gastrointestinal (GI) activity and secretions.

8. **Answer: a**
   RATIONALE: Donepezil has a 70-hour half-life and is usually given in a once-a-day dosing. Galantamine and rivastigmine are usually taken twice a day. Tacrine must be taken four times a day.

9. **Answer: c**
   RATIONALE: There is an increased risk of GI bleeding if indirect-acting cholinergic agonists such as rivastigmine are used with nonsteroidal anti-inflammatory drugs (NSAIDs) such as ibuprofen because of the combination of increased GI secretions and GI mucosal erosion associated with the use of NSAIDs. Fecal incontinence, abdominal cramps, and diarrhea are adverse effects associated with indirect-acting cholinergic agonists.

10. **Answer: b**
    RATIONALE: Atropine should be readily available to counteract the severe effects of an indirect-acting cholinergic agonist. Edrophonium is used as the antidote for nondepolarizing neuromuscular junction (NMJ) blockers. Phentolamine is used to as treatment for extravasation of intravenous norepinephrine or dopamine. Naloxone is used to treat narcotic overdose.

11. **Answer: c**
    RATIONALE: Pyridostigmine is available in oral and parenteral forms; the parenteral form can be used if the patient is having trouble swallowing. In addition, the drug has a longer half-life than neostigmine and thus can be given less frequently. Ambenonium is available only in oral form and would be inappropriate for a patient who is having difficulty swallowing. Rivastigmine is used to treat Alzheimer's disease, not myasthenia gravis.

12. **Answer: a, b, e**
    RATIONALE: Possible adverse effects related to anticholinesterase agents include urinary urgency, blurred vision, flushing, diarrhea, and hypotension.

13. **Answer: b**
    RATIONALE: Although respiratory status and mental status would be important areas to monitor, it would be most important to evaluate serum theophylline levels because these levels can be increased up to twofold when combined with tacrine, placing the patient at high risk for theophylline toxicity.

14. **Answer: c**
    RATIONALE: Intestinal obstruction would be a contraindication to the use of anticholinesterase inhibitors. Asthma, peptic ulcer disease, and parkinsonism would require cautious use and close monitoring.

15. **Answer: a**
    RATIONALE: Direct-acting cholinergic agonists usually stimulate muscarinic receptors within the parasympathetic nervous system. Alpha and beta receptors are found in the sympathetic nervous system and are affected by adrenergic agents.

CHAPTER 33

■ ASSESSING YOUR UNDERSTANDING

FILL IN THE BLANKS

1. Belladonna
2. Anticholinergic
3. Atropine
4. Mydriasis
5. Cholinergic
6. Physostigmine
7. Increase
8. Decreased

MATCHING

1. b	2. c	3. e	4. d	5. a

■ APPLYING YOUR KNOWLEDGE

CASE STUDY

a. The patient is black, so he may require an additional length of time for the mydriatic effect of atropine to occur. Or, the patient may require a larger dose to achieve mydriasis. The patient also is taking a tricyclic antidepressant, which may interact with atropine and increase possible anticholinergic effects. However, systemic absorption of the atropine is less likely when given ophthalmically.

b. Instillation of the eye drops would lead to localized adverse effects such as blurred vision, pupil dilation, and subsequent photophobia. However, the nurse would need to be alert for systemic adverse effects as well. Inadvertent systemic absorption may occur with the instillation of eye drops. Thus, the nurse would need to assess the patient for systemic adverse effects, such as weakness, dizziness, mental confusion, dry mouth, constipation, tachycardia, urinary retention, and decreased sweating. These effects may be exacerbated by the interaction of the atropine (absorbed systemically) with the tricyclic antidepressant.

■ PRACTICING FOR NCLEX

1. Answer: c
RATIONALE: Atropine toxicity is dose related. Typically, slight cardiac slowing, inhibition of sweating, and dry mouth are seen with 0.5 mg of atropine. Cough would not be associated with atropine toxicity.

2. Answer: c
RATIONALE: Scopolamine blocks only the muscarinic effectors in the parasympathetic nervous system and those few cholinergic receptors in the sympathetic nervous system. It does not block the nicotinic receptors and has little or no effect at the neuromuscular junction.

3. Answer: b
RATIONALE: Only scopolamine is available as a transdermal system.

4. Answer: a
RATIONALE: Propantheline is available only in oral form.

5. Answer: d
RATIONALE: A patient with hypertension who receives an anticholinergic is at risk for additive hypertensive effects due to the dominance of the sympathetic system with parasympathetic blockage. Bladder obstruction, paralytic ileus, and increased intraocular pressure are contraindications for the use of an anticholinergic agent.

6. Answer: a
RATIONALE: Flavoxate may be ordered to provide symptomatic relief of dysuria, urgency, nocturia, suprapubic pain, frequency, and incontinence associated with cystitis. Dicyclomine is used to treat irritable or hyperactive bowel. Glycopyrrolate is used to decrease secretions before surgery or intubation and as an adjunct for treatment of ulcers. Methscopolamine is used as an adjunct treatment for peptic ulcers.

7. Answer: b
RATIONALE: The patient should avoid temperature extremes and exertion in warm temperatures because of possible heat intolerance, which could be more severe in older patients. Drinking fluids is important to maintain hydration and prevent heat intolerance. Avoiding driving is an appropriate safety measure. Constipation may occur with an anticholinergic; therefore, increased fiber intake would be appropriate.

8. Answer: b
RATIONALE: If atropine toxicity is due to ingestion, immediate gastric lavage is performed to limit absorption of the drug. Physostigmine would then be given as an antidote. Diazepam may be used if the patient experiences seizures. Cool sponge baths would be used as additional support measure to relieve fever and hot skin.

9. Answer: d
RATIONALE: When used with anticholinergic agents, increased anticholinergic effects can occur with antihistamines, antiparkinson agents, and monoamine oxidase inhibitors. Nonsteroidal anti-inflammatory drugs are not known to interact with anticholinergic agents.

10. Answer: b
RATIONALE: When given intramuscularly, atropine peaks in approximately 30 minutes; for this situation, the peak effects would be noted at approximately 9:30 AM.

11. Answer: a, b, c, e
RATIONALE: Glycopyrrolate can be given orally, intramuscularly, subcutaneously, and intravenously.

12. Answer: d
RATIONALE: Excitement is a possible adverse central nervous system effect associated with anticholinergic agents. Pupil dilation, constipation, and tachycardia are other adverse effects.

13. Answer: c
RATIONALE: The patch should be applied to a clean, dry, intact, and hairless area of the body. The area should not be shaved, as this could abrade the skin and lead to increased absorption. Hair may be clipped if necessary. The backing is peeled off without touching the adhesive side of the patch, and the patch is placed at a new site each time to avoid skin irritation or degradation. The old patch is removed and the area is cleaned before a new patch is applied.

14. Answer: d
RATIONALE: Hyoscyamine acts more specifically on the receptors of the gastrointestinal tract. Ipratropium and tiotropium act more specifically to decreased respiratory secretions and cause bronchodilation. Trospium acts more specifically on the smooth muscle of the urinary tract.

15. Answer: b
RATIONALE: A scopolamine patch is changed every 3 days.

CHAPTER 34

■ ASSESSING YOUR UNDERSTANDING

LABELING

Hypothalamus	Anterior Pituitary	Posterior Pituitary
Gonadotropin-releasing hormone Somatostatin Thyroid-releasing hormone	Adrenocorticotropic hormone (ACTH) Follicle-stimulating hormone Growth hormone Luteinizing hormone Melanocyte-stimulating hormone Prolactin Thyroid-stimulating hormone	Antidiuretic hormone Oxytocin

MATCHING

1. d	**2.** e	**3.** f	**4.** a	**5.** c
6. h	**7.** g	**8.** b		

■ APPLYING YOUR KNOWLEDGE

CASE STUDY

a. The tumor pressing on a small portion of the patient's hypothalamus can result in numerous hormonal problems because the hypothalamus is considered the master gland. It acts as the coordinating center. Hormonally, the secretion of the various releasing hormones may be affected, thereby disrupting the function of the pituitary gland and eventually the target organ function. In addition, this disruption would also interfere with the functioning of the hypothalamic-pituitary axis and the negative feedback system that maintains homeostasis. Depending on the areas of the hypothalamus that are involved, the patient may experience too much secretion of certain releasing hormones and not

Copyright © 2011 by Wolters Kluwer Health | Lippincott Williams & Wilkins. *Study Guide for Focus on Nursing Pharmacology*.

enough of others. In turn, the secretion of hormones by the pituitary also would be altered.

b. The hypothalamus also plays a role in neurologic function and is the site of various neurocenters. Depending on the neurocenters that may be affected by the tumor, the patient may experience problems with the regulation of various body functions such as body temperature, thirst, hunger, water balance, blood pressure, respirations, reproduction, and emotional reactions. It also receives input from virtually all other areas of the brain, including the limbic system and cerebral cortex. Alterations in limbic system function can affect the neurotransmitters of epinephrine, norepinephrine, and serotonin, which in turn could affect the patient's expression of emotion. Additionally, the hypothalamus plays a role in the autonomic nervous system, which could lead to alterations in the sympathetic and parasympathetic nervous system control of body functions. The tumor's extension toward the cerebrum could impact the patient's sensory capabilities and motor function along with speech and communication.

■ PRACTICING FOR NCLEX

1. **Answer: b**
   RATIONALE: Hormones are chemical substances that are produced in small quantities, are secreted directly into the bloodstream, travel through the blood to specific receptor sites, and are immediately broken down.

2. **Answer: c**
   RATIONALE: Although traditionally the pituitary gland was considered the master gland, current thought is that the hypothalamus is the master gland because it is responsible for coordinating the nervous and endocrine responses to internal and external stimuli.

3. **Answer: d**
   RATIONALE: A hormone that takes a while to produce its effect is most likely entering the cell and reacting with a receptor site inside the cell to change messenger RNA, ultimately affecting cellular DNA and the cell's function. Reaction with a receptor on the cell membrane usually results in an immediate hormonal effect. Hormones do not react with a cell as it travels through the bloodstream or in a specialized target area of the body.

4. **Answer: a**
   RATIONALE: The hypothalamus secretes the releasing and inhibiting hormones such as somatostatin, or growth hormone inhibiting factor. ACTH, luteinizing hormone, and prolactin are secreted by the anterior pituitary gland.

5. **Answer: d**
   RATIONALE: Oxytocin and antidiuretic hormone are delivered by the neurologic network that connects the hypothalamus to the pituitary gland. The releasing hormones are delivered by the vascular network.

6. **Answer: d**
   RATIONALE: Plasma osmolality affects the release of antidiuretic hormone from the posterior pituitary gland. Central nervous system activity, hypothalamic hormones, and drugs can affect the release of hormones from the anterior pituitary gland.

7. **Answer: b**
   RATIONALE: Endorphins and enkephalins are released by the intermediate lobe of the pituitary gland. Oxytocin and antidiuretic hormone are released by the posterior pituitary gland. Melanocyte-stimulating hormone is released from the anterior pituitary gland.

8. **Answer: a**
   RATIONALE: Diurnal rhythm occurs when the hypothalamus begins secretion of corticotropin-releasing factor in the evening.

9. **Answer: c**
   RATIONALE: Oxytocin stimulates uterine smooth muscle contraction in late pregnancy and also causes the milk release or letdown reflex in lactating women. Prolactin is the hormone responsible for milk production. Follicle-stimulating hormone and luteinizing hormone are responsible for the initial events of the menstrual cycle.

10. **Answer: a**
    RATIONALE: Prolactin and growth hormone are two anterior pituitary hormones that do not have a target organ to produce hormones for regulation by a negative feedback mechanism. Thyroid hormone, follicle-stimulating hormone, and ACTH are regulated by a negative feedback mechanism.

11. **Answer: b**
    RATIONALE: Parathormone release is regulated by calcium levels. Acid in the gastrointestinal (GI) tract helps regulate GI hormones. Blood pressure aids in the regulation of erythropoietin release by the juxtaglomerular cells of the kidneys. Blood glucose levels regulate the release of insulin, glucagon, and somatostatin from the pancreas.

12. **Answer: c**
    RATIONALE: Activation of the sympathetic nervous system directly causes the release of ACTH. Aldosterone is released in response to ACTH and also is released directly in response to high potassium levels. Prostaglandins are released in response to local stimuli in the tissues that produce them. Calcitonin is released in response to serum calcium levels.

13. **Answer: b**
    RATIONALE: The initiating event in the hypothalamic-pituitary axis is the hypothalamic secretion of releasing factors, which leads to the anterior pituitary secreting the stimulating hormone, which in turn leads to the secretion of the hormone by the gland. Rising levels of the hormone cause the hypothalamus to cease secretion of the releasing hormone.

14. **Answer: c**
    RATIONALE: Aldosterone leads to sodium retention and thus increasing serum sodium levels and increased potassium excretion. Increased glucose levels result from cortisol secretion; increased red blood cell production results from secretion of erythropoietin.

15. **Answer: b**
    RATIONALE: Thyroid hormone secretion stimulates the basal metabolic rate. Gastrin stimulates stomach acid production; testosterone stimulates male secondary sex characteristics. Secretin and cholecystokinin stimulate pancreatic juice and bile secretion.

CHAPTER 35

■ ASSESSING YOUR UNDERSTANDING
CROSSWORD

```
            ¹H
            Y           ²D W A R F I S M
            P           I
³A C R O M E G A L Y    B
            P           E
            I           T           ⁴H
            T           E           Y
            U           S           P
            I           ⁵G I G A N T I S M
            T           N           H
            A           S           A
            R           I           L
            I           P           A
            S           I           M
            M           D           U
                        U           S
                        S
```

SHORT ANSWER

1. Hypothalamic hormones are not all available for pharmacologic use. Ones that are available are used mostly for diagnostic testing, for treating some forms of cancer, or as adjuncts in fertility programs.
2. Gigantism is due to hypersecretion of growth hormone that occurs before the epiphyseal plates of the long bones fuse, causing an acceleration in linear skeletal growth; acromegaly is used to describe the onset of excessive growth hormone secretion that occurs after puberty and epiphyseal plate closure.
3. The prototype growth hormone antagonist is bromocriptine mesylate.
4. Signs of water intoxication include drowsiness, lightheadedness, headache, coma, and convulsions related to the shift to water retention and resulting electrolyte imbalance; and tremor, sweating, vertigo, and headache related to water retention.
5. Growth hormone antagonists include octreotide and bromocriptine.

■ APPLYING YOUR KNOWLEDGE
CASE STUDY

a. The nurse needs to use a nonjudgmental and empathetic approach with the child, encouraging the child to verbalize his feelings about being the "shortest one" in the class.

This information might help to provide clues from which the nurse could plan specific measures to assist the child in coping with the upcoming changes. The nurse also can gain insight into coping mechanisms that the child has used in the past, encouraging the child to use the ones that were effective in dealing with this situation.

b. Growth hormone does promote growth, and this is a benefit that the child is expecting. However, the child will also need to learn how to cope with the changes that will be occurring in his body because the changes can happen suddenly. In addition, there are times when growth may not occur, which could cause significant upset for the child who is expecting growth. Somatropin is associated with thyroid dysfunction manifested by thinning hair and puffy skin. The nurse needs to address these possibilities with the child so that he is aware that they may occur and is prepared if they do happen.

■ PRACTICING FOR NCLEX

1. **Answer: b**
   RATIONALE: Nafarelin is given in nasal form.
2. **Answer: c**
   RATIONALE: Hypothalamic agonists are associated with impaired healing, fluid retention, elevated glucose levels, and electrolyte imbalance. Hypothalamic antagonists can lead to a decrease in testosterone levels leading to a loss of energy.
3. **Answer: b**
   RATIONALE: Leuprolide causes hot flashes, not chills. Other adverse effects include hematuria, peripheral edema, and constipation.
4. **Answer: a**
   RATIONALE: Corticotropin-releasing hormone is used to diagnose Cushing's disease. Gonadorelin is used to evaluate the functional capacity and response of gonadotropes of the anterior pituitary gland. Goserelin is used as an antineoplastic agent, and sermorelin is used to diagnose hypothalamic or pituitary dysfunction in short children.
5. **Answer: c**
   RATIONALE: Somatropin is considered a growth hormone agonist. Bromocriptine, octreotide, and pegvisomant are growth hormone antagonists.
6. **Answer: c**
   RATIONALE: Signs of glucose intolerance include thirst, hunger, and voiding pattern changes. Injection site pain is an adverse effect of the therapy. Fatigue and cold intolerance suggest thyroid dysfunction.
7. **Answer: b**
   RATIONALE: Octreotide must be administered subcutaneously.
8. **Answer: d**
   RATIONALE: Pegvisomant may lead to increased incidence of infection, nausea, diarrhea, and changes in liver function. Gastrointestinal upset, drowsiness, and postural hypotension are associated with bromocriptine.
9. **Answer: d**
   RATIONALE: Octreotide is associated with the development of acute cholecystitis; bromocriptine and pegvisomant are not. Somatropin is a growth hormone agonist.

Copyright © 2011 by Wolters Kluwer Health I Lippincott Williams & Wilkins. *Study Guide for Focus on Nursing Pharmacology.*

10. Answer: a

RATIONALE: Chorionic gonadotropin would be used to induce ovulation in females with functioning ovaries. Corticotropin and cosyntropin are used to diagnose adrenal function. Thyrotropin alfa is used as adjunctive treatment for radioiodine ablation of thyroid tissue for thyroid cancer.

11. Answer: b

RATIONALE: Oxytocin is a posterior pituitary hormone that is used to promote uterine contractions. Desmopressin is used to treat diabetes insipidus. Menotropins and chorionic gonadotropin alfa are fertility agents.

12. Answer: d

RATIONALE: Desmopressin is a synthetic antidiuretic hormone.

13. Answer: b

RATIONALE: Intravenous desmopressin has an onset of action of 30 minutes, or in this case, the drug would begin to work at approximately 10:30 AM.

14. Answer: c

RATIONALE: Corticotropin-releasing hormone is administered as an intravenous infusion of the drug diluted in 500 mL of 5% dextrose in water (D5W) over 8 hours.

15. Answer: c

RATIONALE: Goserelin is a gonadotropin-releasing hormone agonist, actually an analog of gonadotropin-releasing hormone. Leuprolide, ganirelix, and abarelix are gonadotropin-releasing hormone antagonists.

CHAPTER 36

■ ASSESSING YOUR UNDERSTANDING

LABELING

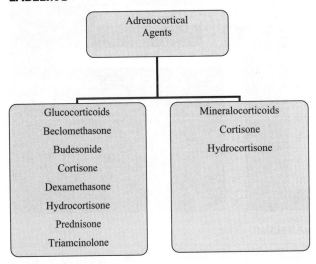

SHORT ANSWER

1. Diurnal rhythm is the response of the hypothalamus and then the pituitary and adrenal glands to wakefulness and sleeping. Normally, the hypothalamus begins secretion of corticotropin-releasing factor (CRF) in the evening, peaking at about midnight; adrenocortical peak response is between 6 and 9 AM; and levels fall during the day until evening, when the low level is picked up by the hypothalamus and CRF secretion begins again.

2. The adrenal medulla is actually part of the sympathetic nervous system (SNS). It is a ganglion of neurons that releases the neurotransmitters norepinephrine and epinephrine into circulation when the SNS is stimulated. The secretion of these neurotransmitters directly into the bloodstream allows them to act as hormones, traveling from the adrenal medulla to react with specific receptor sites throughout the body.

3. The three types of corticosteroids are androgens, glucocorticoids, and mineralocorticoids.

4. People with adrenal insufficiency are exposed to extreme stress such as a motor vehicle accident, a surgical procedure, or a massive infection. Because they are not able to supplement the energy-consuming effects of the sympathetic reaction, they enter an adrenal crisis, which can include physiologic exhaustion, hypotension, fluid shift, shock, and even death.

5. Prolonged use of corticosteroids suppresses the normal hypothalamic–pituitary axis and leads to adrenal atrophy from lack of stimulation.

6. Glucocorticoids stimulate an increase in glucose levels for energy. They also increase the rate of protein breakdown and decrease the rate of protein formation from amino acids, which is another way of preserving energy. Glucocorticoids also cause lipogenesis, or the formation and storage of fat in the body. This stored fat will then be available to be broken down for energy when needed.

■ APPLYING YOUR KNOWLEDGE

CASE STUDY

a. Systemically administered corticosteroids are associated with weight gain, increased appetite, and sodium and fluid retention. They cause lipogenis (formation and storage of fat in the body), which might be seen as an increase in size, primarily in the abdominal area. The round face is most likely due to changes in fluid balance. His friends' comment about "mega Jon" most likely reflects the fluid retention and weight gain associated with corticosteroid use.

b. The child has taken corticosteroids before, so he probably has experienced various adverse effects, especially with his previous history of hospitalizations for exacerbations. The nurse also should remember that the child is a preadolescent, and body image and peers are extremely important to him. The nurse should encourage the child to talk about how he feels and what he has used in the past to cope with his disorder and the effects of drug therapy. The nurse also needs to teach the child about how the corticosteroid acts so that he can have a better understanding for why he needs the medication. The nurse can help the child develop effective strategies for dealing with the therapy and for dealing with his friends' statements. The nurse also needs to reinforce with the child that he needs to take the medication exactly as prescribed and not to stop the drug abruptly to prevent adrenal insufficiency. Rather, the dose needs to be tapered over a period of time.

■ PRACTICING FOR NCLEX

1. **Answer: b**

RATIONALE: The adrenal medulla secretes the neurotransmitters epinephrine and norepinephrine. Androgens, glucocorticoids, and mineralocorticoids are secreted by the adrenal cortex.

Copyright © 2011 by Wolters Kluwer Health | Lippincott Williams & Wilkins. *Study Guide for Focus on Nursing Pharmacology.*

2. Answer: c

RATIONALE: A peak response of increased adrenocorticotropic hormone and adrenocortical hormones occurs sometime early in the morning, about 6 AM to 9 AM. The corticosteroid levels fall to low levels by evening. Then, the hypothalamus and pituitary sense low levels of the hormones and begin the production and release of corticotropin-releasing hormone usually during sleep, around midnight.

3. Answer: c

RATIONALE: Dexamethasone exerts the greatest glucocorticoid effects followed by triamcinolone, prednisone, and then cortisone.

4. Answer: b

RATIONALE: Covering the area with a dressing or diaper would increase the risk for systemic absorption of the drug and should be avoided. Topical corticosteroids should be used sparingly and should not be applied to any open lesions or excoriated areas to reduce the risk for systemic absorption.

5. Answer: a

RATIONALE: Prednisone is available for oral use only.

6. Answer: d

RATIONALE: Long-term systemic corticosteroid therapy in children can increase the child's risk for growth retardation; therefore, this would be most important to assess. Weight gain is associated with corticosteroid use but would not be as critical to monitor as the child's growth pattern. Rectal bleeding can occur with corticosteroids administered via a retention enema. Epistaxis can occur with the use of intranasal corticosteroids.

7. Answer: b

RATIONALE: Prednisone peaks in 1 to 2 hours after administration. In this situation, peak effects would occur between 8 and 9 AM.

8. Answer: c

RATIONALE: Glucocorticoids interfere with the immune and inflammatory reactions of the body, increasing a patient's risk for infection. Thus, fever would need to be reported immediately. Weight gain, abdominal distention, and increased appetite are adverse effects that can occur and do not need to be reported immediately.

9. Answer: a

RATIONALE: Typically, a glucocorticoid is taken in the morning around 8 or 9 AM to mimic the normal peak diurnal concentration levels and thereby minimize suppression of the hypothalamic-pituitary axis.

10. Answer: d

RATIONALE: Glucocorticoids are contraindicated in patients with acute infection because the infection could become serious or even fatal if the immune and inflammatory responses are blocked. Cautious use is necessary in patients with diabetes because glucose control can be upset or peptic ulcer disease because steroid use is associated with the development of peptic ulcers.

11. Answer: b

RATIONALE: Prednisolone exerts some mineralocorticoid effects. Triamcinolone, dexamethasone, and betamethasone exert no mineralocorticoid effects.

12. Answer: c

RATIONALE: Mineralocorticoids increase sodium reabsorption in the renal tubules, leading to sodium and water retention and increased potassium excretion. Calcium is not affected by mineralocorticoids.

13. Answer: a

RATIONALE: Shortness of breath may be a sign of heart failure and needs to be reported. Headache and weakness are general signs and common adverse effects. The nurse would report these if the patient complained that they were getting worse or interfering with the patient's activities of daily living. Slight pedal edema may or may not be significant.

14. Answer: a

RATIONALE: Fludrocortisone can lead to hypokalemia. A serum potassium level less than 3.0 mEq/L would suggest hypokalemia.

15. Answer: b

RATIONALE: Adrenocortical hormones cause the release of glucose for energy, increase the blood volume (aldosterone effect), slow the rate of protein production, and block the activities of the inflammatory and immune systems.

CHAPTER 37

■ ASSESSING YOUR UNDERSTANDING
CROSSWORD

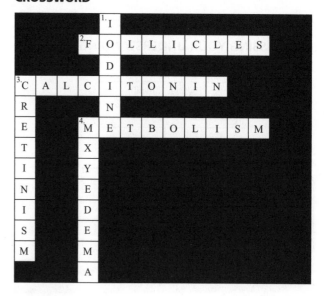

LABELING

Thyroid Hormone Deficiency	Thyroid Hormone Excess
Coarse, dry skin	Tachycardia
Lethargy	Diffuse goiter
Emotional dullness	Fine, soft hair
Weight gain	Intolerance to heat

■ APPLYING YOUR KNOWLEDGE

CASE STUDY

a. The nurse needs to explain to the patient that with the removal of part or all of the thyroid gland, hormone production will be deficient. This is unlike what she experienced before when her thyroid gland was producing too much hormone. In addition, the nurse needs to emphasize that adequate levels of the hormone are necessary to maintain normal body function and metabolism.

b. The patient needs information about how to take the drug, as a single dose before breakfast each day. Doing so will help to maintain consistent therapeutic levels. The nurse should also encourage the patient to take the dose with a full glass of water to prevent any difficulty in swallowing the drug. Additionally, the nurse should teach the patient about the delicate balance between deficient and excess amounts of the hormone and the possibility that symptoms of hyperthyroidism (similar to what she experienced when she was first diagnosed) may occur until the patient's dose is regulated. The nurse also needs to provide information about periodic follow-up testing of thyroid function and hormone levels to evaluate the patient's condition and effectiveness of therapy.

■ PRACTICING FOR NCLEX

1. **Answer: a**
   RATIONALE: Levothyroxine would be used to treat a deficiency of thyroid hormone or hypothyroidism. Methimazole and propylthiouracil are antithyroid agents used to treat hyperthyroidism. Calcitriol is an anithypocalcemic agent used to treat hypoparathyroidism.

2. **Answer: c**
   RATIONALE: Patients with hyperthyroidism typically exhibit flushed, warm skin; hyperactive deep tendon reflexes; tachycardia; and intolerance to heat.

3. **Answer: b**
   RATIONALE: The parafollicular cells of the thyroid produce calcitonin. Parathormone is produced by the parathyroid glands. Levothyroxine and liothyronine are produced by the thyroid gland and stored in the follicular cells.

4. **Answer: b**
   RATIONALE: The initial substance responsible for thyroid hormone release is thyrotropin-releasing hormone from the hypothalamus. This hormone then stimulates the anterior pituitary to release thyroid-stimulating hormone, which in turn causes the release of thyroid hormones. Levothyroxine is one of the thyroid hormones. Iodine is needed to produce the thyroid hormones.

5. **Answer: c**
   RATIONALE: Levothyroxine is a synthetic salt of T4; desiccated thyroid contains both T3 and T4. Liothyronine contains T3. Iodine is an antithyroid agent. Calcitriol is a form of vitamin D.

6. **Answer: d**
   RATIONALE: Methimazole can cause thyroid suppression leading to signs and symptoms of hypothyroidism such as decreased appetite. Nervousness, tachycardia, and weight loss would suggest hyperthyroidism.

7. **Answer: b**
   RATIONALE: Tetany is an indication of hypocalcemia. Lethargy, muscle weakness, and personality changes occur with hypercalcemia.

8. **Answer: c**
   RATIONALE: Calcitriol increases serum calcium levels; therefore, periodic monitoring is important to ensure effectiveness of therapy without causing hypercalcemia. Antacids containing magnesium should be avoided due to the increased risk for hypermagnesemia. Calcitriol is often combined with dietary supplementation of calcium. Dairy products are a good source of calcium and should not be limited. The drug can cause nausea, vomiting, and dry mouth. Taking the drug with food may help alleviate these effects.

9. **Answer: d**
   RATIONALE: Pamidronate is an example of a bisphosphonate. Teriparatide and dihydrotachysterol are antihypocalcemic agents. Calcitonin-salmon is a calcitonin used to treat hypercalcemia.

10. **Answer: c**
    RATIONALE: Ibandronate is taken once a month on the same day each month.

11. **Answer: d**
    RATIONALE: Alendronate can interact with a multivitamin, decreasing the absorption of the bisphosphonate. Therefore, the drugs should be separated by at least a half hour. The multivitamin does not need to be stopped. The alendronate should be taken on arising in the morning before anything else. Antacids also can decrease the absorption of alendronate, and these should also be separated by at least a half hour.

12. **Answer: b**
    RATIONALE: Calcitonin is administered subcutaneously, intramuscularly, or intranasally.

13. **Answer: a**
    RATIONALE: Lethargy would suggest hypercalcemia. Paresthesias, muscle cramps, and carpopedal spasms suggest hypocalcemia.

14. **Answer: c**
    RATIONALE: Signs and symptoms of iodism include sore teeth and gums, metallic taste and burning in the mouth, diarrhea, cold symptoms, and stomach upset. Rash is an adverse effect that is not indicative of iodism.

15. **Answer: b**
    RATIONALE: Teriparatide is administered subcutaneously.

CHAPTER 38

■ ASSESSING YOUR UNDERSTANDING

MATCHING

1. c	**2.** f	**3.** b	**4.** g	**5.** a
6. d	**7.** h	**8.** e		

SHORT ANSWER

1. The pancreas is both an endocrine gland, producing hormones, and an exocrine gland, releasing sodium bicarbonate and pancreatic enzymes directly into the common bile duct to be released into the small intestine, where they

neutralize the acid chyme from the stomach and aid digestion. The endocrine part of the pancreas produces hormones in collections of tissue called the islets of Langerhans. These islets contain endocrine cells that produce specific hormones. The alpha cells release glucagon in direct response to low blood glucose levels. The beta cells release insulin in direct response to high blood glucose levels. Delta cells produce somatostatin in response to very low blood glucose levels. Somatostatin blocks the secretion of both insulin and glucagon.

2. Glucagonlike polypeptide-1 (GLP-1) increases insulin release and decreases glucagon release (in preparation for the nutrients that will soon be absorbed). GLP-1 also slows gastrointestinal (GI) emptying to allow more absorption of nutrients and stimulates the satiety center in the brain to decrease the desire to eat since food is already in the GI tract.

3. Disorders that may result from diabetes include atherosclerosis, retinopathy, neuropathies, and nephropathy.

4. The glycosylated hemoglobin level (HbA1c) test provides a 3-month average of glucose levels.

5. Type 1 diabetes (insulin-dependent diabetes) involves pancreatic beta cells that are no longer functioning.

6. Clinical signs and symptoms include fatigue, lethargy, irritation, glycosuria, polyphagia, polydipsia, and itchy skin (from accumulation of wastes that the liver cannot clear).

■ APPLYING YOUR KNOWLEDGE

CASE STUDY

a. The nurse would need to reinforce the benefits of activity and exercise in maintaining health. However, the nurse would need to emphasize consistency in administering the insulin and ensuring adequate nutrition as well as being alert to the signs and symptoms of hypoglycemia and knowing how to prevent and/or properly intervene if they occur. The nurse would work with the patient and family to develop an appropriate schedule to reduce the child's risks. A referral to a dietician or nutritionist would be helpful in devising an appropriate plan for nutritional intake, especially at times when the child will be participating in the sports activity. The nurse would encourage the child and parents to talk with child's coaches to ensure that they too are knowledgeable of the child's condition, signs and symptoms that require intervention, and appropriate emergency treatment measures.

b. The child is an adolescent and as such can pose a challenge to managing diabetes. The desire to be "normal" often leads to a resistance to dietary restrictions and insulin injections. The child may feel a need to exert independence. The metabolism of the teenager is also in flux, leading to complications in regulating insulin dosage. A team approach, including the child, family members, teachers, coaches, and even friends, may be the best way to help the child deal with the disease and the required therapy. New delivery methods for insulin may help this age group cope with the drug therapy in the future.

■ PRACTICING FOR NCLEX

1. **Answer: a**
   RATIONALE: Glyburide is an example of a sulfonylurea. Metformin is classified as a biguanide. Acarbose and miglitol are alpha-glucosidase inhibitors.

2. **Answer: b**
   RATIONALE: Rosiglitazone would be administered as a single oral dose. Repaglinide is used orally before meals. Exenatide is administered by subcutaneous injection within 60 minutes before morning and evening meals. Miglitol is given with the first bite of each meal.

3. **Answer: d**
   RATIONALE: Fruity breath odor would be noted as ketones build up in the system and are excreted through the lungs. Dehydration would be noted as fluid and electrolytes are lost through the kidneys. Blurred vision and hunger would be associated with hypoglycemia.

4. **Answer: c**
   RATIONALE: Insulin detemir cannot be mixed in solution with any other drug, including other insulins. Regular, lente, and lispro can be mixed.

5. **Answer: a**
   RATIONALE: Regular insulin peaks in 2 to 4 hours, so the nurse would be alert for signs and symptoms of hypoglycemia at this time, which would be between 10:00 AM and 12:00 PM. If insulin lispro were administered, peak effects would occur in 30 to 90 minutes or between 8:30 AM and 9:30 AM. If insulin detemir were given, peak effects would occur in 6 to 8 hours, or between 2:00 PM and 4:00 PM. If NPH insulin were given, peak effects would occur in 4 to 12 hours, or between 12:00 PM and 8:00 PM.

6. **Answer: d**
   RATIONALE: Gentle pressure should be applied to the injection after the needle is withdrawn. Massaging could contribute to erratic or unpredictable absorption.

7. **Answer: b**
   RATIONALE: To ensure therapeutic effectiveness and appropriate suspension of the mixed insulin, the nurse would need to administer the injection within 15 minutes of mixing the insulins in the syringe.

8. **Answer: a**
   RATIONALE: Glipizide is a second-generation sulfonylurea that binds to potassium channels on the pancreatic beta cells to improve insulin binding to insulin receptors and increase the number of insulin receptors. Acarbose and miglitol inhibit alpha-glucosidase, thereby delaying the absorption of glucose. Metformin increases the uptake of glucose. Thiazolidinediones such as rosiglitazone decrease insulin resistance.

9. **Answer: b**
   RATIONALE: Metformin peaks in approximately 2 to 2½ hours; thus, the patient should be alert for possible signs and symptoms of hypoglycemia.

10. **Answer: a**
    RATIONALE: Insulin is needed in type 1 diabetes because the beta cells of the pancreas are no longer functioning. With type 2 diabetes, insulin is produced, but perhaps not enough to maintain glucose control or the insulin receptors are not sensitive enough to insulin.

11. **Answer: c**
    RATIONALE: Incretins increase insulin release, decrease glucagon release, slow GI emptying, and stimulate the satiety center. Growth hormone increases protein building.

12. **Answer: d**
    RATIONALE: Although other delivery systems are available for insulin administration such as the jet injector, insulin pen, and external pump, subcutaneous injection remains the primary delivery system.

Copyright © 2011 by Wolters Kluwer Health I Lippincott Williams & Wilkins. *Study Guide for Focus on Nursing Pharmacology*.

13. Answer: b

RATIONALE: The patient is significantly hypoglycemic and needs emergency treatment. Glucagon would be the agent of choice to raise the patient's glucose level because it can be given intravenously and has an onset of approximately 1 minute. Diazoxide can be used to elevate blood glucose levels, but it must be given orally. Lispro and regular insulin would be used to treat hyperglycemia.

14. Answer: c

RATIONALE: The buttocks would be an inappropriate site for administering insulin subcutaneously. The best sites include the upper arm, abdomen, and upper thigh.

15. Answer: a

RATIONALE: Pramlintide is administered subcutaneously immediately before major meals. Numerous antidiabetic drugs are taken orally, often once a day in the morning. Exenatide is given subcutaneously within 1 hour before the morning and evening meals. Miglitol should be taken orally with the first bite of each meal.

CHAPTER 39

■ ASSESSING YOUR UNDERSTANDING

LABELING

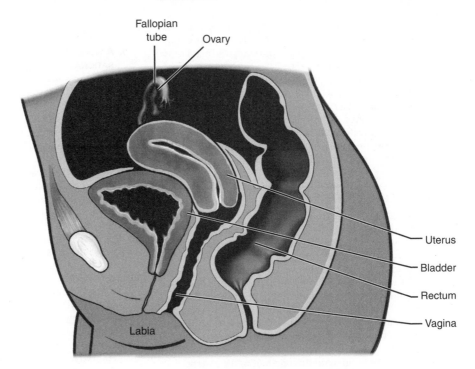

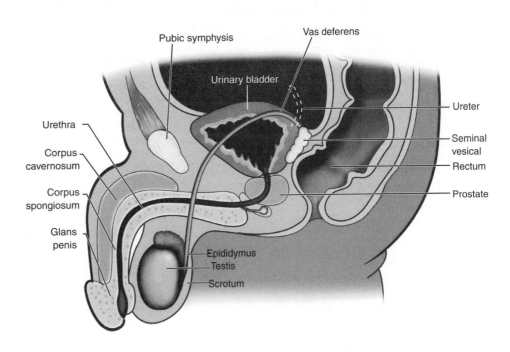

■ APPLYING YOUR KNOWLEDGE

CASE STUDY

a. The nurse would need to provide a review of the various structures involved in reproduction, including the ovaries, fallopian tubes, and uterus, and the hormones involved in the everyday function of the female reproductive system. The nurse also would need to explain the menstrual cycle, correlating the hormones involved with the events that occur, such as ovulation and menstruation. In addition, the nurse would need to review what happens with the system during pregnancy, beginning with fertilization and ending with the birth of the fetus.

b. The girls are adolescents, many of whom have already experienced menarche. So, rather than providing a straight lecture-type presentation on the menstrual cycle, it might be helpful for the nurse to engage the students in a discussion of the topic, either as a class or in small groups, or role-play different scenarios. The nurse could also incorporate visual methods, such as slide shows, videos, posters, or handouts to describe the structures of the system and the events of pregnancy. Independence is a key issue for adolescents. Therefore, the nurse should use methods that foster this independence while at the same time provide the girls with important information so that they are well informed.

■ PRACTICING FOR NCLEX

1. Answer: c
RATIONALE: The gonadotropin-releasing hormone (GnRH) is the hormone responsible for the sequence of events that eventually lead to hormonal secretion from the ovaries and testes. GnRH released from the hypothalamus stimulates the release of follicle-stimulating hormone (FSH) and luteinizing hormone (LH; sometimes referred to as the interstitial cell-stimulating hormone in males) from the anterior pituitary gland. These in turn stimulate the male and female glands to secrete their hormones.

2. Answer: b
RATIONALE: An ovum contains one-half of the genetic material to produce a whole cell. At birth, a female's ovaries contain all of the ova that a woman will have. The fallopian tube is a muscular tube that lies very near to each ovary but is not connected directly to it. The ovaries are responsible for producing estrogen and progesterone.

3. Answer: d
RATIONALE: Progesterone's effects on body temperature are monitored in the rhythm method of birth control to indicate that ovulation has occurred. Estradiol, estrone, and estriol are estrogens produced by the ovaries.

4. Answer: a
RATIONALE: Although progesterone plays a role in breast growth to prepare for lactation, estrogen plays a major role in breast growth overall. Progesterone is responsible for thickened cervical mucus, increased body temperature, and increased appetite.

5. Answer: b
RATIONALE: Progesterone is the hormone responsible for maintaining pregnancy.

6. Answer: d
RATIONALE: A massive release of luteinizing hormone or its surge causes one of the developing follicles to burst and release the ovum. This is called ovulation.

7. Answer: c
RATIONALE: Fertilization of the ovum and implantation in the uterine wall results in the production of human chorionic gonadotropin, which stimulates the corpus luteum to continue to produce estrogen and progesterone until the placenta develops and becomes functional, producing these hormones at a level high enough to sustain the pregnancy. If pregnancy does not occur, the corpus luteum involutes and becomes a white scar on the ovary, called the *corpus albicans*.

8. Answer: d
RATIONALE: Increased light exposure has been found to boost the release of FSH and LH through earlier GnRH release by the hypothalamus. Stress, starvation, and extreme exercise are associated with a decrease in reproductivity related to the controls of the hypothalamus.

9. Answer: b
RATIONALE: The onset of the menstrual cycle at puberty is called *menarche*. Puberty refers to the point at which the hypothalamus starts releasing gonadotropin-releasing hormone to stimulate the release of FSH and LH and begins sexual development. Andropause refers to a decrease in gonadal function in males. Menopause refers to the cessation of menstruation in a female when female ova are depleted.

10. Answer: c
RATIONALE: Prostaglandins in the uterus stimulate uterine contraction to clamp off vessels as the lining sheds away during menstruation. This causes menstrual cramps. High levels of plasminogen in the uterus prevent clotting of the lining as the vessels shear off. Lowered estrogen and progesterone levels trigger the release of FSH and LH and cause the inner lining of the uterus to slough off because it is no longer stimulated by the hormones.

11. Answer: b
RATIONALE: The placenta serves as a massive endocrine gland during pregnancy, maintaining high levels of estrogen and progesterone to support the uterus and developing fetus. The umbilical cord is important for nutrient and oxygen exchange between the fetus and the mother. The embryo implants in the wall of the uterus and becomes the developing fetus. The uterus provides the area for implantation of the embryo and growth of the fetus.

12. Answer: a
RATIONALE: The seminiferous tubules produce sperm. The Leydig cells produce testosterone. The vas deferens stores the produced sperm and carries it from the testes for ejaculation. The prostate gland produces enzymes to stimulate sperm maturation and lubricating fluid.

13. Answer: b, c, d
RATIONALE: Testosterone leads to the following: thickening of the vocal cords, increased hematocrit, and facial hair growth. Increased high-density lipoprotein levels and skin elasticity are associated effects of estrogen.

14. Answer: c
RATIONALE: The human sexual response cycle begins with stimulation, which is followed by a plateau stage, climax, and then recovery or resolution.

15. Answer: a
RATIONALE: During andropause, the seminiferous tubules and insterstitial cells atrophy. The hypothalamus and anterior pituitary gland put out larger amounts of GnRH, FSH, and LH in an attempt to stimulate the gland. If no increase in testosterone or inhibin occurs, levels of GnRH, FSH, and LH return to normal.

CHAPTER 40

■ ASSESSING YOUR UNDERSTANDING

FILL IN THE BLANKS

1. Progestins
2. Secretory
3. Nicotine
4. Raloxifene
5. Clomiphene
6. Oxytoxics

SHORT ANSWER

1. Female sex hormones are used to replace hormones that are missing or to act on the control mechanisms of the endocrine system to decrease the release of endogenous hormones.
2. Women without primary ovarian failure who cannot get pregnant after 1 year of trying may be candidates for the use of fertility drugs.
3. Menotropins also stimulate spermatogenesis in men with low sperm counts and otherwise normally functioning testes.
4. A woman with ovarian cysts who uses a fertility drug may experience an increase in the size of the cysts due to stimulation from the drugs.
5. Oxytocin is available in a nasal form to stimulate the letdown reflex in a lactating woman.

■ APPLYING YOUR KNOWLEDGE

CASE STUDY

a. The nurse needs to listen to the patient's complaints and provide nonjudgmental acceptance and support. While talking with the patient, the nurse may note areas in which clarification or correction is needed because of myths and misconceptions that the patient may relate. These areas provide opportunities for teaching to help the patient better understand what is happening in her body. The nurse also needs to emphasize that they will work together to find a suitable solution. Doing so helps to alleviate any feelings that the patient may have about being alone in dealing with these changes.

b. First, the nurse needs to assess the patient's concerns about hormone replacement therapy. Then, the nurse would address these concerns and provide the patient with information about hormone replacement therapy, including the risks and benefits. The nurse also would need to obtain a complete family and personal history of cancer and coronary artery disease risk factors as well as the use of any other medications or herbal therapies to provide additional information for the patient to weigh the pros and cons about therapy. Once the information has been obtained and the patient understands it, then the patient can make an informed decision about the therapy with the support and guidance from the nurse.

■ PRACTICING FOR NCLEX

1. **Answer: d**
   RATIONALE: The vaginal ring formulation of estradiol is applied once every 3 months.
2. **Answer: c**
   RATIONALE: Progestins are contraindicated in patients with pelvic inflammatory disease because progestins affect the vasculature of the uterus. Cautious use is necessary for women with migraine headaches, asthma, and epilepsy due to possible exacerbation of these conditions with the use of progestins.
3. **Answer: d**
   RATIONALE: Drospirenone used in combination contraceptives has antimineralocorticoid activity and can block aldosterone, leading to increased potassium levels. Irritation is associated with transdermal or vaginal use. Headache is associated with vaginal gel use. Abdominal pain may be due to intrauterine system administration.
4. **Answer: b**
   RATIONALE: Orange juice does not need to be avoided with estrogen hormonal therapy. However, St. John's wort, smoking, and grapefruit juice should be avoided.
5. **Answer: a**
   RATIONALE: Raloxifene is administered only by the oral route.
6. **Answer: c**
   RATIONALE: Clomiphene is administered orally. Cetrorelix, follitropin alfa, and ganirelix are administered parenterally.
7. **Answer: d**
   RATIONALE: Terbutaline, a beta-2 selective adrenergic agonist, is used as a uterine motility agent to relax the gravid uterus to prolong pregnancy and prevent premature labor and delivery. Ergonovine and oxytocin would be used to stimulate uterine contractions. Dinoprostone would be used to terminate a pregnancy of 12 to 20 weeks.
8. **Answer: b**
   RATIONALE: Oxytocin can cause severe water intoxication, which is thought to occur because of related effects of antidiuretic hormone, which may be released in response to oxytocin activity. Oxytocin does stimulate neuroreceptor sites but this is not the reason for the development of water intoxication. Ergonovine and methylergonovine can produce ergotism. Blockage of estrogen receptor sites occurs with estrogen receptor modulators.
9. **Answer: b**
   RATIONALE: Oral contraceptives are started on the fifth day of the cycle for 21 days; the inert tablets, or no tablets, are taken for the next 7 days. Then, a new course of 21 days is started.
10. **Answer: b**
    RATIONALE: Certain drugs such as tetracyclines and penicillins can reduce the effectiveness of progestins. Therefore, the patient needs to use an alternative means of contraception while taking the tetracycline. There is no need to separate administration times of the drug. Reducing the oral contraceptive to every other day further reduces the drug's effectiveness. An increase in adverse effects is not associated with the use of tetracyclines and oral contraceptives.
11. **Answer: d**
    RATIONALE: Estrogens are associated with the development of thrombi and emboli. Complaints of shortness of breath may indicate a possible pulmonary embolism necessitating emergency treatment. Abdominal bloating, weight gain, and dizziness are common adverse effects of estrogen therapy that should be reported, but it is not necessary to report them immediately.
12. **Answer: a**
    RATIONALE: Cetrorelix inhibits premature luteinizing hormone (LH) surges in women undergoing controlled ovarian stimulation by acting as a gonadotropin-releasing hormone (GnRH) antagonist. Chorionic gonadotropin acts like GnRH. Follitropin alfa is a follicle-stimulating molecule. Menotropins are a purified gonadotropin similar to follicle-stimulating hormone and LH.

Copyright © 2011 by Wolters Kluwer Health I Lippincott Williams & Wilkins. *Study Guide for Focus on Nursing Pharmacology.*

13. Answer: b
RATIONALE: Lutropin alfa is a fertility drug that is administered subcutaneously with follitropin alfa.

14. Answer: b
RATIONALE: Dinoprostone begins to act in 10 minutes, reaching a peak action in 15 minutes with a duration of action of 2 to 3 hours.

15. Answer: d
RATIONALE: With emergency contraception, the first dose is started within 72 hours after unprotected intercourse; then, a follow-up dose of the same dosage must be taken 12 hours after the first dose.

CHAPTER 41

■ ASSESSING YOUR UNDERSTANDING

FILL IN THE BLANKS

1. Androgens
2. Hypogonadism
3. III
4. Hirsutism
5. Athletic

SHORT ANSWER

1. Anabolic steroids promote body tissue–building processes, reverse catabolic or tissue-destroying processes, and increase hemoglobin and red blood cell mass.
2. Androgens are male sex hormones and include testosterone produced in the testes and the androgens produced in the adrenal glands.
3. Androgenic effects include acne, edema, hirsutism (increased hair distribution), deepening of the voice, oily skin and hair, weight gain, decrease in breast size, and testicular atrophy.
4. When injected directly into the cavernosum, alprostadil acts locally to relax the vascular smooth muscle and allows filling of the corpus cavernosum, causing penile erection.
5. Patients using PDE5 inhibitors should avoid drinking grapefruit juice when taking the drug as well as avoid taking the drug with or just after a high-fat meal.

■ APPLYING YOUR KNOWLEDGE

CASE STUDY

a. The nurse needs to maintain a nonjudgmental approach with the patient and allow him to verbalize his feelings and concerns, especially in relation to his complaints, his feelings about himself, his sexual ability, and aging (self-esteem, body image, maleness). When responding to the patient, the nurse should be honest with the patient and inform him that the medication may or may not be appropriate for him, depending on a variety of factors. The nurse also needs to review the normal physiologic changes that occur with aging while at the same time reinforce that help is available.

b. The nurse needs to obtain a complete history and physical examination of the patient. It would be essential to find out if there are any underlying medical conditions that may be affecting the patient's status. Information about the use of any medications or herbal therapies also would be important because numerous agents have adverse effects on sexual functioning. In addition, the nurse needs to inquire about other areas, such as stresses that could affect neuroendocrine function and disrupt the hypothalamic-pituitary axis.

■ PRACTICING FOR NCLEX

1. Answer: c
RATIONALE: Androgenic effects include oily skin and hair. Flushing, sweating, and nervousness are antiestrogenic effects.

2. Answer: d
RATIONALE: Testosterone can be administered as a depot injection, transdermal patch, or intramuscular injection. It is not administered orally.

3. Answer: c
RATIONALE: Patients with a history of cardiovascular disease need to be monitored closely when receiving testosterone because the disorder could be exacerbated by the hormone's effect. Prostate or breast cancer would be contraindications to the use of testosterone. Penile implant would be a contraindication for the use of drugs for treating penile erectile dysfunction.

4. Answer: b
RATIONALE: A potentially life-threatening effect associated with long-term testosterone use is hepatocellular cancer. Patients should have liver function studies monitored regularly, before beginning therapy and every 6 months during therapy.

5. Answer: c
RATIONALE: Testosterone is available in a transdermal form. Fluoxymesterone, danazol, and methyltestosterone are administered orally.

6. Answer: d
RATIONALE: Anabolic steroids increase red blood cell mass and hemoglobin, reverse catabolic or tissue-destroying processes, and promote body tissue–building processes.

7. Answer: b
RATIONALE: Postpubertal males may experience priapism, gynecomastia, testicular atrophy, balding, inhibition of testicular function, and change in libido with anabolic steroids.

8. Answer: b
RATIONALE: Elevated liver enzyme levels indicated impaired hepatic function that could be related to the development of hepatocellular cancer—a potential and life-threatening effect associated with androgen therapy. Decreased thyroid function and increased creatinine and creatinine clearance levels are not associated with disease states and can last for up to 2 weeks after discontinuing therapy.

9. Answer: c
RATIONALE: Anabolic steroids are classified as a class III controlled substance.

10. Answer: b
RATIONALE: Sildenafil is a PDE5 inhibitor used to treat penile erectile dysfunction. Alprostadil is a prostaglandin. Oxandrolone is an anabolic steroid. Danazol is an androgen.

11. Answer: b
RATIONALE: Tadalafil is approved for daily use in men who are very sexually active. This drug may be selected if the timing of sexual stimulation is not known and may be several hours away. Sidenafil and vardenafil must be taken approximately 1 hour before sexual stimulation. Alprostadil is injected directly into the cavernosum.

12. Answer: a
RATIONALE: Sildenafil is used in women for the treatment of pulmonary arterial hypertension. It is not used for sexual dysfunction in women. Coronary artery disease and peptic ulcer disease are conditions that require cautious use of the drug in men.

Copyright © 2011 by Wolters Kluwer Health I Lippincott Williams & Wilkins. *Study Guide for Focus on Nursing Pharmacology.*

13. Answer: c
RATIONALE: The PDE5 inhibitors cannot be taken in combination with any organic nitrates or alpha-adrenergic blockers because serious cardiovascular effects may occur, including death. Increased PDE5 inhibitor levels and effects may be seen with ketoconazole, indinavir, and erythromycin; the dosage of the inhibitor would need to be reduced.

14. Answer: d
RATIONALE: Vardenafil should be taken 60 minutes before sexual stimulation.

15. Answer: b
RATIONALE: Transdermal testosterone patches are replaced daily.

CHAPTER 42

■ ASSESSING YOUR UNDERSTANDING

LABELING

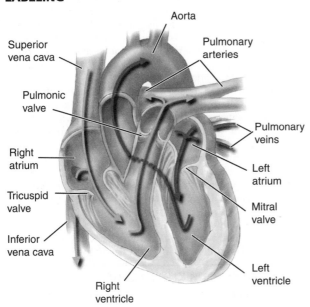

Aorta
Superior vena cava
Pulmonary arteries
Pulmonic valve
Pulmonary veins
Right atrium
Left atrium
Tricuspid valve
Mitral valve
Inferior vena cava
Left ventricle
Right ventricle

SEQUENCING

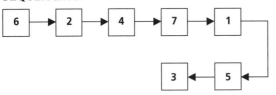

6 → 2 → 4 → 7 → 1
3 ← 5

■ APPLYING YOUR KNOWLEDGE

CASE STUDY

a. If constant and excessive, hypertension can damage the inner fragile lining of the blood vessels and disrupt the flow of blood to the tissues. These vessels can include the coronary vessels. Hypertension also puts a tremendous strain on the heart muscle, increasing myocardial oxygen consumption and putting the heart itself at risk. The patient acknowledges some noncompliance with his antihypertensive medications that could have allowed his blood pressure to rise, causing excess demand on the heart. Blood pressure is a measure of afterload, and the higher the resistance in the system, the harder the heart

will have to contract to pump blood. Chronic hypertension also can overstretch the heart muscle, interfering with the heart's ability to pump effectively. Ultimately, the coronary arteries can be affected.

b. The patient needs to learn to balance activity and rest periods so that he does not overtax the heart. In addition, energy conservation measures would be helpful to minimize the amount of oxygen needed and used to perform certain activities. In addition, measures to control his blood pressure can help to minimize the oxygen demand as well as reduce the workload of the heart.

■ PRACTICING FOR NCLEX

1. Answer: b
RATIONALE: Starling's law of the heart is often compared with the stretching of a rubber band, such that the heart returns to its normal size after it is stretched—the further it is stretched, the stronger is the spring back to normal.

2. Answer: a
RATIONALE: The sinoatrial (SA) node acts as the pacemaker of the heart. The atrioventricular (AV) node, bundle of His, and Purkinje fibers are part of the conduction system.

3. Answer: c
RATIONALE: Automaticity is the cells' ability to generate action potentials or electrical impulses without being excited to do so by external stimuli. Conductivity refers to the ability of the cells to conduct this action potential. Contractility refers to the unified contraction of the atria and ventricles to move blood through the vascular system. Capacitancy refers to the venous system, which is distensible and flexible and able to hold large amounts of blood.

4. Answer: b
RATIONALE: During phase 1, sodium ion concentrations are equal inside and outside the cell. During phase 0, the cell reaches a point of stimulation with sodium rushing into the cell (depolarization). During phase 2, the cell membrane becomes less permeable to sodium, and calcium slowly enters the cell and potassium begins to leave (repolarization). During phase 3, rapid repolarization occurs, as the gates close and potassium rapidly moves out of the cell.

5. Answer: d
RATIONALE: The basic structural unit of cardiac muscle is the sarcomere, which contains the proteins actin and myosin. These proteins are kept apart by the protein troponin.

6. Answer: c
RATIONALE: An electrocardiogram is a recording of the patterns of electrical impulses as they move through the heart. It is a measure of electrical activity and provides no information about the mechanical function of the heart.

7. Answer: b
RATIONALE: The QRS complex represents depolarization of the bundle of His (Q) and the ventricles (RS). The P wave indicates impulses originating in the SA node as they pass through atrial tissue. The T wave represents repolarization of the ventricles. The PR interval reflects the normal delay of conduction at the AV node.

8. Answer: d
RATIONALE: Atrial flutter is characterized by sawtooth-shaped P waves, often with two or three P waves occurring for every QRS complex. Sinus bradycardia would be characterized by a normal-appearing electrocardiogram but with a rate usually less than 60 beats/minute. Paroxysmal atrial tachycardia would be characterized by sporadically occurring runs of rapid heart rate. Atrial fibrillation would be characterized by many irregular

Copyright © 2011 by Wolters Kluwer Health l Lippincott Williams & Wilkins. *Study Guide for Focus on Nursing Pharmacology.*

P waves, depicting bombardment of the AV node in an unpredictable number causing the ventricles to beat in a fast, irregular, and often inefficient heart manner.

9. Answer: c
RATIONALE: Circulation is a closed, high- to low-pressure system that can follow two courses (systemic and pulmonary) and involves a resistance system (arterial) and a capacitance (venous) system.

10. Answer: a
RATIONALE: Hydrostatic pressure regulates the movement of fluids at the arterial end of the capillary; entotic pressure regulates this movement at the venous end of the capillary. It is the pressure that directs flow through the loosely connected endothelial cells of the capillary.

11. Answer: b
RATIONALE: The right coronary artery supplies most of the right side of the heart, including the SA node. The left circumflex artery supplies most of the left ventricle. The left anterior descending artery feeds the septum and anterior areas, including much of the conduction system.

12. Answer: a
RATIONALE: When blood flow to the kidneys is reduced, the cells in the kidney release renin, which then converts angiotensinogen to angiotensin I. This is converted by angiotensin-converting enzyme to angiotensin II, which reacts with specific receptor sites on blood vessels to cause vasoconstriction. Angiotensin II also causes the release of aldosterone.

13. Answer: c
RATIONALE: The superior vena cava brings blood from the head and arms to the right ventricle and the inferior vena cava brings blood from the lower body back to the heart. The aorta delivers blood to the systemic circulation. The pulmonary vein returns blood from the lungs to the left atrium. The triscuspid valve separates the right atrium from the right ventricle.

14. Answer: d
RATIONALE: The Purkinje fibers deliver the impulse to the ventricular cells. The AV node receives the impulse from the atrial bundles and moves it to the bundle of His and then into the bundle branches.

15. Answer: b
RATIONALE: The conduction velocity is the slowest in the AV node and the fastest in the Purkinje fibers.

CHAPTER 43

■ ASSESSING YOUR UNDERSTANDING
LABELING

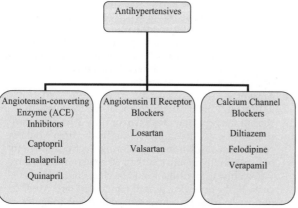

SHORT ANSWER

1. The pressure in the cardiovascular system is determined by heart rate, stroke volume, and total peripheral resistance.
2. Baroreceptors are located in the aortic arch and carotid arteries.
3. The underlying danger of hypertension of any type is the prolonged force on the vessels of the vascular system. The muscles in the arterial system eventually thicken, leading to a loss of responsiveness in the system. The left ventricle thickens because the muscle must constantly work hard to expel blood at a greater force. The thickening of the heart muscle and the increased pressure that the muscle has to generate every time it contracts increase the workload of the heart and the risk of coronary artery disease (CAD) as well. The force of the blood being propelled against them damages the inner linings of the arteries, making these vessels susceptible to atherosclerosis and to narrowing of the lumen of the vessels (see Chapter 46). Tiny vessels can be damaged and destroyed, leading to losses of vision (if the vessels are in the retina), kidney function (if the vessels include the glomeruli in the nephrons), or cerebral function (if the vessels are small and fragile vessels in the brain).
4. Factors that are known to increase blood pressure in some people include high levels of psychological stress, exposure to high-frequency noise, a high-salt diet, lack of rest, and genetic predisposition.
5. Because an underlying cause of hypertension is usually unknown, altering the body's regulatory mechanisms is the best treatment currently available. Drugs used to treat hypertension work to alter the normal reflexes that control blood pressure.
6. A patient with stage 1 hypertension without complicating conditions may receive thiazide diuretics most often. ACE inhibitors, angiotensin receptor blockers, beta blockers, or calcium channel blockers may be used alone or in combination.
7. Lifestyle modifications include weight reduction, smoking cessation, moderation of alcohol intake, reduction of salt in the diet, and increase in physical activity.

■ APPLYING YOUR KNOWLEDGE
CASE STUDY

a. The patient may be describing what is known as "white coat syndrome"—a condition in which the patient is hypertensive only when in the doctor's office having the blood pressure measured. This has been correlated to a sympathetic stress reaction and a tendency to tighten the muscles while waiting to be seen and during the blood pressure measurement. Although this may be occurring to some degree with the patient, his blood pressure has been elevated for a sustained period, which has led to his diagnosis of hypertension. In addition, the patient also has a history of left ventricular hypertrophy, which has caused the heart muscle to be stretched, ultimately causing the heart to work harder to contract. Also, blood pressure machines in grocery stores and pharmacies are not always accurate and can mislead patients. Thus, the nurse would need to address these issues when responding to the patient.

b. The nurse would need to explain that the quinapril is an ACE inhibitor that is relatively well tolerated and not associated with as many adverse effects as other drugs in this class. However, the nurse still needs to review possible adverse effects such as reflex tachycardia, gastrointestinal irritation, constipation, renal problems, and photosensitivity. In addition, the nurse needs to address possible effects

Copyright © 2011 by Wolters Kluwer Health I Lippincott Williams & Wilkins. *Study Guide for Focus on Nursing Pharmacology.*

related to the combination of carvedilol, an alpha- and beta blocker. These might include orthostatic hypotension, dizziness, or the development of possible arrhythmias. Instructions on safety measures and danger signs and symptoms to report would be important.

■ PRACTICING FOR NCLEX

1. Answer: d
RATIONALE: The area of highest pressure in the system is always the left ventricle during systole. This pressure propels the blood out of the aorta and into the system.

2. Answer: a
RATIONALE: The small arterioles are thought to be the most important factor in determining peripheral resistance. Because they have the smallest diameter, they are able to almost stop blood flow into the capillary beds when they constrict, building up tremendous pressure in the arteries behind them as they prevent the blood from flowing through.

3. Answer: c
RATIONALE: The baroreceptor reflex functions continually to maintain blood pressure within a predetermined range of normal. Input from the baroreceptors is received by the medulla in the cardiovascular center. Baroreceptors are located in the carotid arteries.

4. Answer: d
RATIONALE: Enalaprilat is an ACE inhibitor that is administered intravenously. Captopril, enalapril, and lisinopril are administered orally.

5. Answer: b
RATIONALE: Benazepril is associated with an unrelenting cough. Ramipril, lisinopril, and quinapril are not associated with this adverse effect.

6. Answer: c
RATIONALE: Captopril is associated with a sometimes fatal pancytopenia, so it would be most important for the nurse to monitor the patient's complete blood count for changes. Monitoring the electrocardiogram would be important to detect arrhythmias but not as important as monitoring for bone marrow suppression. Nutritional status and liver function studies would be lower priorities for monitoring.

7. Answer: b
RATIONALE: Losartan is an example of an angiotensin II receptor blocker. Moexipril is an ACE inhibitor. Minoxidil is a vasodilator. Amlodipine is a calcium channel blocker.

8. Answer: d
RATIONALE: Calcium channel blockers slow cardiac impulse formation in the conductive tissues, depress myocardial contractility, and relax and dilate arteries, leading to a fall in blood pressure and a decrease in venous return.

9. Answer: c
RATIONALE: Diltiazem, like other calcium channel blockers, should be swallowed whole with a large glass of water. The tablet should not be split in half, crushed, or chewed.

10. Answer: b
RATIONALE: Verapamil, like other calcium channel blockers, interacts with grapefruit juice, increasing the concentration of calcium channel blockers and leading to toxicity. Calcium channel blockers do not interact with ibuprofen. Splitting or crushing the pills could lead to a release of the drug all at once, but this is more common when the drug is first taken. Asking about the time the patient last took the drug might be important, but it

would not address the problem associated with the significant adverse effects.

11. Answer: b
RATIONALE: Manifestations of cyanide toxicity include absent reflexes, dilated pupils, dyspnea, headache, vomiting, dizziness, ataxia, loss of consciousness, imperceptible pulse, pink color, distant heart sounds, and shallow breathing. Hair growth is an adverse effect of minoxidil. Chest pain is an adverse effect associated with vasodilator therapy related to changes in blood pressure.

12. Answer: a
RATIONALE: Prazosin is an alpha-1 blocker that is used to treat hypertension. Labetolol and guanabenz are alpha- and beta blockers used to treat hypertension. Nadolol is a beta blocker used to treat hypertension.

13. Answer: c
RATIONALE: Midodrine is an alpha-specific adrenergic agent that is used to treat orthostatic hypotension. Dopamine is a sympathomimetic agent that is used to treat shock. Methyldopa and clonidine are alpha-2 blockers used to treat hypertension.

14. Answer: d
RATIONALE: Hydrochlorothiazide is a thiazide diuretic that promotes the loss of sodium as well as potassium from the body. Subsequently, the patient is at risk for hypokalemia. Amiloride, spironolactone, and triamterene are potassium-sparing diuretics. The patient using these diuretics would need to be monitored for hyperkalemia because potassium is not lost along with sodium.

15. Answer: b
RATIONALE: Aliskiren is a renin inhibitor. Mecamylamine is a ganglionic blocker. Candesartan is an angiotensin II receptor blocker; captopril is an ACE inhibitor.

CHAPTER 44

■ ASSESSING YOUR UNDERSTANDING

MATCHING

1. c	**2.** f	**3.** d	**4.** e	**5.** g
6. a	**7.** h	**8.** b		

FILL IN THE BLANKS

1. Cardiotonic
2. Pulmonary edema
3. Rapid
4. Fluid
5. Decreased
6. Jugular
7. Nocturia
8. Inotropic

■ APPLYING YOUR KNOWLEDGE

CASE STUDY

a. The patient is experiencing signs and symptoms of both right-sided heart failure and left-sided heart failure. Right-sided heart failure is evidenced by the pitting edema, jugular vein distention, and nocturia. Left-sided heart failure is evidenced by the patient's tachypnea, rales, third heart sound, and orthopnea (the need to sleep on two pillows).

b. The nurse would need to instruct the patient to take the digoxin at the same time each day on an empty stomach to ensure adequate absorption of the drug. In addition, the nurse needs to teach the patient about signs and symptoms of digoxin toxicity especially because digoxin interacts with amiodarone, which could lead to an increase in

Copyright © 2011 by Wolters Kluwer Health I Lippincott Williams & Wilkins. *Study Guide for Focus on Nursing Pharmacology.*

digoxin levels. The combination of digoxin and the thiazide diuretic increases the risk for arrhythmias, so the nurse needs to teach the patient to report if he notices any changes in his heart rhythm, such as palpitations. The patient also needs to have his serum potassium levels checked periodically because the thiazide diuretic can lead to excess potassium loss (hypokalemia) further contributing to the risk for arrhythmias and digoxin toxicity. The patient also needs instruction in how to monitor his apical pulse rate and to hold the drug if the pulse rate is less than 60 beats/minute and notify the prescriber.

■ PRACTICING FOR NCLEX

1. **Answer: a, b, e, f**
   RATIONALE: Left-sided heart failure would be indicated by tachypnea, hemoptysis, orthopnea, increased urine output (polyuria), nocturia, dyspnea, and cough. Peripheral edema and hepatomegaly suggest right-sided heart failure.

2. **Answer: b**
   RATIONALE: Vasodilators decrease cardiac workload, relax vascular smooth muscle to decrease afterload, and allow pooling in the veins thereby decreasing preload. Decreased blood volume results from the use of diuretics.

3. **Answer: c**
   RATIONALE: Digoxin increases the force of myocardial contraction, increases cardiac output and renal perfusion, and slows the heart rate.

4. **Answer: d**
   RATIONALE: Therapeutic digoxin levels range from 0.5 ng/mL to 2.0 ng/mL. A level above 2.0 ng/mL would indicate toxicity.

5. **Answer: d**
   RATIONALE: Intravenous digoxin must be administered slowly over at least 5 minutes to prevent cardiac arrhythmias and adverse effects.

6. **Answer: d**
   RATIONALE: Food and antacids interfere with the absorption of the drug. Digoxin should be taken on an empty stomach at approximately the same time each day. *If the patient takes an antacid, the patient should separate the dose of antacid and digoxin by 2 to 4 hours.

7. **Answer: b**
   RATIONALE: If the pulse rate is below 60 beats/minute, the patient should hold the dose and recheck his pulse in 1 hour. Then, if the pulse is still low, he make a note of it, withhold the drug, and notify the prescriber. The prescriber can then determine the next action.

8. **Answer: d**
   RATIONALE: Inamrinone is administered only by the intravenous route.

9. **Answer: b**
   RATIONALE: Although renal function studies may be appropriate to monitor and evaluate the need for possible dosage changes, inamrinone is associated with thrombocytopenia. Therefore, it would be most important for the nurse to monitor the patient's platelet count. Inamrinone is not associated with changes in pulmonary function or white blood cell counts.

10. **Answer: c**
    RATIONALE: After the initial bolus dose of inamrinone, the dose may be repeated in 30 minutes as needed.

11. **Answer: a**
    RATIONALE: Digoxin is the drug most often used to treat heart failure. Human B-type natriuretic peptide, nitrate,

or furosemide also may be used, but these drugs are not the ones most commonly used.

12. **Answer: b**
    RATIONALE: Renal failure would be least likely to contribute to the development of heart failure. Coronary artery disease, valvular disease, hypertension, and cardiomyopathy are commonly associated with heart failure.

13. **Answer: d**
    RATIONALE: If a patient's pulse rate is less than 60 beats/minute, the drug should be withheld and the pulse retaken in 1 hour. If the pulse is still below 60 beats/minute, the dose is held and the prescriber should be notified.

14. **Answer: c**
    RATIONALE: Digoxin is a cardiac glycoside. Inamrinone and milrinone are phosphodiesterase inhibitors. Captopril is an angiotensin-converting enzyme inhibitor.

15. **Answer: b**
    RATIONALE: Peripheral edema would be noted in patients with right-sided heart failure. Wheezing, hemoptysis, and dyspnea would suggest left-sided heart failure.

CHAPTER 45

■ ASSESSING YOUR UNDERSTANDING

LABELING

Class I	Class II	Class III	Class IV
Disopyramide Flecainide Lidocaine Mexiletine Propafenone Quinidine	Acebutolol Propranolol	Amiodarone Sotalol	Diltiazem Verapamil

SEQUENCING

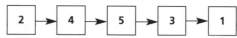

■ APPLYING YOUR KNOWLEDGE

CASE STUDY

a. Atrial fibrillation is associated with the development of blood clots due to the uncoordinated pumping, which leads to blood stagnating in the auricles. If the atria would contract properly, these clots would then travel to the lungs, brain, or periphery. Initially, heparin is used to initiate coagulation because warfarin is an oral agent that takes several days to reach therapeutic level.

b. The patient most definitely needs electrocardiogram monitoring to evaluate the current rhythm status and to determine if the amiodarone is effective in converting the arrhythmia. In addition, this monitoring is important to evaluate for the development of other arrhythmias (proarrhythmic effect) that may pose danger to the patient. Amiodarone also interacts with oral anticoagulants, so the nurse needs to assess the patient for signs and symptoms of bleeding once warfarin therapy is initiated. The nurse would need to inspect the patient for bruising and petechiae, check invasive device insertion sites for oozing, and urge the patient to report any frank or occult blood in his urine or stool. The nurse would also need to institute bleeding precautions to reduce the patient's risk for bleeding.

■ PRACTICING FOR NCLEX

1. Answer: c
RATIONALE: Antiarrhythmic agents alter the conductivity or suppress automaticity of the heart.

2. Answer: d
RATIONALE: Heart block is an arrhythmia related to an alteration in conduction through the muscle. Premature atrial contraction, atrial flutter, and ventricular fibrillation are arrhythmias due to stimulation from an ectopic focus.

3. Answer: b
RATIONALE: Procainamide is a class Ia antiarrhythmic agent. Lidocaine and mexiletine are classified as class Ib antiarrhythmics. Flecainide is a class 1c antiarrhythmic.

4. Answer: a
RATIONALE: Class I antiarrhythmics stabilize the cell membrane by binding to sodium channels, depressing phase 0 of the action potential.

5. Answer: a
RATIONALE: Disopyramide is administered orally.

6. Answer: b
RATIONALE: Quinidine interacts with digoxin, possibly leading to increased digoxin levels and digoxin toxicity. The effects of digoxin, not quinidine, are increased. Bleeding may occur if class I antiarrhythmics are given with oral anticoagulants such as warfarin. Renal dysfunction is unrelated to the use of both drugs.

7. Answer: d
RATIONALE: Quinidine requires a slightly acidic urine for excretion. Patients receiving quinidine should avoid foods that alkalinize the urine, such as citrus juices, antacids, milk products, and vegetables.

8. Answer: a
RATIONALE: Lidocaine, when given by intramuscular injection, has an onset of action between 5 to 10 minutes and peaks in 5 to 15 minutes.

9. Answer: b
RATIONALE: Class II antiarrhythmics are beta-adrenergic blockers that block the beta receptor sites in the heart and kidneys. Membrane stabilization and phase 0 depression occurs with class I antiarrhythmics. Blockage of potassium channels during phase 3 of the action potential occurs with class III antiarrhythmics. Blockage of calcium ion movement occurs with class IV antiarrhythmics.

10. Answer: c
RATIONALE: Esmolol, a class II agent, is administered intravenously.

11. Answer: a
RATIONALE: Class II antiarrhythmics are contraindicated in sinus bradycardia but should be used cautiously in patients with diabetes, thyroid dysfunction, and hepatic dysfunction.

12. Answer: d
RATIONALE: Bronchospasm is a possible adverse effect of acebutolol, a class II antiarrhythmic. Other effects include hypotension, decreased libido, and decreased exercise tolerance.

13. Answer: d
RATIONALE: Dofetilide is a class III antiarrhythmic that blocks potassium channels and slows the outward movement of potassium during phase 3 of the action potential.

14. Answer: b
RATIONALE: Sotalol absorption is decreased by the presence of food, so it should be taken on an empty stomach to maximize absorption. There is no need to sit up after taking the drug. Antacids would interfere with the absorption.

Holding the drug if the pulse rate is less than 60 beats/minute applies to digoxin.

15. Answer: b
RATIONALE: Adenosine slows conduction through the atrioventricular node, prolongs the refractory period, and decreases automaticity through the atrioventricular node. Digoxin used as an antiarrhythmic slows calcium from leaving the cell, prolonging the action potential and slowing conduction and heart rate.

CHAPTER 46

■ ASSESSING YOUR UNDERSTANDING

MATCHING

1. g	**2.** d	**3.** e	**4.** b	**5.** h
6. f	**7.** c	**8.** a		

SHORT ANSWER

1. Coronary artery disease is the leading cause of death in the Western world.
2. Unlike other tissues in the body, the heart muscle receives its blood supply during diastole while it is at rest. This is important because when the heart muscle contracts, it becomes tight and clamps the blood vessels closed, rendering them unable to receive blood during systole, which is when all other tissues receive fresh blood.
3. The person with atherosclerosis has a classic supply-and-demand problem. The heart may function without problem until increases in activity or other stresses place a demand on it to beat faster or harder. Normally, the heart would stimulate the vessels to deliver more blood when this occurs, but the narrowed vessels are not able to respond and cannot supply the blood needed by the working heart. The heart muscle then becomes hypoxic.
4. Antianginal drugs can work to improve blood delivery to the heart muscle in one of two ways: by dilating blood vessels (i.e., increasing the supply of oxygen) or by decreasing the work of the heart (i.e., decreasing the demand for oxygen).
5. Nitrates act directly on smooth muscle to cause relaxation and to depress muscle tone. Because the action is direct, these drugs do not influence any nerve or other activity, and the response is usually quite fast.

■ APPLYING YOUR KNOWLEDGE

CASE STUDY

a. Nitroglycerin sublingual tablets should be kept in the original dark container in which they were dispensed because the drugs need to be protected from light. Otherwise, they will lose their potency. In addition, keeping the tablets in the original container allows the nurse and the patient to check the expiration date to ensure that the tablets are still usable. The tablets also need to be stored in a cool, dry place. The patient's back pants pocket is not such a place.

b. The nurse needs to teach the patient about proper storage of the drug, including the need to keep the drug in its dark container to protect it from light and to store the drug in a cool, dry place. The nurse also needs to emphasize that the patient check the expiration date so that the patient has access to medication that is still potent. Since there is no way to tell if the tablets have expired and since they have not been protected from light and heat, it would be appropriate for the nurse to obtain a new prescription for the patient so that he can have a fresh supply should he need them. The nurse could also instruct the patient to note if the tablet fizzles or burns when he uses them, as this would indicate potency.

■ PRACTICING FOR NCLEX

1. Answer: a

RATIONALE: Angina is most accurately described as the body's response to a lack of oxygen in the heart muscle. It commonly is manifested as chest pain, but it can occur at rest or with activity. Angina does not necessarily indicate damage to the heart muscle. Ischemia leads to damage. Prinzmetal's angina is a type of angina that is due to vessel spasm.

2. Answer: b

RATIONALE: Unstable angina is chest pain that occurs when the patient is at rest. Stable angina is chest pain that occurs with activity and is relieved by rest. Prinzmetal's angina is chest pain due to vessel spasm. Myocardial infarction indicates ischemia and subsequent necrosis of the heart muscle.

3. Answer: b

RATIONALE: Most of the deaths caused by myocardial infarction occur as a result of fatal arrhythmias.

4. Answer: d

RATIONALE: Isosorbide is classified as a nitrate. Metoprolol is a beta-blocker. Amlodipine and nicardipine are calcium channel blockers.

5. Answer: c

RATIONALE: Isosorbide dinitrate is available as an oral agent, sublingual tablet, and chewable tablet. It cannot be given intravenously.

6. Answer: c

RATIONALE: Nitrates would be contraindicated in patients with cerebral hemorrhage because the relaxation of the cerebral vessels could cause intracranial bleeding. Cardiac tamponade, hypotension, and hepatic disease require cautious use of nitrates.

7. Answer: b

RATIONALE: Nitroglycerin sublingual spray begins to act in approximately 2 minutes.

8. Answer: a

RATIONALE: A fizzing or burning sensation indicates that the tablet is potent. The patient should place the tablet under his tongue and away from any lesions or abrasions. If needed, the patient can take a sip of water to moisten the mucous membranes so that the tablet will dissolve quickly. After placing the tablet under the tongue, the patient should close his mouth and wait until the table has dissolved.

9. Answer: b

RATIONALE: Nitroglycerin can be repeated every 5 minutes if relief is not felt for a total of three doses.

10. Answer: a

RATIONALE: Phosphodiesterase 5 inhibitors, such as sildenafil, tadalafil, or vardenafil used to treat erectile dysfunction, should be avoided if the patient is taking nitrates due to the risk of severe hypotension and cardiovascular events. Beta-blockers in combination with nitrates may cause hypotension and should be used cautiously together. Nitrates do not interact with nonsteroidal anti-inflammatory drugs or cardiac glycosides.

11. Answer: b

RATIONALE: Nadolol is a beta-blocker used as an antianginal agent. Amlodipine and verapamil are calcium channel blocker antianginal agents. Ranolazine is classified as a piperazine acetamide.

12. Answer: c

RATIONALE: Propranolol is used after a myocardial infarction to prevent reinfarction. The drug could cause vasospasm and as such would not be indicated for the treatment of Prinzmetal's angina.

13. Answer: d

RATIONALE: Calcium channel blockers such as amlodipine are indicated as treatment for Prinzmetal's angina because they relieve coronary artery vasospasm. Nitroglycerin is indicated for acute angina attacks. Metoprolol and nadolol would be contraindicated for patients with Prinzmetal's angina.

14. Answer: b

RATIONALE: Although the exact mechanism of action of the drug is not understood, it does prolong the QT interval. It does not decrease heart rate or blood pressure but does decrease myocardial workload, bringing the supply and demand for oxygen back into balance.

15. Answer: c

RATIONALE: Transdermal nitroglycerin is applied once daily. The patch has a duration of 24 hours. Isosorbide dinitrate can be used before an activity that may cause chest pain. Sublingual, translingual spray, or buccal nitroglycerin is used with episodes of acute angina.

CHAPTER 47

■ ASSESSING YOUR UNDERSTANDING

LABELING

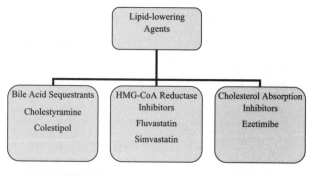

SHORT ANSWER

1. Metabolic syndrome is characterized by increased insulin resistance, high blood pressure, altered lipid levels, abdominal obesity, proinflammatory state, and prothrombotic state.

2. Nonmodifiable risk factors for coronary artery disease include family history, age, and gender.

3. Gout increases uric acid levels, which seem to injure vessel walls.

4. Black Americans have lower serum cholesterol levels, higher high-density lipoprotein (HDL) levels, and lower low-density lipoprotein (LDL) levels, and their HDL to cholesterol level is less when compared with white Americans.

5. Ways to modify risk factors include decreasing dietary fats, losing weight, eliminating smoking, increasing exercise levels, and decreasing stress as well as treating hypertension, gout, and diabetes.

6. Chylomicrons are a package of fats and proteins on which micelles are carried to allow absorption.

Copyright © 2011 by Wolters Kluwer Health I Lippincott Williams & Wilkins. *Study Guide for Focus on Nursing Pharmacology.*

■ APPLYING YOUR KNOWLEDGE

CASE STUDY

a. First, the nurse would need to investigate exactly what types of fruit juices the patient is drinking. Grapefruit juice should be avoided in patients who are taking HMG-CoA inhibitors because it alters the metabolism of the drug, leading to an increased serum drug level and increased risk for adverse effects, including rhabdomyolysis.

b. The patient may be experiencing early signs of rhabdomyolysis, especially if the patient has been drinking grapefruit juice while taking the drug. She needs to have some laboratory testing done to determine if she is experiencing problems with any liver or renal dysfunction and to evaluate for possible rhabdomyolysis. It would be important to obtain specimens to evaluate muscle and liver enzyme levels for increases that may suggest rhabdomyolysis. Muscle and liver enzymes such as creatine kinase, lactic dehydrogenase, aspartate aminotransferase, and alanine aminotransferase levels may be elevated to three times the normal level with rhabdomyolysis. In addition, renal function studies would be important because the breakdown of muscle results in the waste products injuring the glomerulus leads to renal failure.

■ PRACTICING FOR NCLEX

1. **Answer: b, c**
   RATIONALE: Characteristics of metabolic syndrome include waist measurement over 40 inches in men; triglyceride levels greater than 150 mg/dL or HDL levels less than 40 mg/dL in men or less than 50 mg/dL in women; fasting blood glucose levels greater than 110 mg/dL; blood pressure greater than 130/85 mm Hg; increased plasminogen activator levels; and increased macrophages, levels of interleukin-6, and tumor necrosis factor.

2. **Answer: d**
   RATIONALE: A triglyceride level of 180 mg/dL is considered borderline high (normal or desirable would be less than 150 mg/dL). A total cholesterol of 160 mg/dL and an LDL cholesterol of 110 mg/dL would be considered normal or desirable. An HDL level of 45 mg/dL would be considered normal; levels above 60 mg/dL would be considered high.

3. **Answer: a**
   RATIONALE: Bile acids act like a detergent in the small intestine and break up fats into small units. These small units are called *micelles*. High levels of cholesterol are part of bile acids. Chylomicrons are carriers for micelles.

4. **Answer: b**
   RATIONALE: HDLs are loosely packed lipids that are used for energy and to pick up remnants of fats and cholesterol left in the periphery by the breakdown of LDLs. LDLs are tightly packed cholesterol, triglycerides, and lipids that are carried by proteins that enter the circulation to be broken down for energy or stored for future use as energy.

5. **Answer: c**
   RATIONALE: Cholestyramine is classified as a bile acid sequestrant. Lovastatin is a HMG-CoA reductase inhibitor. Ezetimibe is a cholesterol absorption inhibitor. Gemfibrozil is classified as a fibrate.

6. **Answer: d**
   RATIONALE: The absorption of thiazide diuretic can be decreased or delayed with colestipol, a bile acid sequestrant. Therefore, the diuretic should be taken 1 hour before or 4 to 6 hours after the colestipol.

7. **Answer: b**
   RATIONALE: Cholestyramine should not be mixed with carbonated beverages. Soups, fruit juices, cereals, liquids, or pulpy fruit are acceptable alternatives.

8. **Answer: c**
   RATIONALE: The drug is administered at bedtime because the highest rates of cholesterol synthesis occur between 12 and 5 AM, and the drug should be taken when it will be most effective.

9. **Answer: d**
   RATIONALE: Ezetimibe is a cholesterol absorption inhibitor that works in the brush border of the small intestine to decrease absorption of dietary cholesterol from the small intestine. HMG-CoA reductase inhibitors block the enzyme involved in cholesterol synthesis. Bile acid sequestrants block bile acids to form insoluble complexes for excretion in the feces. Fibrates stimulate the breakdown of lipoproteins from the tissues and their removal from the plasma.

10. **Answer: d**
    RATIONALE: Increased serum levels and resultant toxicity can occur if a statin is combined with warfarin, an oral anticoagulant. This would increase the patient's risk for bleeding. Abdominal pain and cataract development are related to the use of atorvastatin alone. Liver failure also is associated with atorvastatin use alone.

11. **Answer: d**
    RATIONALE: To ensure the need for the drug therapy, the patient needs to have attempted lifestyle modifications including a cholesterol-lowering diet and exercise program for at least 3 to 6 months.

12. **Answer: b**
    RATIONALE: The initial effect on lipid levels is usually seen within 5 to 7 days of starting niacin therapy.

13. **Answer: a**
    RATIONALE: Niacin acts to inhibit the release of free fatty acids from adipose tissue, increases the rate of triglyceride removal from the plasma, and generally reduces LDL and triglyceride levels and increases HDL levels. Fenofibrate inhibits triglyceride synthesis in the liver, resulting in a reduction of LDL levels. Gemfibrozil inhibits the peripheral breakdown of lipids, reduces the production of triglycerides and LDLs, and increases HDL concentrations. Fenofibric acid activates a specific hepatic receptor that results in increased breakdown of lipids, elimination of triglyceride-rich particles from the plasma, and reduction in the production to an enzyme that naturally inhibits lipid breakdown.

14. **Answer: c**
    RATIONALE: Although any combinations may be used, niacin is often combined with bile acid sequestrants for increased effects.

15. **Answer: b**
    RATIONALE: The presence of fatty acids, lipids, and cholesterol in the duodenum stimulates contraction of the gallbladder and the release of bile, which contains bile acids. Once their action is completed, they are reabsorbed and recycled to the gallbladder, where they remain until the gallbladder is stimulated again.

CHAPTER 48

■ ASSESSING YOUR UNDERSTANDING

MATCHING

1. e   **2.** h   **3.** f   **4.** b   **5.** i
6. d   **7.** a   **8.** g   **9.** c   **10.** j

LABELING

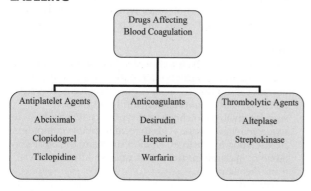

■ APPLYING YOUR KNOWLEDGE

CASE STUDY

a. The patient had an acute embolism or blood clot that had traveled to the lungs. The alteplase was used to dissolve the clot and restore blood flow.

b. Heparin was used to prevent the formation of any new clots. Warfarin also was used to prevent blood clots. The patient was receiving both drugs because warfarin's onset of action typically takes approximately 3 days. Once therapeutic levels of warfarin are achieved (prothrombin time [PT] 1.5 to 2.5 times the control or international normalized ratio [INR] of 2 to 3), then the heparin is stopped.

c. The patient needs instructions about the following: appropriate administration, including the need to use the same formulation of the drug and possible dosage adjustments; follow-up laboratory testing of coagulation status; bleeding precautions; safety measures, including ways to avoid injury that could lead to bruising; measures to stop bleeding, such as ice and direct pressure; importance of reporting any blood in urine or stool; the use of a Medic-alert bracelet; foods containing vitamin K such as green leafy vegetables and the importance of maintaining consistent use of these foods to prevent decreasing the effectiveness of warfarin; and measures to prevent recurrent deep vein thrombosis and pulmonary embolism.

■ PRACTICING FOR NCLEX

1. Answer: a
RATIONALE: Thrombin is a topical hemostatic agent. Protamine sulfate is the antidote for heparin. Pentoxifylline is a hemorheologic agent (one that can induce hemorrhage). Urokinase is a thrombolytic agent.

2. Answer: b
RATIONALE: The first reaction to a blood vessel injury is local vasoconstriction. In addition, injury then exposes blood to the collagen and other substances under the endothelial lining of the vessel, causing platelet aggregation. Release of factor XI occurs in response to activation of the Hageman factor. Thrombin formation occurs at the end of the intrinsic pathway.

3. Answer: a
RATIONALE: Clopidogrel is administered orally.

4. Answer: c
RATIONALE: Anagrelide decreases the production of platelets in the bone marrow, necessitating close monitoring of platelet levels for thrombocytopenia.

5. Answer: a
RATIONALE: Warfarin is administered orally.

6. Answer: a
RATIONALE: Heparin's effectiveness is monitored by the results of the partial thromboplastin time. The INR and PT are used to monitor warfarin. Vitamin K is the antidote for warfarin, and levels are not monitored to evaluate the effects of any anticoagulant.

7. Answer: d
RATIONALE: Fondaparinux inhibits factor Xa and blocks the clotting cascade to prevent clot formation. Heparin and argatroban block the formation of thrombin from prothrombin. Warfarin decreases the production of vitamin K–depending clotting factors in the liver.

8. Answer: b
RATIONALE: Protamine sulfate is the antidote for heparin overdose. Vitamin K is the antidote for warfarin overdose. Urokinase is a thrombolytic. Drotrecogin alfa is a C reactive protein that has anticoagulant effects.

9. Answer: c
RATIONALE: When combined with phenytoin, warfarin leads to a decrease in anticoagulant effect, which would necessitate an increase in the dosage of the warfarin. Clofibrate, quinidine, and cefoxitin increase the risk of bleeding with warfarin; thus, a decreased dose of warfarin would be indicated.

10. Answer: d
RATIONALE: Treatment with a thrombolytic must be instituted within 6 hours of the onset of symptoms of an acute myocardial infarction to achieve maximum therapeutic effectiveness. In this case, 4 PM would be the latest.

11. Answer: c
RATIONALE: When used for hip surgery, enoxaparin typically is administered for 7 to 10 days to prevent deep vein thrombosis that may lead to pulmonary embolism after hip replacement.

12. Answer: c
RATIONALE: Therapeutic range for heparin would be 1.5 to 2.5 times the patient's baseline. For a baseline value of 32 seconds, this would range from 48 to 80 seconds. A value of 64 seconds would be considered therapeutic.

13. Answer: d
RATIONALE: Drotrecogin alfa is approved for use in adults with severe sepsis who are at high risk for death. The usual dose is given by intravenous infusion for a total of 96 hours. It is associated with a high risk for bleeding, which requires extremely close patient monitoring. It is a very expensive drug, which may be a factor in limiting its use.

14. Answer: a
RATIONALE: Antihemophilic factor is factor VIII, which is the factor missing in classic hemophilia. Coagulation factors VIIa and IX are separate clotting factors. Factor IX complex contains plasma fractions of many of the clotting factors and increases blood levels of factors II, VII, IX, and X.

15. Answer: b
RATIONALE: Aminocaproic acid is the only systemic hemostatic agent available. Absorbable gelatin, human fibrin sealant, and thrombin are topical hemostatic agents.

Copyright © 2011 by Wolters Kluwer Health I Lippincott Williams & Wilkins. *Study Guide for Focus on Nursing Pharmacology.*

CHAPTER 49

■ ASSESSING YOUR UNDERSTANDING

MATCHING

1. e   **2.** a   **3.** d   **4.** f   **5.** b
6. c

SHORT ANSWER

1. Erythropoietin is released from the kidneys in response to decreased blood flow or decreased oxygen tension in the kidneys. Under the influence of erythropoietin, an undifferentiated cell in the bone marrow becomes a hemocytoblast. This cell uses certain amino acids, lipids, carbohydrates, vitamin B_{12}, folic acid, and iron to turn into an immature red blood cell (RBC). In the last phase of RBC production, the cell loses its nucleus and enters the circulation. This cell, called a *reticulocyte*, finishes its maturing process in the circulation.

2. The average life span of an RBC is 120 days.

3. The bone marrow must have adequate amounts of iron, which is used in forming hemoglobin rings to carry the oxygen; minute amounts of vitamin B_{12} and folic acid to form a strong supporting structure that can survive being battered through blood vessels for 120 days; and essential amino acids and carbohydrates to complete the hemoglobin rings, cell membrane, and basic structure.

4. A deficiency anemia occurs when the diet cannot supply enough of a nutrient or enough of the nutrient cannot be absorbed; fewer RBCs are produced, and the ones that are produced are immature and inefficient iron carriers. Megaloblastic anemia involves decreased production of RBCs and ineffectiveness of those RBCs that are produced (they do not usually survive for the 120 days that is normal for the life of an RBC). Hemolytic anemia involves a lysing of RBCs because of genetic factors or from exposure to toxins.

5. Pernicious anemia occurs when the gastric mucosa cannot produce intrinsic factor and vitamin B_{12} cannot be absorbed.

■ APPLYING YOUR KNOWLEDGE

CASE STUDY

a. Epoetin alfa is indicated for the treatment of anemia associated with cancer chemotherapy when the bone marrow is suppressed. It acts like the natural glycoprotein erythropoietin to stimulate production of the RBCs in the bone marrow.

b. Epoetin alfa is associated with a possible decrease in the normal levels of erythropoietin. Administration to a patient with normal renal function can actually cause a more severe anemia if endogenous levels fall and no longer stimulate RBC production. The patient's blood count needs to be monitored closely because of the risk for developing pure red cell aplasia secondary to erythropoietin; neutralizing antibodies can occur. In addition, the drug should not be used if the patient's hemoglobin is above 12 g/dL because of the risk of cardiovascular events and increased rates of tumor progression death in cancer patients. Other areas that need close monitoring include the patient's cardiovascular and central nervous system status for possible adverse effects.

■ PRACTICING FOR NCLEX

1. **Answer: c**
   RATIONALE: Anemias are disorders that involve too few or ineffective RBCs that alter the ability of the blood to carry oxygen. White blood cells are associated with the immune response. Plasma proteins are important in the immune response and blood clotting. Lack of vitamin B_{12} is associated with a specific type of anemia.

2. **Answer: d**
   RATIONALE: Sickle cell anemia is an example of a hemolytic anemia that involves lysing of RBCs because of genetic factors or from exposure to toxins. Iron deficiency anemia is a deficiency anemia. Pernicious anemia and folic acid deficiency anemia are examples of megaloblastic anemia.

3. **Answer: c, d, e**
   RATIONALE: Folic acid is found in green leafy vegetables such as broccoli, milk, liver, and eggs. Fruits and fish are not good sources of folic acid.

4. **Answer: c**
   RATIONALE: Hydroxocobalamin is administered intramuscularly for 5 to 10 days and then monthly.

5. **Answer: a**
   RATIONALE: Hydroxyurea is indicated for the treatment of sickle cell anemia to increase the amount of fetal hemoglobin produced in the bone marrow and to dilute the formation of abnormal hemoglobin S in adults who have sickle cell anemia. Epoetin alfa is indicated for treatment of anemia associated with renal failure and those on dialysis and for patients with anemia associated with AIDS therapy and cancer chemotherapy. Ferrous sulfate and iron dextran are indicated for the treatment of iron deficiency anemia.

6. **Answer: a**
   RATIONALE: Darbepoetin alfa is administered once a week. Epoetin alfa is administered three times/week. Methoxy polyethylene glycol–epoetin alfa is administered once every 2 weeks or once a month.

7. **Answer: c**
   RATIONALE: Iron dextran is administered by intramuscular injection using the Z-track technique. Ferrous gluconate, fumarate, and sulfate are administered orally. Iron sucrose and sodium ferric gluconate complex are given intravenously.

8. **Answer: a**
   RATIONALE: Iron is not absorbed if taken with antacids, so the patient should avoid this combination. Adequate iron intake is necessary to assist in regaining a positive iron balance. It can take 2 to 3 weeks to see an improvement and up to 6 to 10 months to return to a stable iron level once a deficiency exists. Iron absorption also is altered if it is taken with milk, eggs, coffee, or tea. These substances should be avoided.

9. **Answer: b**
   RATIONALE: The patient needs to be informed that his stools may become dark or green. Small frequent meals with snacks can help minimize nausea. The patient may take the drug with meals as long as those meals do not include eggs, milk, coffee, or tea. Constipation is possible, so the patient needs to increase the fiber in his diet.

10. **Answer: a**
    RATIONALE: Vitamin B_{12} is important for maintaining the myelin sheath. Folic acid is important in preventing neural tube defects and is essential for cell division in all types of tissues. RBCs are important for transporting oxygen to the tissues.

11. **Answer: a, b, d**
    RATIONALE: The bone marrow uses iron, carbohydrates, amino acids, folic acid, and vitamin B_{12} to produce healthy, efficient RBCs.

12. **Answer: b**
    RATIONALE: Epoetin alfa has a duration of effect of usually 24 hours.

Copyright © 2011 by Wolters Kluwer Health l Lippincott Williams & Wilkins. *Study Guide for Focus on Nursing Pharmacology.*

13. Answer: c
RATIONALE: Deferoxamine is the antidote for iron toxicity. Dimercaprol is used for arsenic, gold, or mercury poisoning. Succimer and edetate calcium disodium can be used to treat lead poisoning.

14. Answer: b
RATIONALE: Leucovorin is used as a rescue following methotrexate therapy. Cyancobalamin is used to treat megaloblastic anemia. Hydroxyurea is used to treat sickle cell anemia. Iron sucrose is indicated for treatment of iron deficiency anemia.

15. Answer: d
RATIONALE: Oral liquid iron solution can stain the teeth; therefore, it should be taken through a straw to prevent this from occurring. Orange juice is acidic, and although it may enhance the absorption of the medication, it should not be used concurrently. The risk of staining would still be present. Drinking a big glass of water after swallowing the solution would not reduce the risk of staining the teeth. The dose should not be mixed with other foods, especially dairy products such as yogurt, which can interfere with absorption.

CHAPTER 50

■ ASSESSING YOUR UNDERSTANDING
LABELING

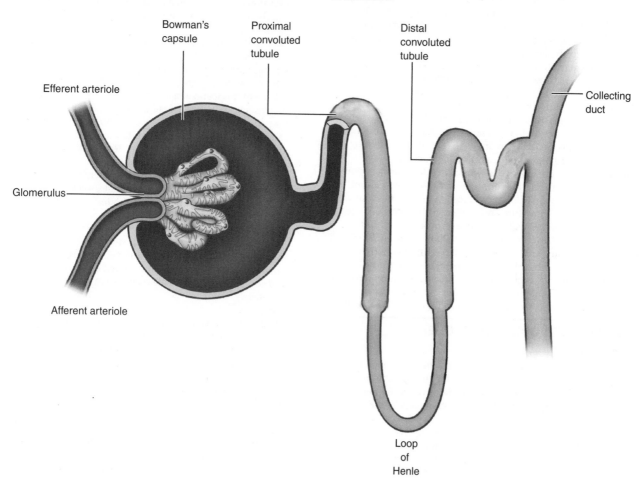

MATCHING
1. c **2.** f **3.** b **4.** g **5.** a
6. e **7.** h **8.** d

■ APPLYING YOUR KNOWLEDGE
CASE STUDY

a. The students would need to demonstrate glomerular filtration, tubular secretion, and tubular reabsorption. The students could arrange themselves as the glomerulus, Bowman's capsule, proximal convoluted tubule, descending loop of Henle, loop of Henle, ascending loop of Henle, distal convoluted tubule, and collecting duct. The students could be connected by rope, tubing, or other item to illustrate the "tubule," such as a noodle commonly found in swimming pools. Other props could be used to represent sodium, water, calcium, potassium, chloride, aldosterone, and antidiuretic hormone. These props could then be moved back and forth along the "tubule" to illustrate secretion and reabsorption.

b. The students would need to address water, sodium, chloride, potassium, and calcium. When demonstrating the movement of sodium, chloride would need to go hand in hand with the sodium. The students could use the props identified above to act out the movement of the various electrolytes along the tubule and the countercurrent mechanism.

Copyright © 2011 by Wolters Kluwer Health I Lippincott Williams & Wilkins. *Study Guide for Focus on Nursing Pharmacology.*

PRACTICING FOR NCLEX

1. **Answer: b**
   RATIONALE: The renal system consists of the kidneys and structures of the urinary tract: ureters, bladder, and urethra. The kidneys have three protective layers. The system has four major functions: maintaining the volume and composition of body fluids, regulating vitamin D activation, regulating blood pressure, and regulating red blood cell production. Most of the fluid that is filtered by the kidneys is returned to the body.

2. **Answer: c**
   RATIONALE: All nephrons filter and make urine, but only the medullary nephrons can concentrate or dilute urine. The renal pelvises drain the urine into the ureters. The renal arteries come directly off the aorta. Erythropoietin is produced by a small group of cells called the *juxtaglomerular apparatus*.

3. **Answer: c**
   RATIONALE: The kidneys receive approximately 25% of the cardiac output.

4. **Answer: d**
   RATIONALE: It is estimated that only about 25% of the total number of nephrons are necessary to maintain healthy renal function. This means that the renal system is well protected from failure with a large backup system. However, it also means that by the time a patient manifests signs and symptoms suggesting failure of the kidneys, extensive kidney damage has already occurred.

5. **Answer: b**
   RATIONALE: Tubular secretion involves the active movement of substances from the blood into the renal tubule. Movement of fluid and other elements through the glomerulus into the tubule describes glomerular filtration. The movement of substances from the tubule back into the vascular system describes tubular reabsorption. The process of concentrating or diluting urine refers to the countercurrent mechanism.

6. **Answer: b**
   RATIONALE: Approximately 1% of the filtrate or less than 2 L of fluid is excreted each day in the form of urine.

7. **Answer: d**
   RATIONALE: The glomerulus acts as an ultrafine filter for all of the blood that flows into it. The semipermeable membrane keeps lipids, proteins, and blood cells inside the vessel, whereas the hydrostatic pressure from the blood pushes water and smaller components of the plasma into the tubule.

8. **Answer: a**
   RATIONALE: Sodium is filtered through the glomerulus and enters the renal tubule, where it is actively reabsorbed in the proximal convoluted tubule to the peritubular capillaries.

9. **Answer: c**
   RATIONALE: Aldosterone is released into the circulation in response to angiotensin III, high potassium levels, or sympathetic stimulation. Aldosterone stimulates a sodium–potassium exchange pump in the cells of the distal tubule, causing reabsorption of sodium in exchange for potassium. As a result of aldosterone stimulation, sodium is reabsorbed into the system and potassium is lost in the filtrate. Natriuretic hormone causes a decrease in sodium reabsorption from the distal tubules with a resultant dilute urine or increased volume. Natriuretic hormone is released in response to fluid overload or hemodilution.

10. **Answer: b**
    RATIONALE: The fluid in the ascending loop of Henle is hypotonic in comparison to the hypertonic situation in the peritubular tissues. The filtrate in the descending loop is highly concentrated in comparison to the rest of the filtrate.

11. **Answer: a**
    RATIONALE: About 65% of the potassium that is filtered at the glomerulus is reabsorbed at Bowman's capsule and the proximal convoluted tubule. Another 25% to 30% is reabsorbed in the ascending loop of Henle.

12. **Answer: d**
    RATIONALE: Parathyroid hormone stimulates the reabsorption of calcium in the distal convoluted tubule to increase serum calcium levels when they are low. Aldosterone is important in adjusting sodium levels. Antidiuretic hormone is important in maintaining fluid balance and is released in response to falling blood volume, sympathetic stimulation, or rising sodium levels. Vitamin D regulates the absorption of calcium from the gastrointestinal tract.

13. **Answer: b**
    RATIONALE: Whenever blood flow or oxygenation to the nephron is decreased (due to hemorrhage, shock, congestive heart failure, or hypotension), renin is released from the juxtaglomerular cells. Calcium is not involved. Renin activates angiotensinogen. After subsequent conversions, angiotensin III ultimately stimulates the release of aldosterone from the adrenal gland.

14. **Answer: b**
    RATIONALE: Urine is usually a slightly acidic fluid; this acidity helps to maintain the normal transport systems and to destroy bacteria that may enter the bladder. The acidity does not play a role in maintaining fluid balance or affect sphincter control. Peristaltic movement is necessary to push urine down from the ureters into the bladder.

15. **Answer: c**
    RATIONALE: In the female, the urethra is a very short tube that leads from the bladder to an area populated by normal flora, including *Escherichia coli*, which can cause frequent bladder infections or cystitis. In the male, the urethra is much longer and passes through the prostate gland, a small gland that produces an alkaline fluid that is important in maintaining the sperm and lubricating the tract. Neither the prostate nor the fluid has any effect on the development of cystitis. The urinary bladder does stretch, but the amount of stretch is highly variable.

CHAPTER 51

ASSESSING YOUR UNDERSTANDING
LABELING

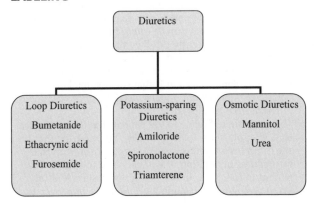

SHORT ANSWER

1. Diuretic agents are commonly thought of simply as drugs that increase the amount of urine produced by the kidneys. Most diuretics do increase the volume of urine produced to some extent, but the greater clinical significance of diuretics is their ability to increase sodium excretion. Most diuretics prevent the cells lining the renal tubules from reabsorbing an excessive proportion of the sodium ions in the glomerular filtrate. As a result, sodium and other ions (and the water in which they are dissolved) are lost in the urine instead of being returned to the blood, where they would cause increased intravascular volume and therefore increased hydrostatic pressure, which could result in leaking of fluids at the capillary level.

2. Fluid rebound is a reflex reaction of the body to the loss of fluid or sodium; the hypothalamus causes the release of antidiuretic hormone, which retains water, and stress related to fluid loss combines with decreased blood flow to the kidneys to activate the renin-angiotensin-aldosterone system, leading to further water and sodium retention.

3. Heart failure can cause edema as a result of several factors. The failing heart muscle does not pump sufficient blood to the kidneys, causing activation of the renin-angiotensin system and resulting in increases in blood volume and sodium retention. Because the failing heart muscle cannot respond to the usual reflex stimulation, the increased volume is slowly pushed out into the capillary level as venous pressure increases because the blood is not being pumped effectively.

4. Thiazide and thiazidelike diuretics act to block the chloride pump. Chloride is actively pumped out of the tubule by cells lining the ascending limb of the loop of Henle and the distal tubule. Sodium passively moves with the chloride to maintain an electrical neutrality. (Chloride is a negative ion, and sodium is a positive ion.) Blocking of the chloride pump keeps the chloride and the sodium in the tubule to be excreted in the urine, thus preventing the reabsorption of both chloride and sodium in the vascular system. Because these segments of the tubule are impermeable to water, there is little increase in the volume of urine produced, but it will be sodium rich, which is a saluretic effect.

5. The prototype loop diuretic is furosemide.

6. Most often, carbonic anhydrase inhibitors are used to treat glaucoma because the inhibition of carbonic anhydrase results in decreased secretion of aqueous humor of the eye.

■ APPLYING YOUR KNOWLEDGE

CASE STUDY

a. It would be important to investigate if the patient is continuing to take her potassium supplement even though the furosemide has been stopped. It would also be important to ask the patient about the foods that she is eating. For example, she may still be eating foods that are high in potassium, inadvertently thinking that she still needs to do so. The nurse also needs to determine the patient's understanding of her current drug therapy. It is possible that the patient understands that she is still taking a "diuretic" but does not understand that spironolactone is different from furosemide.

b. The nurse should relate to the patient that the spironolactone is a potassium-sparing diuretic, emphasizing that she is not losing potassium like she had been with the furosemide. In addition, the nurse needs to instruct the patient to watch her intake of high-potassium foods to avoid raising her potassium level too high. Moreover, the nurse should make sure that the patient is no longer using the potassium supplement. Other teaching should address the signs and symptoms of hypo- and hyperkalemia so that the patient can contact the health care provider should any occur. Hyperkalemia can cause lethargy, confusion, ataxia, muscle cramps, and cardiac arrhythmias, the latter being especially problematic for the patient with a history of hypertension and heart failure.

■ PRACTICING FOR NCLEX

1. **Answer: b**
   RATIONALE: If a patient decreases his fluid intake to decrease the number of trips to the bathroom, the patient is at risk for fluid rebound, which leads to water retention. Fluid retention, leading to weight gain, would occur. Hypokalemia and dehydration would not be associated effects.

2. **Answer: a**
   RATIONALE: Metolazone is an example of a thiazidelike diuretic. Chlorothiazide is a thiazide diuretic; furosemide is a loop diuretic; and triamterene is a potassium-sparing diuretic.

3. **Answer: d**
   RATIONALE: Hydrochlorothiazide is administered intravenously. Only chlorothiazide can be given by intravenous infusion.

4. **Answer: c**
   RATIONALE: Indapamide would be contraindicated in a patient with hypokalemia because any fluid and electrolyte imbalance could be potentiated by the changes caused by the diuretic. Indapamide would be used cautiously in patients with diabetes, systemic lupus erythematosus, or gout.

5. **Answer: b**
   RATIONALE: Chlorthalidone is a thiazidelike diuretic that may lead to hypercalcemia (due to decreased calcium excretion), hyperuricemia (increased levels of uric acid due to decreased uric acid secretion), and hypokalemia. Anemia is not associated with this drug.

6. **Answer: b**
   RATIONALE: Hydrochlorothiazide has an onset of action of 2 hours, peaking in 4 to 6 hours, and lasting approximately 6 to 12 hours.

7. **Answer: b**
   RATIONALE: Bumetanide is a loop diuretic that blocks the chloride pump in the ascending loop of Henle. It also has a similar effect in the descending loop and in the distal convoluted tubule.

8. **Answer: c**
   RATIONALE: Use of furosemide can lead to hypotension due to fluid loss, alkalosis due to loss of bicarbonate, hypocalcemia due to loss of calcium, and hyperglycemia (with long-term use) due to diuretic effect on glucose levels.

9. **Answer: b**
   RATIONALE: Furosemide, when given intravenously, begins to act in 5 minutes, reaching peak effects in 30 minutes. In this case, this would be 8:30 AM.

10. **Answer: a**
    RATIONALE: Furosemide is less powerful than bumetanide and torsemide and therefore has a larger margin of safety for home use (see the Critical Thinking Scenario in this chapter for additional information about using furosemide in heart failure). Ethacrynic acid is used less frequently in the clinical setting because of the improved potency and reliability of the newer drugs.

Copyright © 2011 by Wolters Kluwer Health | Lippincott Williams & Wilkins. *Study Guide for Focus on Nursing Pharmacology.*

11. **Answer: b**
    RATIONALE: Metabolic acidosis is a relatively common and potentially dangerous effect that occurs when bicarbonate is lost due to the action of carbonic anhydrase inhibitors. Metabolic alkalosis would occur if bicarbonate were retained. No respiratory acid-base imbalances are associated with this drug.

12. **Answer: d**
    RATIONALE: Spironolactone acts as an aldosterone antagonist blocking the actions of aldosterone in the distal tubule. Amiloride and triamterene block potassium secretion through the tubule. Carbonic anhydrase inhibitors slow the movement of hydrogen ions. Loop diuretics block the chloride pump.

13. **Answer: a, b, d**
    RATIONALE: Foods high in potassium should be avoided. These would include bananas, prunes, and broccoli.

14. **Answer: b**
    RATIONALE: Instructions for a patient taking a diuretic include taking the drug with food or meals if gastrointestinal upset occurs, taking the dose early in the morning to prevent interfering with sleep, implementing safety precautions if dizziness or weakness is a problem, and ensuring adequate fluid intake to prevent fluid rebound. It is not necessary to lie down after taking the drug.

15. **Answer: a**
    RATIONALE: Mannitol is a powerful osmotic diuretic that is used to treat increased intracranial pressure. It is given intravenously and begins to work in 30 to 60 minutes. Furosemide, amiloride, and bumetanide are not indicated for the treatment of increased intracranial pressure.

CHAPTER 52

■ ASSESSING YOUR UNDERSTANDING

MATCHING

1. b   2. d   3. c   4. e   5. a

SHORT ANSWER

1. Cystitis is an infection of the bladder. Blockage anywhere in the urinary tract can lead to backflow problems and the spread of bladder infections into the kidneys resulting in pyelonephritis.

2. The two types of urinary anti-infectives include antibiotics that are particularly effective against the gram-negative bacteria that cause most urinary tract infections (UTIs) and drugs that work to acidify the urine.

3. The urinary tract antispasmodics relieve these spasms by blocking parasympathetic activity, thus suppressing overactivity, which leads to relaxation of the detrusor and other urinary tract muscles.

4. Pentosan polysulfate sodium is used specifically to decrease the pain and discomfort associated with interstitial cystitis.

5. Two types of drugs are currently used to relieve the symptoms of benign prostatic hyperplasia (BPH). These drugs include the alpha-adrenergic blockers and drugs that block testosterone production.

6. Saw palmetto is an herbal therapy that has been used very successfully for the relief of symptoms associated with BPH.

■ APPLYING YOUR KNOWLEDGE

CASE STUDY

a. Trospium is an anticholinergic that relieves the overactive bladder by blocking parasympathetic activity, thereby suppressing overactivity. As a result, the detrusor and other urinary tract muscles relax. The drug specifically blocks muscarinic receptors and reduces bladder muscle tone.

b. Patient teaching should include how to take the drug (at least 1 hour before meals, usually twice a day); possible adverse effects including anticholinergic effects such as dry mouth, dizziness, photophobia (due to pupil dilation), nausea, constipation, decreased sweating, and tachycardia and palpitations as well as measures to address these, such as using sugarless hard candy and frequent sips of water (for dry mouth), safety measures (for dizziness and photophobia), increased fiber intake (for constipation), avoidance of overactivity or heat extremes (for decreased sweating); importance of adequate fluid intake to prevent urinary stasis and possible UTIs; and the need to check with her health care provider before using any over-the-counter cold remedies or antihistamines, as these could increase the risk of anticholinergic effects.

■ PRACTICING FOR NCLEX

1. **Answer: d**
   RATIONALE: Nitrofurantoin is considered a urinary tract anti-infective. Flavoxate is an antispasmodic; phenazopyridine is a urinary tract analgesic; and doxazosin is an alpha-adrenergic blocker used for treating BPH.

2. **Answer: c**
   RATIONALE: Methenamine works to acidify the urine. Cinoxacin, fosfomycin, and co-trimoxazole act against the gram-negative bacteria that cause most UTIs.

3. **Answer: b**
   RATIONALE: Nitrofurantoin does not need a dosage adjustment when used for patients with renal dysfunction. Dosage adjustments would be necessary for cinoxacin, norfloxacin, and co-trimoxazole.

4. **Answer: b**
   RATIONALE: Fosfomycin is administered as one packet dissolved in water. It is used as a one-time dose, so it does not need to be continued for 7 to 14 days like most anti-infectives. Citrus juices and milk should be avoided because these cause the urine to be alkaline and promote bacterial growth. Rather, the patient should drink fluids that make the urine more acidic.

5. **Answer: a**
   RATIONALE: Oxybutynin is available as a transdermal patch as well as in an oral form. Flavoxate, tolterodine, and darifenacin are available only in oral form.

6. **Answer: b**
   RATIONALE: Trospium interacts with digoxin, leading to increased serum levels of digoxin. Therefore, the nurse would need to monitor the patient for signs and symptoms of digoxin toxicity. Levels of trospium would not increase, so increased central nervous system effects or excess anticholinergic effects would most likely not occur. The combination of tropsium and digoxin does not change the color of urine.

7. **Answer: d**
   RATIONALE: Phenazopyridine can cause the urine to turn a reddish-orange. Nitrofurantoin can cause the urine to change to brown or dark yellow. Methylene blue can cause the urine to become blue-green.

8. **Answer: c**
   RATIONALE: When given by the transdermal patch, oxybutynin has a duration of 96 hours; thus, the patch should be replaced every 4 days.

9. **Answer: a**

RATIONALE: Pentosan should be used cautiously in patients with splenic dysfunction because of the drug's heparinlike actions. The drug is contraindicated in patients with conditions involving an increased risk for bleeding, such as use of anticoagulants, thrombocytopenia, and recent surgery.

10. **Answer: b**

RATIONALE: Dutasteride blocks testosterone production by inhibiting the intracellular enzyme that converts testosterone to a potent androgen, DHT, on which the prostate gland depends for its development and maintenance. Doxazosin, tamsulosin, alfuzosin, and terazosin are alpha-adrenergic blockers used to treat BPH. Pentosan, a urinary bladder protectant acts as a buffer to control cell permeability. Urinary anti-infectives such as norfloxacin interfere with DNA replication in susceptible gram-negative bacteria leading to cell death.

11. **Answer: c**

RATIONALE: Tamsulosin should be taken one-half hour after the same meal each day.

12. **Answer: d**

RATIONALE: Dutasteride is associated with impotence, decreased libido, and sexual dysfunction, all of which are related to decreased levels of DHT. Hypotension and tachycardia are associated with the use of alpha-adrenergic blockers such as alfuzosin, doxazosin, or terazosin.

13. **Answer: d**

RATIONALE: Periodically, a patient receiving an agent for BPH should have his prostate-specific antigen level evaluated to reconfirm that the enlargement is not due to cancer. Other testing such as a complete blood count, serum electrolyte levels, and renal functions studies would not be as important.

14. **Answer: b**

RATIONALE: Flank pain, chills, fever, and tenderness are indicative of pyelonephritis. Urinary frequency, dysuria, and urgency are associated with cystitis.

15. **Answer: c**

RATIONALE: Tolterodine is a urinary antispasmodic used to treat overactive bladder. Nalidixic acid and methylene blue are urinary anti-infectives used to treat UTIs. Terazosin is an alpha-adrenergic blocker used to treat BPH.

CHAPTER 53

■ ASSESSING YOUR UNDERSTANDING

LABELING

Upper Respiratory Tract	Lower Respiratory Tract
Larynx	Alveoli
Mouth	Bronchiole
Nose	Bronchus
Pharynx	Lung
Sinuses	
Trachea	

MATCHING

1. e	**2.** g	**3.** f	**4.** d	**5.** c
6. b	**7.** j	**8.** h	**9.** a	**10.** i

■ APPLYING YOUR KNOWLEDGE

CASE STUDY

a. The patient is most likely experiencing atelectasis based on the decreased aeration of the lungs at the bases, crackles, decreased oxygen saturation levels, and lack of coughing. In addition, the patient has had anesthesia for surgery and is receiving morphine for pain, which can also depress respiratory function. The lack of coughing also is impairing the patient's ability to move secretions, which are preventing air from entering the alveoli.

b. Since pain is interfering with his ability to cough and move, administering the morphine would be appropriate so that the patient can accomplish these actions with minimal discomfort. Although morphine can lead to respiratory depression, its use here would facilitate measures to help move secretions and thus be beneficial to the patient. In addition, the nurse can have the patient splint his incision to assist in coughing. Frequent turning, deep breathing, and the use of incentive spirometry to maximize lung expansion would be helpful. Elevating the head of the bed also would allow for increased chest expansion with each breath. Depending on his oxygen saturation levels, oxygen administration may be needed to ensure adequate tissue oxygenation.

■ PRACTICING FOR NCLEX

1. **Answer: b**

RATIONALE: Asthma is characterized by reversible bronchospasm, inflammation, and hyperactive airways. Sometimes an infection may be a trigger, but it is not always associated with asthma. Alveolar collapse refers to atelectasis, which might occur with asthma if the airways become blocked with secretions. Progressive loss of lung compliance is associated with acute respiratory distress syndrome.

2. **Answer: c**

RATIONALE: Ventilation refers to the movement of air in and out of the body. Perfusion refers to the delivery of oxygen via the blood to tissues and cells. Respiration refers to the act of breathing to allow gas exchange and to the exchange of gases at the alveolar level.

3. **Answer: d**

RATIONALE: The respiratory membrane is made up of the capillary endothelium, capillary basement membrane, interstitial space, alveolar basement membrane, alveolar epithelium, and surfactant layer. Cilia, goblet cells, and mast cells are found along the upper respiratory tract.

4. **Answer: c**

RATIONALE: Sympathetic stimulation leads to an increased rate and depth of respiration and bronchodilation. Parasympathetic stimulation including the vagus nerve would lead to stimulation of diaphragmatic contraction, bronchoconstriction, and inspiratory movement.

5. **Answer: c**

RATIONALE: With the common cold, numerous viruses can invade the tissue, initiating the release of histamine and prostaglandins causing an inflammatory response. The mucous membranes become engorged with blood, the tissues swell, and goblet cells increase the production of mucus.

6. Answer: b

RATIONALE: Seasonal rhinitis, or hay fever, is a condition of the upper respiratory tract that involves a response to an antigen such as pollen or dust. Asthma affects the lower respiratory tract and can be associated with a response to an antigen. Sinusitis results from inflammation of the sinus cavities due to irritation or infection. Pharyngitis involves a bacterial or viral infection.

7. Answer: a

RATIONALE: The left lung consists of two lobes, and the right lung consists of three lobes.

8. Answer: b

RATIONALE: At the alveolar level, oxygen and carbon dioxide move via diffusion. Active transport involves the use of energy to move substances. Facilitated diffusion requires the use of a carrier molecule. Osmosis refers to the movement of water.

9. Answer: a, c, d, f

RATIONALE: Disorders affecting the lower respiratory tract such as atelectasis, bronchitis, respiratory distress syndrome, and cystic fibrosis all involve, to some degree, an alteration in the ability to move gases in and out of the lungs. The common cold and sinusitis are upper respiratory tract disorders that typically are not associated with altered gas exchange.

10. Answer: c

RATIONALE: Although an inflammatory reaction occurs leading to swelling and increased blood flow with bronchitis, it is the change in the capillary permeability that allows proteins to leak into the area.

11. Answer: b

RATIONALE: Bronchiectasis is a chronic disease characterized by dilation of the bronchial tree and chronic inflammation of the bronchial passages. The chronic inflammation leads to replacement of the bronchial epithelial cells by fibrous scar tissue. Asthma is an obstructive disorder characterized by reversible bronchospasm, inflammation, and hyperactive airways. Bronchitis is an acute inflammation of the bronchi. Pneumonia is an inflammation of the lungs.

12. Answer: c

RATIONALE: With respiratory distress syndrome, there is a surfactant deficiency necessitating the use of surfactant replacement. Anti-infectives would be used to treat infections; bronchodilators would be used to relieve bronchospasm; and antihistamines may be used to address allergic reactions.

13. Answer: d

RATIONALE: Cigarette smoking is most commonly associated with chronic obstructive pulmonary disease. The patient may be at greater risk for infection, but infection is not an underlying factor contributing to the disorder. Allergen exposure is more commonly related to seasonal rhinitis or asthma. Genetic inheritance is associated with cystic fibrosis.

14. Answer: b

RATIONALE: The bronchospasm associated with asthma is due to the immediate release of histamine.

15. Answer: a, b, c

RATIONALE: Mast cells release histamine, serotonin, adenosine triphosphate, and other chemicals to ensure a rapid and intense inflammatory reaction to any cell injury. Release of epinephrine and dopamine are not associated with mast cells.

CHAPTER 54

■ ASSESSING YOUR UNDERSTANDING

LABELING

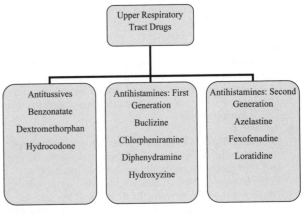

MATCHING

1. c   **2.** a   **3.** b   **4.** d

■ APPLYING YOUR KNOWLEDGE

CASE STUDY

a. Nasal steroids typically are ordered for patients with allergic rhinitis who are no longer getting a response with other decongestants. The patient stopped taking his fexofenadine, which he admits to being effective. So it would be appropriate to restart the fexofenadine rather than add another drug to the regimen. Also, this type of agent does not work immediately; it may take up to 1 week before effects are seen. The patient needs fairly prompt relief.

b. The patient needs instructions in how to use the nasal spray properly (sitting upright with a finger over one of the nares, holding the bottle upright and placing the tip about ½ inch into the open nares, and firmly squeezing the bottle to deliver the drug but not too forcefully), to use the spray exactly as recommended, not to use the spray for longer than recommended to prevent rebound congestion, general respiratory hygiene measures, and measures to reduce the risk of exposure to allergens.

■ PRACTICING FOR NCLEX

1. Answer: b

RATIONALE: Codeine, a centrally acting antitussive, works directly on the medullary cough center. Benzonatate provides local anesthetic action on the respiratory passages, lungs, and pleurae. Ephedrine and tetrahydrozoline are topical nasal decongestants.

2. Answer: c

RATIONALE: Antitussives are used cautiously in patients with asthma because cough suppression can lead to accumulation of secretion and a loss of respiratory reserve. Airway maintenance is important for patients who have had surgery and need a cough to maintain the airway. Antitussives such as codeine and hydrocodone must be used cautiously in patients with a history of addiction. Increased sedation can be problematic for patients who need to drive or be alert.

Copyright © 2011 by Wolters Kluwer Health | Lippincott Williams & Wilkins. *Study Guide for Focus on Nursing Pharmacology.*

3. Answer: b

RATIONALE: Measures to assist with cough control when using antitussives include cool temperatures, humidification, lozenges, and increased fluids.

4. Answer: a

RATIONALE: Pseudoephedrine is the only oral decongestant. Phenylephrine, tetrahydrozoline, and xylometazoline are topical decongestants.

5. Answer: d

RATIONALE: Topical decongestants are sympathomimetic, imitating the effects of the sympathetic nervous system to cause vasoconstriction. Pseudoephedrine has adrenergic properties. Topical decongestants are not anticholinergics or antihistamines.

6. Answer: c

RATIONALE: Parents should use the children's, pediatric, or infant formulations of the drug. Over-the-counter cough and cold preparations should not be used in children under the age of 2 years. The parents need to read the label carefully to determine the dosage and frequency, and they need to use the device that comes with the drug to ensure a proper dosage.

7. Answer: a

RATIONALE: Adverse effects related to the sympathomimetic effects of pseudoephedrine are more likely to occur, including feelings of anxiety, restlessness, hypertension, sweating, tenseness, tremors, arrhythmias, and pallor.

8. Answer: c

RATIONALE: The onset of nasal steroids is not immediate, and it may take up to 7 days before any changes occur. If no effect occurs within 21 days, the drug should be discontinued.

9. Answer: d

RATIONALE: Loratadine is a second-generation antihistamine. Brompheniramine, promethazine, and meclizine are considered first-generation antihistamines.

10. Answer: d

RATIONALE: The adverse effects most often seen with antihistamine use are drowsiness and sedation. However, second-generation antihistamines are less sedating in many people. The anticholinergic effects associated with both generations include drying of the respiratory and gastrointestinal mucous membranes, gastrointestinal upset and nausea, arrhythmias, dysuria, urinary hesitancy, and skin eruption and itching associated with dryness.

11. Answer: a

RATIONALE: The onset of oral diphenhydramine is 15 to 30 minutes.

12. Answer: b

RATIONALE: Guaifenesin should not be used for more than 1 week; if the cough persists, encourage the patient to seek health care.

13. Answer: b

RATIONALE: Meclizine is used to relieve the nausea and vomiting associated with motion sickness. Clemastine, cyproheptadine, and hydroxyzine are used to provide relief of seasonal and perennial allergic rhinitis.

14. Answer: c

RATIONALE: In treating cystic fibrosis, acetylcysteine splits apart the disulfide bonds that are responsible for holding the mucus material together. When used to treat acetaminophen toxicity, the drug protects liver cells from damage because it normalizes hepatic glutathione levels and binds with a reactive hepatotoxic metabolite of acetaminophen.

Dornase alfa selectively breaks down respiratory tract mucus by separating extracellular DNA from proteins. Expectorants liquefy secretions.

15. Answer: c

RATIONALE: Patients receiving dornase alfa should be cautioned to store the drug in the refrigerator, protected from light. The nurse also needs to review how to administer the drug using a nebulizer.

CHAPTER 55

■ ASSESSING YOUR UNDERSTANDING

LABELING

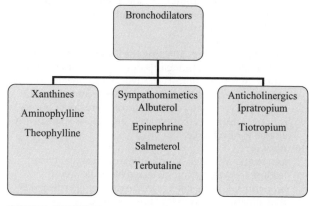

SHORT ANSWER

1. The first step for treatment of pulmonary obstructive diseases includes reducing environmental exposure to irritants such as stopping smoking, filtering allergens from the air, and avoiding exposure to known irritants and allergens.

2. The obstruction of respiratory distress syndrome in the neonate is related to a lack of the lipoprotein surfactant, which leads to an inability to maintain an open alveolus. Surfactant is essential in decreasing the surface tension in the tiny alveolus, allowing it to expand and remain open. If surfactant is lacking, the alveoli collapse and gas exchange cannot occur. Pharmacologic therapy for respiratory distress syndrome involves instilling surfactant into the alveoli.

3. Xanthines have a relatively narrow margin of safety, and they interact with many other drugs. Therefore, they are no longer considered the first-choice bronchodilators.

4. Most of the sympathomimetics used as bronchodilators are beta-2 selective adrenergic agonists. That means that at therapeutic levels, their actions are specific to the beta-2 receptors found in the bronchi. This specificity is lost at higher levels.

5. Anticholinergics are used as bronchodilators because of their effect on the vagus nerve, which is to block or antagonize the action of the neurotransmitter acetylcholine at vagal-mediated receptor sites. Normally, vagal stimulation results in a stimulating effect on smooth muscle, causing contraction. By blocking the vagal effect, relaxation of smooth muscle in the bronchi occurs, leading to bronchodilation.

6. A mast cell stabilizer prevents the release of inflammatory and bronchoconstricting substances when the mast cells are stimulated to release these substances because of irritation or the presence of an antigen.

Copyright © 2011 by Wolters Kluwer Health I Lippincott Williams & Wilkins. *Study Guide for Focus on Nursing Pharmacology.*

7. Administration of lung surfactants requires proper placement of an endotracheal tube, suctioning the infant before administration (but not for 2 hours after administration unless necessary), and careful monitoring and support of the infant to ensure lung expansion and proper oxygenation.

■ APPLYING YOUR KNOWLEDGE

CASE STUDY

a. Albuterol is a sympathomimetic agent that is used to provide relief for acute bronchospasm. It is a beta-2 selective adrenergic agent that will dilate the bronchi and increase the rate and depth of respiration. The drug is absorbed rapidly into the lungs, so it would be helpful in a relatively short period of time.

b. The patient needs to understand that he may experience increased sympathomimetic effects related to the use of the albuterol in combination with his usual maintenance inhaler, which includes formoterol—also a sympathomimetic agent. Although little of the drug is absorbed, the patient is receiving two drugs of the same class, increasing his risk for possible adverse effects. These effects may include central nervous system stimulation, gastrointestinal upset, cardiac irregularities, hypertension, sweating, pallor, and flushing. The patient also needs to understand that if the albuterol does not relieve his symptoms, he needs to seek medical care to prevent further bronchoconstriction, which would compromise his airflow.

■ PRACTICING FOR NCLEX

1. **Answer: d**
   RATIONALE: Mast cell stabilizers work at the cellular level to inhibit the release of histamine and the release of slow-reacting substance of anaphylaxis. Epinephrine is not affected by mast cell stabilizers. Xanthines are thought to work by directly affecting the mobilization of calcium within the cell by stimulating two prostaglandins.

2. **Answer: c**
   RATIONALE: Xanthines were once the main treatment choices for asthma and bronchospasm; however, due to their narrow range of safety and interaction with many other drugs, they are no longer considered first-line bronchodilators.

3. **Answer: d**
   RATIONALE: A serum theophylline level greater than 20 mcg/mL is considered toxic.

4. **Answer: b**
   RATIONALE: Nicotine increases the metabolism of xanthines; therefore, an increased dosage would be necessary. Hyperthyroidism, gastrointestinal, upset or alcohol intake requires cautious use of the drug because these conditions may be exacerbated by the systemic effects of the drug. The drug dosage may need to be decreased in these situations.

5. **Answer: c**
   RATIONALE: Levalbuterol is administered only as an inhalant by nebulizer.

6. **Answer: b**
   RATIONALE: The patient should use the inhaler approximately 15 minutes before exercising to achieve the maximum therapeutic effects.

7. **Answer: d**
   RATIONALE: When given intravenously, epinephrine peaks in approximately 20 minutes. It would be at this time that the drug is most effective.

8. **Answer: b**
   RATIONALE: Metaproterenol is mixed with saline in the nebulizer chamber for administration. The child should sit upright or be in a semi-Fowler's position. He should breathe slowly and deeply during the treatment. The treatment is completed when all of the solution (liquid) is gone from the chamber.

9. **Answer: c**
   RATIONALE: The use of ipratropium is contraindicated in the presence of known allergy to the drug or to peanuts or soy products because the vehicle used to make ipratropium, an aerosol, contains a protein associated with peanut allergies.

10. **Answer: a**
    RATIONALE: Inhaled steroids, such as triamcinolone, can take from 2 to 3 weeks to reach effective levels, so the patient should be encouraged to take them to reach and then maintain the effective levels. The drug is not effective for acute attacks. It can cause hoarseness and sore throat. The patient should rinse his mouth after using the inhaler to decrease the risk of systemic absorption and decrease gastrointestinal upset and nausea.

11. **Answer: c**
    RATIONALE: With ipratropium, the usual dosage is 2 inhalations four times/day for a total of 8 inhalations. However, the patient can use up to 12 inhalations if needed in 1 day.

12. **Answer: b**
    RATIONALE: Montelukast selectively and competitively blocks receptors for the production of leukotrienes D4 and E4, which are components of slow-reacting substance of anaphylaxis. As a result, the drug blocks many of the signs and symptoms of asthma, such as neutrophil and eosinophil migration, neutrophil and monocyte aggregation, leukocyte adhesion, increased capillary permeability, and smooth muscle contraction.

13. **Answer: d**
    RATIONALE: A beta-2 selective adrenergic agonist or sympathomimetic would be most appropriate because these agents are rapidly distributed after injection and rapidly absorbed after inhalation. An inhaled steroid would require 2 to 3 weeks to reach effective levels. Leukotriene receptor antagonists and mast cell stabilizers do not have immediate effects.

14. **Answer: b**
    RATIONALE: Beractant is a lung surfactant. Cromolyn is a mast cell stabilizer. Zileuton is a leukotriene receptor antagonist. Theophylline is a xanthine.

15. **Answer: a, c, e**
    RATIONALE: Before administering calfactant, it would be important to ensure proper endotracheal tube placement because the drug is instilled directly into the trachea. In addition, lung sounds and oxygen saturation levels would be important as a baseline to evaluate effectiveness of the drug.

Copyright © 2011 by Wolters Kluwer Health l Lippincott Williams & Wilkins. *Study Guide for Focus on Nursing Pharmacology.*

CHAPTER 56

■ ASSESSING YOUR UNDERSTANDING
LABELING

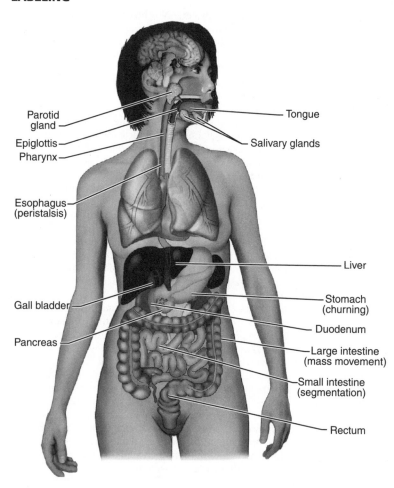

Parotid gland
Epiglottis
Pharynx
Esophagus (peristalsis)
Gall bladder
Pancreas

Tongue
Salivary glands
Liver
Stomach (churning)
Duodenum
Large intestine (mass movement)
Small intestine (segmentation)
Rectum

MATCHING

1. e	**2.** c	**3.** g	**4.** b	**5.** a
6. d	**7.** f	**8.** h		

■ APPLYING YOUR KNOWLEDGE
CASE STUDY

a. The gallbladder stores bile that is produced in the liver. Bile is very important in the digestion of fats and is deposited into the small intestine when the gallbladder is stimulated to contract by the presence of fats. Once bile is delivered to the gallbladder for storage, it is concentrated; water is removed by the walls of the gallbladder. It would be important for the nurse to obtain more information about the types of food eaten during a meal in which the woman then develops pain afterward. In addition, it would be important for the nurse to investigate the patient's history a bit further to gather data about the signs and symptoms that her mother and sister experienced when they had their gallstones.

b. The patient's pain might be related to the contraction of the gallbladder in response to fatty foods that the patient may have ingested. If the patient has gallstones, then the concentrated bile has crystallized. The stones can move down the duct, causing severe pain. If large enough, the stones can block the duct, preventing bile from reaching its intended target.

■ PRACTICING FOR NCLEX

1. Answer: b
   RATIONALE: The exocrine pancreas secretes pancreatin and pancrelipase. Insulin is secreted by the beta cells of the endocrine pancreas. Gastrin and hydrochloric acid are secreted by the stomach.

2. Answer: a
   RATIONALE: Saliva is the fluid produced by the salivary glands in the mouth that makes the food bolus slippery and easier to swallow. Bile is stored in the gallbladder and released to break down fats. Chyme refers to the contents of the stomach containing ingested food and secreted enzymes, water, and mucus. Pancrelipase is a pancreatic enzyme.

3. Answer: b
   RATIONALE: The stomach is responsible for the mechanical and chemical breakdown of foods into useable nutrients. The mouth initiates secretion of saliva that contains water and digestive enzymes to begin the digestive process. The small intestine is responsible for absorption of nutrients.

Copyright © 2011 by Wolters Kluwer Health I Lippincott Williams & Wilkins. *Study Guide for Focus on Nursing Pharmacology*.

The pancreas secretes enzymes and sodium bicarbonate into the beginning of the small intestine to neutralize acid from the stomach and further facilitate digestion.

4. **Answer: a**
   RATIONALE: The mucosal layer is the innermost layer of the gastrointestinal (GI) tract, followed by the circular muscularis layer, the nerve plexus, the longitudinal muscularis, and finally the adventitia.

5. **Answer: c**
   RATIONALE: Pepsin is secreted by the chief cells of the stomach in response to gastrin, which is secreted when the food arrives at the stomach. Gastrin also stimulates the parietal cells of the stomach to secrete hydrochloric acid. Bile is secreted by the gallbladder in response to fats in the bolus.

6. **Answer: d**
   RATIONALE: Amylase is secreted by the pancreas to break down sugars. Chymotrypsin and trypsin break down proteins into amino acids; sodium bicarbonate is secreted to neutralize the acid bolus.

7. **Answer: c**
   RATIONALE: The small intestine uses a process of segmentation with an occasional peristaltic wave to clear the segment. Peristalsis is seen in the esophagus. Churning occurs in the stomach. Mass movement with an occasional peristaltic wave occurs in the large intestine.

8. **Answer: c**
   RATIONALE: Vomiting is a central reflex. Gastroenteric, somatointestinal, and ileogastric are local reflexes.

9. **Answer: b**
   RATIONALE: Absence of bowel sounds or intestinal activity secondary to abdominal surgery indicates a disruption of the intestinointestinal reflex, which occurs due to intense irritation from handling of the intestines. The continued stretch of the ileum with constipation is associated with the ileogastric reflex. The gastroenteric reflex occurs with stimulation of the stomach by stretching, the presence of food, or cephalic stimulation. The gastrocolic reflex involves stimulation of the stomach that also causes increased activity in the colon.

10. **Answer: a**
    RATIONALE: The swallowing reflex is stimulated whenever a food bolus stimulates pressure receptors in the back of the throat and pharynx. These receptors send impulses to the medulla, which stimulates a series of nerves that cause the following actions: The soft palate elevates and seals off the nasal cavity; respirations cease in order to protect the lungs; the larynx rises and the glottis closes to seal off the airway; and the pharyngeal constrictor muscles contract and force the food bolus into the top of the esophagus, where pairs of muscles contract in turn to move the bolus down the esophagus and into the stomach.

11. **Answer: c**
    RATIONALE: The swallowing reflex can be facilitated in a number of ways if swallowing (food or medication) is a problem. Icing the tongue by sucking on an ice pop or an ice cube blocks external nerve impulses and allows this more basic reflex to respond. Icing the sternal notch or the back of the neck, although not as appealing, has also proved effective in stimulating the swallowing reflex. In addition, keeping the head straight (not turned to one side) allows the muscle pairs to work together and helps the process. Providing stimulation of the receptors in the mouth through temperature variations and textured foods helps initiate the reflex.

12. **Answer: b**
    RATIONALE: Once the chemotrigger receptor zone is stimulated, a series of reflexes occurs. Salivation increases, and there is a large increase in the production of mucus in the upper GI tract, which is accompanied by a decrease in gastric acid production. This action protects the lining of the GI tract from potential damage by the acidic stomach contents. The sympathetic system is stimulated, with a resultant increase in sweating, increased heart rate, deeper respirations, and nausea.

13. **Answer: c**
    RATIONALE: The GI system is comprised of one continuous, long tube and is the only body system that is open to the external environment with an opening at the mouth and again at the anus. It is responsible for only a very small part of waste excretion; the kidneys and lungs are responsible for excreting most of the waste products of normal metabolism. It is protected from friction with movement by the peritoneum that lines the abdominal wall and viscera with a small free space between the two layers.

14. **Answer: d**
    RATIONALE: High levels of acid decrease the secretion of gastrin. Alcohol, caffeine, proteins, and calcium increase gastrin secretion.

15. **Answer: c, d**
    RATIONALE: The large intestine absorbs mostly water and sodium. The lower end of the stomach absorbs mostly water and alcohol. The small intestine absorbs drugs, nutrients, anything that is taken into the GI tract, and secretions.

CHAPTER 57

■ ASSESSING YOUR UNDERSTANDING

LABELING

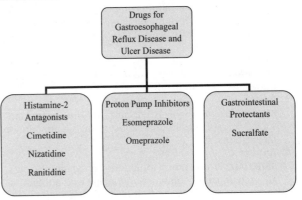

FILL IN THE BLANKS

1. Hydrochloric acid
2. Acute (or stress)
3. Famotidine
4. Rebound
5. Neutralize
6. Constipation, diarrhea
7. Before
8. Sucralfate

■ APPLYING YOUR KNOWLEDGE

CASE STUDY

a. The patient may be experiencing acid rebound because of his frequent use of antacids. The stomach produces more

Copyright © 2011 by Wolters Kluwer Health I Lippincott Williams & Wilkins. *Study Guide for Focus on Nursing Pharmacology.*

acid in response to the alkaline environment. Neutralizing the stomach contents to an alkaline level stimulates gastrin production to cause an increase in acid production and return the stomach to its normal acidic state. In many cases, the acid rebound causes an increase in symptoms, which results in an increased intake of the antacid. This leads to more acid production and an ongoing cycle.

b. When more and more antacid is used, the risk for systemic effects rises. Alkalosis with resultant metabolic changes (nausea, vomiting, neuromuscular changes, headache, irritability, muscle twitching, and even coma) may occur. The use of calcium salts, such as TUMS may lead to hypercalcemia and milk-alkali syndrome (seen as alkalosis, renal calcium deposits, or severe electrolyte disorders). Constipation or diarrhea may result, depending on the antacid being used. The nurse would need to determine the type of liquid antacid used because a magnesium salt antacid would lead to diarrhea, magaldrate may result in alkalosis, and an aluminum salt antacid could lead to hypophosphatemia and altered systemic calcium levels.

c. The patient needs to understand how to use over-the-counter antacids properly and that continued used can lead to a vicious cycle due to acid rebound. In addition, the patient needs to understand that systemic adverse effects are possible if antacids are overused. The nurse should also remind the patient that if his symptoms do not improve after a period of time using the antacid, he should see his health care provider.

■ PRACTICING FOR NCLEX

1. **Answer: d**
RATIONALE: Prostaglandins inhibit the secretion of gastrin and increase the secretion of the mucous lining of the stomach, providing a buffer. Histamine-2 antagonists block the release of hydrochloric acid in response to gastrin; proton pump inhibitors suppress the secretion of hydrochloric acid into the lumen of the stomach, and antacids interact with acids at the chemical level to neutralize them.

2. **Answer: a**
RATIONALE: Cimetidine is considered the prototype histamine-2 receptor antagonist.

3. **Answer: b**
RATIONALE: Omeprazole is available over the counter; lansoprazole, rabeprazole, and esomeprazole are prescription medications.

4. **Answer: c**
RATIONALE: Proton pump inhibitors such as omeprazole are used as part of combination therapy with antibiotics for treatment of *Helicobacter pylori* infection.

5. **Answer: d**
RATIONALE: Aluminum binds dietary phosphates and causes hypophosphatemia, but they do not cause acid rebound like other antacids. Magnesium antacids cause diarrhea; calcium salts cause hypercalcemia.

6. **Answer: a**
RATIONALE: Esomeprazole is available in intravenous preparations and delayed-release oral forms. Omeprazole, rabeprazole, and dexlansoprazole are available in delayed-release oral forms only.

7. **Answer: c**
RATIONALE: The medication should be swallowed whole with a large glass of water. It should not be chewed, crushed, or opened. Antacids, if prescribed, should be taken 1 hour before or 2 hours after the omeprazole.

8. **Answer: b**
RATIONALE: Constipation is the most frequently seen adverse effect; thus, the patient should increase his fiber intake to prevent constipation. Diarrhea is possible, but constipation is more likely. The patient should drink fluids and use sugarless lozenges to help with a dry mouth. Fluid intake also will help to prevent constipation.

9. **Answer: b**
RATIONALE: Pancrelipase is given with meals and snacks so that the enzyme is available when it is needed.

10. **Answer: d**
RATIONALE: Histamine-2 receptor antagonists are used for stress ulcer prophylaxis because the drugs block the production of acid thereby protecting the stomach lining, which is at risk because of decreased mucus production. Reducing the overall acid level is the rationale for use as short-term treatment of active duodenal ulcer. Blocking the overproduction of hydrochloric acid is the rationale for treatment of pathologic hypersecretory conditions. Decreasing the acid being regurgitated into the esophagus is the rationale for treatment of erosive gastroesophageal reflux.

11. **Answer: c**
RATIONALE: Cimetidine was the first drug in this class to be developed and has been associated with antiandrogenic effects including gynecomastia and galactorrhea. Ranitidine, famotidine, and nizatidine are not associated with these effects.

12. **Answer: d**
RATIONALE: Nizatidine is the drug of choice for patients with liver dysfunction because it does not undergo first-pass metabolism in the liver like the other histamine-2 receptor antagonists such as cimetidine, famotidine, or ranitidine.

13. **Answer: a, c, d, e**
RATIONALE: Indications of systemic alkalosis include headache, confusion, irritability, tetany, nausea, and weakness.

14. **Answer: c**
RATIONALE: Alopecia can occur with proton pump therapy, but it is not a common adverse effect. Common adverse effects include dizziness, headache, and cough.

15. **Answer: b**
RATIONALE: Sucralfate has an onset of action of 30 minutes and a duration of 5 hours.

CHAPTER 58

■ ASSESSING YOUR UNDERSTANDING
LABELING

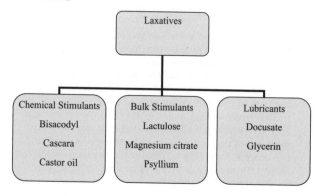

SHORT ANSWER

1. Gastrointestinal (GI) stimulants stimulate parasympathetic activity within the GI tract, resulting in increased GI secretions and motility on a general level throughout the tract. They do not have the local effects of laxatives to increase activity only in the intestines.

2. Antidiarrheal agents slow the motility of the GI tract through direct action on the lining of the GI tract to inhibit local reflexes (bismuth subsalicylate), through direct action on the muscles of the GI tract to slow activity (loperamide), or through action on central nervous system centers that cause GI spasm and slowing.

3. A lubricant is an agent that increases the viscosity of the feces, making it difficult to absorb water from the bolus and easing movement of the bolus through the intestines.

4. Chemical stimulants directly stimulate the nerve plexus in the intestinal wall, causing increased movement and the stimulation of local reflexes. Bulk stimulants (also called *mechanical stimulants*), are rapid-acting, aggressive laxatives that cause the fecal matter to increase in bulk. They increase the motility of the GI tract by increasing the fluid in the intestinal contents, which enlarges bulk, stimulates local stretch receptors, and activates local activity.

5. Cathartic dependence is a reaction that occurs when patients use laxatives over a long period and the GI tract becomes dependent on the vigorous stimulation of the laxative. Without this stimulation, the GI tract does not move for a period of time (i.e., several days), which could lead to constipation and drying of the stool and ultimately to impaction.

6. Docusate has a detergent action on the surface of the intestinal bolus, increasing the admixture of fat and water and making a softer stool.

■ APPLYING YOUR KNOWLEDGE

CASE STUDY

a. Various factors may be contributing to this older adult's constipation. These may include a lack of exercise or activity (the patient lives alone and may not be getting out often), low intake of fiber foods and adequate fluids (the patient is living alone and may not be eating nutritious meals or consuming enough food), prescribed medications being used for other underlying medical conditions, or development of new medical conditions that could be affecting the GI tract.

b. The nurse would need to instruct the patient to drink plenty of fluids with the psyllium to prevent problems that can occur if the drug starts to pull in fluid while still in the esophagus. Additionally, the nurse should recommend that the patient use the pysllium exactly as directed and to check with the health care provider before taking any other over-the-counter products. Other instructions would include teaching the patient about possible adverse effects and making sure that if she is taking any other prescribed medications that she separate their administration by at least 30 minutes to prevent interfering with the timing or absorption of these medications. The nurse would also encourage the patient to increase her fiber intake, providing her with suggestions for high-fiber foods, and to increase her fluid intake (if not contraindicated by underlying medical conditions). Additionally, the nurse would suggest ways that the patient can increase her activity level.

PRACTICING FOR NCLEX

1. **Answer: a**
   RATIONALE: When given intravenously, metoclopramide has an onset of action of 1 to 5 minutes.

2. **Answer: c**
   RATIONALE: Laxative, or cathartic, drugs are indicated to remove ingested poisons from the lower GI tract; as an adjunct in anthelmintic therapy when it is desirable to flush helminths from the GI tract; to prevent straining when it is clinically undesirable (such as after surgery, myocardial infarction, or obstetric delivery); for the short-term relief of constipation; and to evacuate the bowel for diagnostic procedures. Lubricants ease defecation without stimulating the movement of the GI tract. GI stimulants provide more generalized GI stimulation, resulting in an overall increase in GI activity and secretions.

3. **Answer: d**
   RATIONALE: Polycarbophil is an example of a bulk laxative. Bisacodyl and senna are examples of chemical stimulant laxatives. Docusate is an example of a lubricant laxative.

4. **Answer: d**
   RATIONALE: Although bisacodyl can be taken at any time, the drug has an onset of action of 6 to 8 hours, making it preferable for the drug to work overnight and seeing the effects in the morning.

5. **Answer: a**
   RATIONALE: Cascara is administered orally. Senna may be administered orally or as a rectal suppository. Bisacodyl is given orally or rectally. No laxative is given intramuscularly.

6. **Answer: c**
   RATIONALE: Chemical stimulant laxatives are used cautiously in patients with coronary artery disease and heart block because these conditions could be affected by the decrease in absorption and changes in electrolytes that can occur. Acute abdominal disorders such as appendicitis, diverticulitis, and ulcerative colitis would be contraindications to the use of chemical stimulants.

7. **Answer: c**
   RATIONALE: Polyethylene glycol–electrolyte solution is dispensed as 4 L of solution, and the patient is to take 240 mL (8 ounces) of the solution every 10 minutes until the solution is finished. Mixing a packet in a glass of cold water would be appropriate for psyllium.

8. **Answer: b**
   RATIONALE: The patient's symptoms are most likely related to a sympathetic stress reaction due to intense neurostimulation of the GI tract or to the loss of fluid and electrolyte imbalance. Direct stimulation refers to the action of chemical stimulant laxatives. Detergent action is related to the use of docusate. Formation of a slippery coat relates to the use of mineral oil.

9. **Answer: a**
   RATIONALE: Although abdominal cramping, diarrhea, and sweating may occur with lubricant laxatives such as mineral oil, it would be especially important to inform the patient about possible leakage and staining with mineral oil, which occurs because the stool cannot be retained by the external sphincter.

10. **Answer: b**
    RATIONALE: Dexpanthenol works by increasing acetylcholine levels and stimulating the parasympathetic system. Metoclopramide works by blocking dopamine receptors and making the GI cells more sensitive to

Copyright © 2011 by Wolters Kluwer Health l Lippincott Williams & Wilkins. *Study Guide for Focus on Nursing Pharmacology.*

acetylcholine. Bulk laxatives exert an osmotic pull on fluids. Loperamide acts directly on the muscles of the GI tract to slow activity.

11. **Answer: c**
RATIONALE: Bismuth subsalicylate is indicated for the treatment of traveler's diarrhea and in preventing cramping and distention associated with dietary excess and some viral infections. Loperamide is indicated for the short-term treatment of diarrhea associated with dietary problems and some viral infections. Opium derivatives are indicated for the short-term treatment of cramping and diarrhea.

12. **Answer: b**
RATIONALE: Alosetron is classified as a serotonin 5-HT antagonist. Hyoscyamine is an anticholinergic agent that may be used to treat irritable bowel syndrome. Lubiprostone is a locally acting chloride channel activator used for treatment of chronic, idiopathic constipation and for treatment of irritable bowel syndrome with constipation in women. Methylnaltrexone is a selective antagonist to opioid binding at the mu-receptors.

13. **Answer: c**
RATIONALE: Rifaximin is the first antibiotic approved by the Food and Drug Administration specifically for treating traveler's diarrhea, acting against noninvasive strains of *Escherichia coli*, which is the most common cause of traveler's diarrhea.

14. **Answer: d**
RATIONALE: Patients with advanced disease who are receiving palliative care and no longer are responsive to traditional laxatives may receive methylnaltrexone for treatment of opioid-induced constipation. Lubiprostone is a locally acting chloride channel activator used for treatment of chronic, idiopathic constipation and for treatment of irritable bowel syndrome with constipation in women. Psyllium or mineral oil probably would have been tried earlier on and most likely would be ineffective because the patient's constipation is opioid induced.

15. **Answer: b**
RATIONALE: Irritable bowel syndrome is a very common disorder, striking three times as many women as men and reportedly accounting for half of all referrals to GI specialists. The disorder is characterized by abdominal distress, bouts of diarrhea or constipation, bloating, nausea, flatulence, headache, fatigue, depression, and anxiety. No anatomical cause has been found for this disorder. Underlying causes might be stress related.

CHAPTER 59

■ ASSESSING YOUR UNDERSTANDING

LABELING

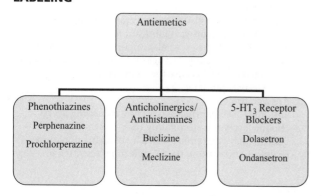

SHORT ANSWER

1. The two phenothiazines used most commonly as antiemetics are prochlorperazine and promethazine.
2. Antiemetics work by reducing the hyperactivity of the vomiting reflex in one of two ways: locally, to decrease the local response to stimuli that are being sent to the medulla to induce vomiting, or centrally, to block the chemoreceptor trigger zone (CTZ) or suppress the vomiting center directly.
3. Cyclizine is an anticholinergic/antihistamine that blocks the transmission of impulses to the CTZ.
4. Aprepitant is given orally in combination with dexamethasone.
5. Dronabinol and nabilone contain the active ingredient of cannabis (marijuana).

■ APPLYING YOUR KNOWLEDGE

CASE STUDY

a. The patient is most likely experiencing intractable hiccups, which occur when the diaphragm is repetitively stimulated, leading to persistent diaphragmatic spasm.
b. The nurse would need to instruct the patient to take the medication as prescribed and to be alert for possible adverse effects, primarily central nervous system (CNS) effects such as drowsiness, dizziness, weakness, headache, and tremor. The risk for drowsiness, dizziness, and headache may be increased because these adverse effects also occur with omeprazole. The nurse should instruct the patient in safety measures to reduce the risk of injury related to CNS effects and to avoid alcohol intake with this drug, which would potentiate the CNS effects. The nurse would also need to inform the patient about dry mouth and relief measures such as frequent sips of fluid, ice chips, and sugarless hard candies. Other adverse effects to address include nasal congestion, sweating, and possible urinary retention. Photosensitivity is possible, so the nurse should encourage the use of protective clothing and sunscreen when outside. Chlorpromazine is associated with the development of neuroleptic malignant syndrome. The nurse should review the signs and symptoms of this disorder (hyperpyrexia, muscle rigidity, altered mental status, irregular pulse or blood pressure, diaphoresis, and arrhythmias) and emphasize the need for immediate medical care.

■ PRACTICING FOR NCLEX

1. **Answer: c**
RATIONALE: Granisetron is classified as a 5-HT$_3$ receptor blocker. Chlorpromazine is a phenothiazine; cyclizine is an anticholinergic/antihistamine; and aprepitant is a substance P/neurokinin-1 receptor antagonist.

2. **Answer: b**
RATIONALE: Phenothiazines are centrally acting antiemetics that block the CTZ in the medulla. Antacids, local anesthetics, absorbents, and gastrointestinal (GI) protectants act locally.

3. **Answer: a**
RATIONALE: Promethazine should be used cautiously in patients with active peptic ulcer disease. The drug would be contraindicated in patients with severe hypotension (possibly interfering with drug metabolism) or patients with brain injury or coma due to the risk of further CNS depression.

4. **Answer: b**
RATIONALE: CNS effects, especially dizziness and drowsiness, are associated with phenothiazines and necessitate safety measures such as assistance with ambulation. GI

Copyright © 2011 by Wolters Kluwer Health | Lippincott Williams & Wilkins. *Study Guide for Focus on Nursing Pharmacology.*

overstimulation could result in diarrhea or additional vomiting, which might require the patient to use the bathroom but not be the basis for assisting the patient. The nurse's actions are not related to urinary abnormalities or endocrine effects.

5. **Answer: a**
   RATIONALE: Offering carbonated drinks can help to promote the patient's comfort. Deep breathing, a quiet restful environment, and frequent mouth care such as every 2 hours or as needed would be appropriate.

6. **Answer: c**
   RATIONALE: When given rectally, prochlorperazine has an onset of action of 60 to 90 minutes. In this situation, the time of 7:15 PM would be most appropriate.

7. **Answer: b**
   RATIONALE: Metoclopramide is given intravenously 30 minutes before chemotherapy.

8. **Answer: d**
   RATIONALE: Cyclizine is indicated for the treatment of motion sickness. Promethazine is used to prevent and control nausea and vomiting associated with anesthesia and surgery. Dolasetron is indicated for treatment of nausea and vomiting associated with emetogenic chemotherapy and for the prevention of postoperative nausea and vomiting. Perphenazine is indicated for the treatment of severe nausea and vomiting and intractable hiccups.

9. **Answer: c**
   RATIONALE: There is an increased risk of sedation if meclizine is combined with other CNS depressants such as alcohol. The patient should be instructed to avoid this combination. Meclizine does not interact with caffeine or chocolate. Aged cheese should be avoided by patients taking monoamine oxidase inhibitors.

10. **Answer: a**
    RATIONALE: Palonosetron cannot be repeated for 7 days. The drug is not a controlled substance. Granisetron is used only on the days that chemotherapy is given. Metoclopramide typically is given as one dose 30 minutes before chemotherapy, then every 2 hours for two doses, then every 3 hours for three doses.

11. **Answer: c, d, e**
    RATIONALE: Aprepitant is associated with constipation, anorexia, headache, diarrhea, gastritis, nausea, and fatigue.

12. **Answer: b**
    RATIONALE: Aprepitant acts directly in the CNS to block receptors associated with nausea and vomiting with little to no effect on serotonin, dopamine, or corticosteroid receptors. Metoclopramide reduces the responsiveness of the nerve cells in the CTZ to circulating chemicals that induce vomiting. Meclizine blocks cholinergic receptors in the vomiting center. Granisetron blocks the 5-HT$_3$ receptors associated with nausea and vomiting in the CTZ and locally.

13. **Answer: d**
    RATIONALE: Palonosetron is available for intravenous use only.

14. **Answer: c**
    RATIONALE: Trimethobenzamide is similar to the antihistamines but is not associated with as much sedation and CNS depression, making it a drug of choice.

15. **Answer: c**
    RATIONALE: Dronabinol is classified as a category C-III controlled substance. Nabilone is a category C-II substance. Both drugs are approved for use only in managing the nausea and vomiting associated with cancer chemotherapy in cases that have not responded to other treatment.

Copyright © 2011 by Wolters Kluwer Health I Lippincott Williams & Wilkins. *Study Guide for Focus on Nursing Pharmacology.*